Informatik aktuell

Herausgegeben
im Auftrag der Gesellschaft für Informatik (GI)

Klaus Hermann Maier-Hein · Thomas M. Deserno
Heinz Handels · Thomas Tolxdorff
Herausgeber

Bildverarbeitung
für die Medizin 2017

Algorithmen – Systeme – Anwendungen

Proceedings des Workshops
vom 12. bis 14. März 2017 in Heidelberg

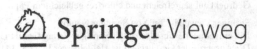

Herausgeber

Klaus Hermann Maier-Hein, geb. Fritzsche
Deutsches Krebsforschungszentrum
Juniorgruppe Medizinische Bildverarbeitung
Im Neuenheimer Feld 280, 69120 Heidelberg
Deutschland

Thomas Martin Deserno, geb. Lehmann
Uniklinik RWTH Aachen
Institut für Medizinische Informatik
Pauwelsstr. 30, 52074 Aachen
Deutschland

Heinz Handels
Universität zu Lübeck
Institut für Medizinische Informatik
Ratzeburger Allee 160, 23562 Lübeck
Deutschland

Thomas Tolxdorff
Charité – Universitätsmedizin Berlin
Institut für Medizinische Informatik
Hindenburgdamm 30, 12200 Berlin
Deutschland

ISSN 1431-472X
Informatik aktuell
ISBN 978-3-662-54344-3   ISBN 978-3-662-54345-0   (eBook)
DOI 10.1007/978-3-662-54345-0

Die Deutsche Nationalbibliothek verzeichnet diese Publikation in der Deutschen Nationalbibliografie; detaillierte bibliografische Daten sind im Internet über http://dnb.d-nb.de abrufbar.

CR Subject Classification (1998): A.0, H.3, I.4, I.5, J.3, H.3.1, I.2.10, I.3.3, I.3.5, I.3.7, I.3.8, I.6.3

Springer Vieweg

Springer Vieweg ist Teil von Springer Nature
Die eingetragene Gesellschaft ist Springer-Verlag GmbH Deutschland
Die Anschrift der Gesellschaft ist Heidelberger Platz 3, 14197 Berlin, Germany

Bildverarbeitung für die Medizin 2017

Veranstalter

MIC   Juniorgruppe Medizinische Bildverarbeitung
                 Deutsches Krebsforschungszentrum (DKFZ), Heidelberg

Unterstützende Fachgesellschaften

BVMI	Berufsverband Medizinischer Informatiker
CURAC	Deutsche Gesellschaft für Computer- und Roboterassistierte Chirurgie
DAGM	Deutsche Arbeitsgemeinschaft für Mustererkennung
DGBMT	Fachgruppe Medizinische Informatik der Deutschen Gesellschaft für Biomedizinische Technik im Verband Deutscher Elektrotechniker
GI	Gesellschaft für Informatik - Fachbereich Informatik in den Lebenswissenschaften
GMDS	Gesellschaft für Medizinische Informatik, Biometrie und Epidemiologie
IEEE	Joint Chapter Engineering in Medicine and Biology, German Section

Tagungsvorsitz

PD Dr. Klaus H. Maier-Hein
Juniorgruppe Medizinische Bildverarbeitung, DKFZ

Tagungssekretariat

Janina Dunning und Stefanie Strzysch
Juniorgruppe Medizinische Bildverarbeitung, DKFZ
Postanschrift: 69121 Heidelberg
Lieferanschrift: Im Neuenheimer Feld 581
Telefon: +49 6221 42 2354 (Dunning)
                +49 6221 42 2327 (Strzysch)
Email: bvm-orga@dkfz-heidelberg.de
Web: http://bvm-workshop.org

Lokales BVM-Komitee

PD Dr. Klaus H. Maier-Hein
Dr. Diana Nabers
Jens Petersen
Sarina Thomas
u.v.m.

Verteilte BVM-Organisation

PD Dr. Klaus H. Maier-Hein, Jens Petersen
Deutsches Krebsforschungszentrum Heidelberg (Anmeldung)

Prof. Dr. Heinz Handels, Dr. Jan-Hinrich Wrage
Universität zu Lübeck (Beitragsbegutachtung)

Prof. Dr. Thomas Tolxdorff, Dr. Thorsten Schaaf
Charité – Universitätsmedizin Berlin (Internetpräsenz)

Prof. Dr. Thomas M. Deserno, Jan Dovermann, Benedikt Bender
Rheinisch-Westfälische Technische Hochschule Aachen (Tagungsband)

Programmkomitee

Prof. Dr. Dr. Johannes Bernarding, Universität Magdeburg
Priv.-Doz. Dr. Jürgen Braun, Charité-Universitätsmedizin Berlin
Prof. Dr. Oliver Burgert, HS Reutlingen
Prof. Dr. Thorsten Buzug, Universität zu Lübeck
Prof. Dr. Thomas Deserno, RWTH Aachen
Prof. Dr. Hartmut Dickhaus, Universität Heidelberg
Dr. Jan Ehrhardt, Universität zu Lübeck
Dr. Ralf Floca, DKFZ Heidelberg
Dr. Nils Forkert, University of Calgary, Canada
Prof. Horst Hahn, Fraunhofer MEVIS Bremen
Prof. Dr. Heinz Handels, Universität zu Lübeck
Priv.-Doz. Dr. Peter Hastreiter, Universität Erlangen
Dr. Tobias Heimann, Siemens Healthcare GmbH Erlangen
Prof. Dr. Joachim Hornegger, Universität Erlangen
Prof. Ron Kikinis, MD, Harvard Medical School Boston USA
Prof. Dr. Andreas Maier, Universität Erlangen
Priv.-Doz. Dr. Klaus Maier-Hein, DKFZ Heidelberg
Prof. Dr. Lena Maier-Hein, DKFZ Heidelberg
Dr. Andre Mastmeyer, Universität zu Lübeck
Prof. Dr. Hans-Peter Meinzer, DKFZ Heidelberg
Prof. Dr. Dorit Merhof, RWTH Aachen
Prof. Jan Modersitzki, Fraunhofer MEVIS, Lübeck
Prof. Dr. Heinrich Müller, Technische Universität Dortmund
Prof. Dr. Henning Müller, Universit Sierre Schweiz
Prof. Dr. Arya Nabavi, INI Hannover
Prof. Dr. Nassir Navab, Technische Universität München
Dr. Marco Nolden, DKFZ Heidelberg
Prof. Dr. Christoph Palm, OTH Regensburg
Prof. Dr. Bernhard Preim, Universität Magdeburg
Priv.-Doz. Dr. Karl Rohr, Universität Heidelberg
Priv.-Doz. Dr. Dennis Säring, FH Wedel
Prof. Dr. Heinz-Peter Schlemmer, DKFZ Heidelberg

Dr. Stefanie Speidel, KIT Karlsruhe
Prof. Dr. Thomas Tolxdorff, Charité-Universitätsmedizin Berlin
Prof. Dr. Klaus Tönnies, Universität Magdeburg
Dr. Gudrun Wagenknecht, Forschungszentrum Jülich
Dr. René Werner, UKE Hamburg
Dr. Stefan Wesarg, Fraunhofer IGD Darmstadt
Prof. Dr. Herbert Witte, Universität Jena
Priv.-Doz. Dr. Thomas Wittenberg, Fraunhofer IIS, Erlangen
Prof. Dr. Ivo Wolf, HS Mannheim
Priv.-Doz. Dr. Stefan Wörz, Universität Heidelberg

Sponsoren des Workshops BVM 2017

Die BVM wäre ohne die finanzielle Unterstützung der Industrie in ihrer so erfolgreichen Konzeption nicht durchführbar. Deshalb freuen wir uns sehr über langjährige kontinuierliche Unterstützung mancher Firmen sowie auch über das neue Engagement anderer.

Sponsoren

ADR AG Advanced Digital Research
Ludwig-Wagner-Str. 19, D-69168 Wiesloch
http://www.dicom-disc.de

Agfa HealthCare GmbH
Konrad-Zuse-Platz 1-3, D-53227 Bonn
http://www.agfahealthcare.de

Chili GmbH
Friedrich-Ebert-Str. 2, D-69221 Dossenheim
http://www.chili-radiology.com

GHG Gotthardt Healthgroup AG
Hauptstraße 90, D-69117 Heidelberg
http://www.gotthardt.com

Haption GmbH
Dennewartstr. 25, 52068 Aachen
http://www.haption.de

Heidelberg Engineering GmbH
Max-Jarecki-Straße 8, D-69115 Heidelberg
http://www.heidelbergengineering.com

Karl Storz GmbH und Co. KG
Mittelstraße 8, D-78532 Tuttlingen
https://www.karlstorz.com

mbits imaging GmbH
Bergheimer Strasse 147, D-69155 Heidelberg
https://mbits.info

Mint Medical GmbH
Friedrich-Ebert-Str. 2, D-69221 Dossenheim
http://www.mint-medical.com

NDI Europe GmbH
Güttinger Str. 37, D-78315 Radolfzell
http://www.ndidigital.com

Dentsply Sirona Sirona Dental Systems GmbH
Fabrikstr. 31, D-64625 Bensheim
http://dentsplysirona.com

Springer Springer-Verlag GmbH
Tiergarten Strasse 17, D-69121 Heidelberg
http://www.springer.com

Visus Technology Transfer GmbH
Universitätsstr. 136, D-44799 Bochum
http://www.visus.com

Preisträger des BVM-Workshops 2016 in Berlin

BVM-Preis 2016 für die beste wissenschaftliche Arbeit (1. Platz)

Heiko Tzschätzsch mit *Jing Guo, Florian Dittmann, Jürgen Braun, Ingolf Sack*
(Charité Berlin)
Tomoelastography by Multifrequency Wave Number Recovery

BVM-Preis 2016 für die beste wissenschaftliche Arbeit (2. Platz)

Tobias Norajitra mit *Sandy Engelhardt, Thomas Held, Sameer Al-Maisary, Raffaele de Simone, Hans-Peter Meinzer, Klaus Maier-Hein* (DKFZ Heidelberg)
3D statistische Formmodelle mit verteilter Erscheinungsmodellierung: Segmentierung per Abstimmung

BVM-Preis 2016 für die beste wissenschaftliche Arbeit (3. Platz)

Harald Hoppe mit *Fabian Seebacher, Martin Klemm* (Hochschule Offenburg)
Nicht modellbasierte Kalibration von Kameras mit Monitoren

BVM-Preis 2016 für den besten Vortrag

Nicole Schubert mit *David Gräsel, Uwe Pietrzyk, Katrin Amunts, Markus Axer*
(Forschungszentrum Jülich)
Visualization of Vector Fields Derived from 3D Polarized Light Imaging

BVM-Preis 2016 für die beste Posterpräsentation

Christian Hintze mit *Johannes Junggeburth, Bernhard Hill, Dorit Merhof*
(RWTH Aachen)
Biometrische Messung der Pupillenreaktion

BVM-Award für eine herausragende Masterarbeit aus dem Bereich der Medizinischen Bildverarbeitung

Florin C. Ghesu
(Friedrich-Alexander Universität Erlangen-Nürnberg)
Efficient Deep Learning Architectures for 3D-4D Medical Image Analysis

Vorwort

In der computergestützten Verarbeitung und automatischen Analyse medizinischer Bilddaten werden momentan erhebliche Fortschritte erzielt und die Grenzen des Machbaren sichtlich erweitert. Der Workshop *Bildverarbeitung für die Medizin (BVM)* bietet ein Forum zur Präsentation und Diskussion der neuesten Algorithmen, Systeme und Anwendungen in diesem Bereich. Ziel ist sowohl die Vertiefung der Interaktion zwischen Wissenschaftlern, Industrie und Anwendern als auch die explizite Einbeziehung von Nachwuchswissenschaftler, die über ihre Bachelor-, Master-, Promotions- und Habilitationsprojekte berichten. Die BVM konnte sich durch erfolgreiche Veranstaltungen in Aachen, Berlin, Erlangen, Freiburg, Hamburg, Heidelberg, Leipzig, Lübeck und München als zentrales interdisziplinäres Forum etablieren.

Für den diesjährigen Workshop konnten neben den spannenden Beiträgen der Teilnehmer fünf hochinteressante eingeladene Vorträge gewonnen werden:

- Professor Wiro Niessen, University Medical Center Rotterdam und Delft University of Technology, zum Thema *Big Data in Medical Image Computing*.

- Dr. Bram Stieltjes, Klinik für Radiologie und Nuklearmedizin in Basel, zum Thema *The future of radiology and cooperation at the interdisciplinary interface*.

- Olaf Ronneberger, Google DeepMind in London, zum Thema *U-Net: Convolutional Networks for Biomedical Image Segmentation*.

- Karlheinz Meier, Kirchhoff-Institut für Physik in Heidelberg, zum Thema *Neuromorphic computing - Principles, achievements and potentials*.

- Dogu Teber, Urologische Klinik in Heidelberg, zum Thema *The operating room of the future*.

Aus insgesamt 77 Einreichungen wurden 30 Vorträge, 41 Poster und zwei Softwaredemonstrationen angenommen. Die besten Arbeiten werden auch in diesem Jahr mit wertvollen BVM-Preisen ausgezeichnet. Die Webseite des Workshops findet sich unter

http://www.bvm-workshop.org

An dieser Stelle möchten wir allen, die bei den umfangreichen Vorbereitungen zum Gelingen des Workshops beigetragen haben, unseren herzlichen Dank für ihr Engagement bei der Organisation des Workshops aussprechen: den Referenten der Gastvorträge, den Autoren der Beiträge, den Referenten der Tutorien, den Industrierepräsentanten, dem Programmkomitee, den Fachgesellschaften, den Mitgliedern des BVM-Organisationsteams und allen Mitarbeitern der Juniorgruppe für Medizinische Bildverarbeitung sowie der Abteilung für Computer-assistierte Medizinische Interventionen am Deutschen Krebsforschungszentrum.

Wir wünschen allen Teilnehmerinnen und Teilnehmern des Workshops BVM 2017 spannende neue Kontakte und inspirierende Eindrücke aus der Welt der medizinischen Bildverarbeitung.

Januar 2017

Klaus H. Maier-Hein (Heidelberg)
Thomas Deserno (Aachen)
Heinz Handels (Lübeck)
Thomas Tolxdorff (Berlin)

Inhaltsverzeichnis

Die fortlaufende Nummer am linken Seitenrand entspricht den Beitragsnummern, wie sie im endgültigen Programm des Workshops zu finden sind. Dabei steht V für Vortrag, P für Poster und S für Softwaredemonstration.

Eingeladene Vorträge

Tutorials

Segmentation

Detection

Reconstruction & Registration

Deep Learning

Poster

Software Demo

Computer-Assisted Diagnosis

Computer-Assisted Interventions

Shape & Visualization

Invited Talk: Big Data in Medical Image Computing

Wiro Niessen

Erasmus MC Rotterdam, The Netherlands
Delft University of Technology, Delft, The Netherlands
Quantib BV, Rotterdam, The Netherlands
w.niessen@erasmusmc.nl

Big data are dramatically increasing the possibilities for prevention, cure and care, and changing the landscape of the healthcare system. Will artificial intelligence make doctors obsolete or give them more possibilities? Will citizens be delivered into the hands of anonymous information systems or will they gain more control over their personal health. It is difficult to predict the speed of change and impact of both big data and artificial intelligence on health care, but it is clear that changes will be tremendous.

In this presentation, I will show examples of possible large benefits. For example how large scale data analytics in longitudinal population neuroimaging studies, especially when combining imaging with other clinical, biomedical and genetic data, provides a unique angle to study the brain, both in normal ageing and disease. And how this can be the basis of new methods for disease detection, diagnosis, and prognosis in clinical practice.

Invited Talk: The Future of Radiology and Cooperation at the Interdisciplinary Interface

Bram Stieltjes

Klinik für Radiologie und Nuklearmedizin, Basel, Switzerland
bram.stieltjes@usb.ch

Despite a tremendous advance in knowledge in informatics and specifically in medical image analysis in the last decades, the mainstay of current imaging-based diagnostics remains an artisan hand-work performed by medical doctors. Clearly, a translational gap is present between basic sciences and diagnostic clinical routine that hampers the process of industrialization and automation that has pervasively changed the face of many other jobs, blue and white collar alike. I will clarify why I believe that the main challenges in this field are not of pure technical nature and aim to outline an environment that I believe would enhance the translation of developed technology into clinical routine. I hope that this presentation will spark a discussion on major hurdles for seamless integration of informatics in a diagnostic environment and may generate ideas on inspiring future models for cooperation in this field.

Invited Talk: U-Net
Convolutional Networks for Biomedical Image Segmentation

Olaf Ronneberger

Google DeepMind, London, UK
olafr@google.com

In the last years, deep convolutional networks have outperformed the state of the art in many visual recognition tasks. A central challenge for its wide adoption in the bio-medical imaging field is the limited amount of annotated training images. In this talk, I will present our u-net for biomedical image segmentation. The architecture consists of an analysis path and a synthesis path with additional shortcut-connections. The network is trained end-to-end from scratch with only approximately 30 annotated images per application. The surprisingly simple strategy to train a network with such a low number of samples is a data augmentation with elastic deformations. Furthermore, the u-net can segment arbitrarily large images with a seamless tiling strategy. For 3D images we have developed a training strategy to learn a full 3D segmentation from a few annotated slices per volume. This can be used in a semi-automated setup to create a dense segmentation from the sparse annotations on the same volume, or in a fully-automated setup, where sparse annotations speed up the training data generation significantly.

Invited Talk: Neuromorphic Computing
Principles, Achievements, and Potentials

Karlheinz Meier

Kirchhoff-Institut für Physik, Heidelberg, Germany
meierk@kip.uni-heidelberg.de

Neural networks have recently taken the field of machine learning by storm. Their success rests upon the availability of high performance computing hardware which allows to train very wide and deep networks. Traditional neural networks have very limited biological realism. Recent work on more brain-like hardware architectures has led to first large-scale implementations of neuromorphic computing systems. In the keynote, guiding design principles of neuromorphic machines, their application and performance as well as future plans are discussed.

Invited Talk: The Operating Room of the Future

Dogu Teber

Urologische Klinik, Universitätsklinikum Heidelberg, Germany
doguteber@googlemail.com

The increasing networking of data systems in medicine leads not only to a modern interdisciplinarity in the sense of a cooperation of different medical disciplines, but also poses new challenges to the concept of the operating room as building infrastructure. The surgical operating room of the future augments its reality, away from pure space characteristics, to an intelligent and communicative interactive platform. In analogy to a smart phone which becomes more a platform for different application beyond the function as a pure telephone device, the operating room of the future serves as sensor and actuator at the same time. A modular architecture with open interfaces for image acquisition and analysis, interaction and visualization, supports the integration and combination of heterogeneous data that are generated in a hospital and operating room environment. Based on this, we aim to describe surgical evolution not only in the context of minimal invasiveness (smaller incisions) but more as "smart surgery"with expandable software applications as ready-to-use applications (apps) especially in the field of image guided surgery and surgical decision support, which are integral part of the infrastructure of a new operating room concept.

Tutorial: Deep Learning
Advancing the State-of-the-Art in Medical Image Analysis

Vincent Christlein[1], Florin C. Ghesu[1], Tobias Würfl[1], Andreas Maier[1],
Fabian Isensee[2], Peter Neher[2], Klaus Maier-Hein[2]

[1]Pattern Recognition Lab, Friedrich-Alexander-Universität, Erlangen, Germany
[2]Junior Group Medical Image Computing, German Cancer Research Center,
Heidelberg, Germany
vincent.christlein@cs.fau.de

Deep Learning (DL) represents a key technological innovation in the field of machine learning. Recent advancements have attracted much attention by showing substantial improvements in a wide range of applications such as image recognition, speech recognition, natural language processing and artificial intelligence. In some cases the performance even surpasses human accuracy, which motivated the introduction of a series of DL-based software products and automatization solutions (for example Apple Siri, Google Now, Google Autonomous Driving etc.). The same success also echoes in the research efforts of the medical imaging community. However, in this case several constraints such as data-availability, inherent data noise or lack of labeled data directly affect the pace of advancements.

We will start the tutorial by introducing the core element of deep learning – the deep neural network, with its distinguishing capability of automatically learning hierarchies of complex features directly from the raw training data without the need for 'manual' feature engineering. Using this knowledge-base we will discuss several state-of-the-art deep architectures. In this context we will also present the algorithms required to train these models as well as a practical analysis of regularization / data-normalization techniques which prove to be essential in achieving high performance.

This technology also addresses inherent limitations faced in typical medical image analysis problems. The most important of these is the task of object recognition / classification which is an important prerequisite for many clinical applications, for example image-to-image registration, advanced biophysical simulations and cell detection or classification problems for cancer diagnosis.

To complement the aforementioned learning techniques for classification problems we will dedicate the third part of our tutorial to applications of deep learning to segmentation problems. Here we will outline the two predominant strategies, namely patch-based and single pass segmentation approaches. For both strategies we will present specific systems from current literature as well as examples of our own work in the areas of DL-based volumetric image parsing.

The last part of the tutorial is focused on the inherent constraints and obstacles we face when using DL methods in the context of medical image analysis and how they can be addressed. Specifically, we will discuss recent developments in reducing and training large models, such as model compression and semi-supervised learning. We will also discuss solutions that address the computational limitations of DL models for 3D data based on our own research. The tutorial will be concluded with an open discussion related to unresolved problems and the future of deep learning in the medical imaging community [1, 2, 3, 4, 5, 6].

References

1. Würfl T, et al. Deep Learning Computed Tomography. MICCAI. 2016.
2. Ghesu FC, et al. An Artificial Agent for Anatomical Landmark Detection. MICCAI. 2016.
3. Ghesu FC, et al. Intelligent Anatomy Parsing. Elsevier(book chapter - in press). 2016.
4. Christlein V, et al. Offline Writer Identification Using CNN Activation Features. GCPR. 2015.
5. Ghesu FC, et al. Marginal Space Deep Learning: Efficient Architecture for Volumetric Image Parsing. TMI (deep learning - special issue). 2015.
6. Ghesu FC, et al. Marginal Space Deep Learning: Efficient Architecture for Detection in Volumetric Image Data. MICCAI. 2015.

Tutorial: Hands-On Workshop Minimal Invasive Chirurgie (MIC)

Felix Nickel, Beat Müller

Klinik für Allgemein-, Viszeral- und Transplantationschirurgie,
Universität Heidelberg
felix.nickel@med.uni-heidelberg.de

In der Minimal Invasiven Chirurgie (MIC), auch Schlüssellochchirurgie oder laparoskopische Chirurgie genannt, wird im Gegensatz zur offenen Chirurgie nur über kleine Schnitte operiert. Über spezielle Zugänge durch die Bauchdecke werden eine Kamera und lange stabförmige Instrumente in den Bauchraum eingeführt. Das Verfahren ist durch den Verzicht auf große Schnittwunden besonders schonend für den Patienten und führt häufig zur schnelleren Erholung von der Operation. Die laparoskopischen Operationstechniken haben sich in den letzten Jahren in immer mehr Bereichen durchgesetzt und gewinnen zunehmend an Bedeutung, Verbreitung und Beliebtheit. Für manche Operationen ist die laparoskopische Technik inzwischen schon der etablierte Standard, wie z.B. für die Gallenblasenentfernung. Die Schwierigkeit der laparoskopischen Chirurgie liegt im Erlernen der Operationstechnik, da diese durch den indirekten Zugang und die indirekte Sicht deutlich anspruchsvoller ist als konventionelle offene Verfahren.

In diesem Tutorial erhalten die Teilnehmer Einblick in die Techniken der MIC. Hierbei werden sowohl physische Simulatoren mit realen Operationsinstrumenten verwendet, als auch Computersimulatoren an denen Operationen in der Virtuellen Realität (VR) geübt werden können. Das MIC Trainingszentrum in Heidelberg ist mit den modernsten Geräten und Instrumenten ausgestattet inklusive High-Definition 3D-Techniken. Im eigens entwickelten Forschungsprojekt „iSurgeon" werden durch Sensoren gestützt (Microsoft Kinect, NDI Polaris, Myo Armbänder) Expertenmodelle aufgenommen und den Trainierenden wird ein Echtzeit Feedback im Abgleich mit den Expertenmodellen gegeben um die Lernkurve zu beschleunigen. Mit Serious Gaming Applikationen können operative Techniken zudem mit spielerischen Elementen in virtuellen Umgebungen gelernt werden. Es werden Übungen zur Kameraführung und zum Umgang mit den Instrumenten durchgeführt um insbesondere die Eigenheiten der speziellen räumlichen Wahrnehmung beim Operieren mit indirekter Sicht über die Kamera kennenzulernen. Das Nähen und Knoten, welches bei der Laparoskopie besonders anspruchsvoll ist, wird ebenfalls an den Geräten geübt. Durch den Einsatz von Tierorganen können Teile, aber auch ganze Operationen sehr realistisch und nachvollzogen werden. Vom Computersimulator gibt es zusätzlich Rückmeldung über den Trainingsfortschritt und es können standardisierte Tests automatisch durchgeführt werden.

Nach einer Kurzen Einleitung und einem Überblick über die MIC Techniken mit Vorstellung des MIC Trainingszentrums und der Projekte lernen die

Teilnehmer des Workshops die MIC Techniken Hands-On selbst durchzuführen. Forschungsprojekte werden vorgestellt und mit den Teilnehmern werden neue Ideen diskutiert.

Tutorial: Medical Image Processing with MITK
Introduction and new Developments

Caspar Goch, Jasmin Metzger, Marco Nolden

Department for Medical and Biological Informatics, DKFZ Heidelberg, Germany
c.goch@dkfz.de

The Medical Imaging Interaction Toolkit (MITK) is a powerful tool for image processing and application development with a long history [1, 2]. It provides an easy-to-use superbuild for a variety of development scenarios and a host of customization options. This very exibility can be intimidating to new users and even more experienced users might miss out on new developments due to the sheer size of the code base. In this tutorial we will give an overview on MITK, the underlying concepts and the usage of the MITK Workbench. Afterwards we will show the attendees how to start their own software development with MITK and what pitfalls to look out for. Due to time constraints this will be in the form of a development demonstration, instead of a hands-on session. This will be followed by an introduction into more advanced usage scenarios, intended to provide a customized Workbench for special work ows or to conform to branding requirements. We will close with newly finished and ongoing developments and the new opportunities which arise based on them.

Literaturverzeichnis

1. Wolf I, Vetter M, Wegner I, et al. The medical imaging interaction toolkit. Med Image Anal. 2005;9(6):594–604.
2. Nolden M, Zelzer S, Seitel A, et al. The medical imaging interaction toolkit: challenges and advances. Int J Comput Assist Radiol Surg. 2013;8(4):607–20.

Fully Automatic Segmentation of Papillary Muscles in 3D LGE-MRI

Tanja Kurzendorfer[1], Alexander Brost[2], Christoph Forman[3],
Michaela Schmidt[3], Christoph Tillmanns[4], Andreas Maier[1]

[1]Pattern Recognition Lab, Friedrich-Alexander University of Erlangen-Nuremberg,
Erlangen, Germany
[2]Siemens Healthcare GmbH, Forchheim, Germany
[3]Siemens Healthcare GmbH, Erlangen, Germany
[4]Diagnostikum Berlin, Kardiologie, Berlin, Germany
tanja.kurzendorfer@fau.de

Abstract. Cardiac resynchronization therapy is a treatment option for patients suffering from symptomatic heart failure. The problem with this treatment option is, that 30 % to 40 % of the patients do not respond. One reason might be the inappropriate placement of the left ventricular lead via the coronary sinus. Therefore, endocardial pacing systems have been developed. Nonetheless, the implantation of these devices requires in addition to the knowledge of the anatomy and scar of the left ventricle (LV), the information of the papillary muscles. As pacing in a papillary muscles may lead to severe problems. To overcome this issue, a fully automatic papillary muscle segmentation in 3D LGE-MRI is presented. First, the left ventricle is initialized using a registration based approach, afterwards the short axis view of the LV is estimated. In the next step, the blood pool is segmented. Finally, the papillary muscles are extracted using a threshold based approach. The proposed method was evaluated on six 3D LGE-MRI data sets and were compared to gold standard annotations from clinical experts. This comparison resulted in a Dice coefficient of 0.72.

1 Introduction

Patients suffering from heart failure (HF) may be candidates for implantation of a cardiac-resynchronization-therapy (CRT) device. CRT devices require one lead to be positioned in the coronary vein system for pacing the left ventricle (LV). Nonetheless, about 30 % to 40 % of the patients do not benefit from such a system. There are various issues raised in medical literature. One reason is the confined placement in the venous system [1, 2]. To overcome this issue, current research focuses on developing endocardial pacing systems, which allow for free and unrestricted placement of a wireless lead inside the LV. For the implantation of such an endocardial CRT pacing systems, the information about the left ventricle's anatomy, scar and in particular the papillary muscles and the chordae tendineae are highly important. Placing an endocardial lead inside the

LV in a papillary muscle may lead to complications. However, information about the propagation of papillary muscles is difficult to obtain. In current clinical practice, scar quantification is performed by segmenting the left ventricle in 2D late gadolinium enhanced (LGE) MRI. Recently, 3D LGE-MRI acquisitions are developed that allow a full coverage of the entire heart within a single acquisition and a high isotropic resolution [3]. Besides technological improvements regarding image acquisition and the clear clinical demand, the challenge arises in the fast and accurate image analysis. A first semi-automatic solution for myocardial segmentation using solely 3D LGE-MRI was proposed by Kurzendorfer et al. [4]. In this work, a fully automatic segmentation of the papillary muscles within the left ventricle is presented in 3D LGE-MRI.

2   Method

The papillary muscles segmentation pipeline consists of four major steps: First, a two-step registration is performed for an initialization of the left ventricle. Second, the principal components of the left ventricle are computed and a pseudo short axis view is estimated. In the third step, the blood pool is segmented in polar space. In the final step, the papillary muscles are segmented using a threshold based approach. Fig. 1 provides an overview of the segmentation pipeline.

2.1   Left ventricle initialization

The left ventricle is initialized using a two stage registration [5] with an atlas volume $\mathbf{A} \in \mathbb{R}^{I \times J \times K}$, where I, J and K are the image image dimensions. The segmentation of the atlas volume $\mathbf{A}$ was done manually resulting in a labeled mask $\mathbf{L}$. First, a similarity transform is performed, which allows scaling, rotation and translation. To match the complex deformations of cardiac images a non-rigid registration is applied afterwards. For the matching of the transformation

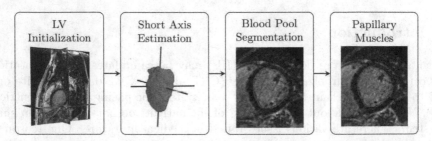

Fig. 1. Overview of the papillary muscles segmentation pipeline. First, the left ventricle is initialized using a registration based approach. In the next step, the short axis view is estimated with the help of principal component analysis. In the third step, the blood pool is segmented in polar space. In the final step, the papillary muscles are extracted using a threshold based approach.

a mutual information based similarity measure is used [6]. After the registration, the transformation is applied to the atlas label map $\mathbf{L}$ of the atlas volume $\mathbf{A}$, resulting in a registered mask $\mathbf{M} \in \mathbb{R}^{I \times J \times K}$.

2.2 Short axis estimation

After the location of the left ventricle is known, the short axis view is estimated using principle component analysis [7]. Therefore, the vertices of the surface of mask $\mathbf{M}$ are extracted using the marching cubes algorithm [8], resulting in $\mathbf{C} \in \mathbb{R}^{N \times 3}$, where N is the number of vertices. Subsequently, the covariance matrix $\boldsymbol{\Sigma}$ of the contour points is calculated. Having the covariance matrix $\boldsymbol{\Sigma}$ the singular value decomposition (SVD) is applied, which results in $\boldsymbol{\Sigma} = \mathbf{U}\mathbf{S}\mathbf{V}^T$ where $\mathbf{U}$ is a 3×3 matrix where the columns are orthogonal unit vectors. The first column corresponds to the largest variation, i.e. the short axis view. The second box of Fig. 1 shows the three unit vectors of $\mathbf{M}$, with the first marked in blue. In the next step, the offset to the center of rotation is calculated. Then, the affine transformation around the unit vectors, considering the offset can be applied to the image volume. The short axis view is needed for the segmentation of the LV, as prior knowledge such as circularity and convexity can be applied.

2.3 Blood pool segmentation

As the rough outline of the blood pool is known through the atlas registration, the volume can be cropped to the region of interest. The refinement of the blood pool starts with the slice that corresponds to the center of mass of the contour points $\mathbf{C}$, see Fig. 2 (a) for an example. The polar image of the slice is calculated, where the origin of the polar image corresponds to the center of the found contours, as depicted in Fig. 2 (b). The segmentation is performed in polar space for several reasons: The contours have a roughly circular shape in the short axis view, therefore, in polar space they all have a similar horizontal length. Furthermore, the size of the polar image is smaller, which allows for a faster processing. Through this mapping the Cartesian coordinates (x, y) are converted to polar coordinates (r, ρ). The contours $\mathbf{C}_s$ from the transformed mask $\mathbf{M}$ are converted to polar space, where s corresponds to the current slice index. Fig 2 (c) shows an example of the polar image with the transformed contours. These contours are used to refine the boundaries of the blood pool. For the refinement the edge information is extracted using the Canny edge detector.

To extract minor edges, the standard deviation σ_G of the Gaussian smoothing is set to 2.5, as depicted in Fig. 2 (d). Having the edge image $\mathbf{E}$, a minimal cost path (MCP) search is initialized using six equally spread points from $\mathbf{C}_s$. The MCP finds the distance weighted minimal path through the edge image $\mathbf{E}$. The costs for one move from point $\mathbf{p}_i$ to point $\mathbf{p}_j$ is calculated as follows

$$c(\mathbf{p}_i, \mathbf{p}_j) = \frac{d}{2}\mathbf{E}(\mathbf{p}_i) + \frac{d}{2}\mathbf{E}(\mathbf{p}_j) \qquad (1)$$

where $d = ||\mathbf{p}_i - \mathbf{p}_j||_2$. The diagonal moves vs. the axial moves are of different length and therefore, the path costs c are weighted accordingly. The cost path is calculated as the sum of the costs at each point of the path. The result of the MCP is visualized in Fig. 2 (e). The contours from the MCP are converted back to Cartesian coordinates, see Fig. 3 (a). As papillary muscles close to the endocardial border may be included, the convex hull is calculated, as depicted in Fig. 3 (b). After the first contour is refined, these steps are repeated for the subsequent slices in the pseudo SA view until the base and apex are reached. In addition, the information about the shape, radius and center is used to garantee for inter-slice smoothness.

2.4   Papillary muscles segmentation

In the next step, the papillary muscles can be segmented. In the first step, morphological erosion is applied to the blood pool contour with a radius of 2 pixels. Afterwards, Otsu thresholding is applied to the blood pool region only. All the pixels that are less than the Otsu threshold θ_O are defined as possible candidates for the papillary muscles. However, if there are not more than 7 pixels connected, it is declared as noise and they are not considered as candidates for the papillary muscles. The final result of the segmented papillary muscles for one slice is visualized in Fig. 3 (c).

After the segmentation is finished, the segmentation mask of the blood pool and the papillary muscles are exported as 3D surface meshes and can be used for further procedure planning and guidance. See Fig. 3 (d) for an example, with the papillary muscles visualized in blue and the surface of the blood pool in red.

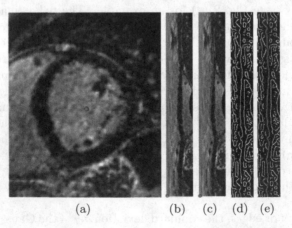

(a)   (b)   (c)   (d)   (e)

Fig. 2. (a) Slice in short axis orientation, which corresponds to the center of mass of the mask **M** marked as a red dot. (b) Corresponding image in polar space, where the origin (red dot) corresponds to the center of mass in Cartesian coordinates. (c) Polar image with the transformed contour points $\mathbf{C}_s$ in polar space. (d) Edge information from the Canny edge detector with a Gaussian smoothing of $\sigma = 2.5$. (e) Final result of the MCP.

3   Evaluation and results

The fully automatic segmentation of the papillary muscles was evaluated on six clinical LGE-MRI data sets (sparse GRE prototype sequence and reconstruction, spatial resolution $(1.3\,\text{mm})^3$) from individual patients. The data was acquired with a 3T MAGNETOM Skyra scanner (Siemens Healthcare GmbH, Erlangen, Germany). Gold standard annotations of the papillary muscles were provided by two clinical experts. The annotations were performed using MITK. Given the gold standard annotations, the segmentation was evaluated using the Dice coefficient (DC) and the Jaccard index (JI). The DC is a quantitative measure for the segmentation quality, as it measures the proportion of the true positives in the segmentation. The JI measures the union overlap between two segmentation masks. Both scores range from 0 to 1, with 1 corresponding to perfect overlap. For both scores the whole 3D volume was considered. The segmentation of the papillary muscles resulted in a DC of 0.72 ± 0.08. The best segmentation result had a DC of 0.85 and the worst a DC of 0.61. For the Jaccard index similar observations could be made, with a mean JI of 0.57 ± 0.10. The best JI had a value of 0.74 and the worst of 0.44.

The evaluation was performed on an Intel i7 with 2.80GHz equipped with 16 GB RAM. The whole segmentation pipeline needs less than 4 minutes implemented with Python, single-threaded.

4   Discussion and conclusion

The results are summarized in Tab. 1. The proposed method achieved a DC of 0.72 and a JC of 0.57. The relatively low Dice coefficient can be attributed to the fact, that in one data set the papillary muscles were scarred and sometimes in addition some parts of the chordae tendineae were included in the segmentation.

In sum this work presents a simple and efficient approach for papillary muscle segmentation in 3D LGE-MRI. The segmented papillary muscles as well as

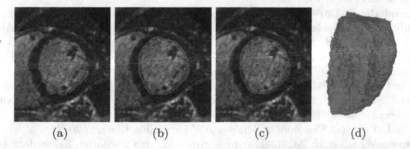

(a)   (b)   (c)   (d)

Fig. 3. Final steps of the segmentation pipeline. (a) Contour points after the MCP in Cartesian coordinates. (b) Convex hull of the MCP, resulting in the final result for the blood pool refinement. (c) Final result showing the blood pool contour in red and the papillary muscles in blue. (d) Result in 3D, the blood pool is visualized in red and the papillary muscles in blue.

Table 1. Papillary muscles segmentation results using the Dice coefficient and the Jaccard index.

Description	Mean ± Std	Min	Max	Inter-Obs
Dice	0.72 ± 0.08	0.61	0.85	0.96 ± 0.06
Jaccard	0.57 ± 0.10	0.44	0.74	0.93 ± 0.11

the information about myocardial scarring and the anatomy of the left ventricle can be extracted from one sequence and then be used to plan the procedure. In addition, the papillary muscles can be overlaid onto the fluoroscopic images and used during the intervention for guidance. Future work will include the investigation of scarred myocardium and papillary muscles for further improvement of the segmentation algorithm. A clear benefit of this approach is that all relevant information for a CRT procedure can be extracted from a single LGE-MRI data set.

Disclaimer. The methods and information presented in this paper are based on research and are not commercially available.

References

1. Shetty A, Duckett S, Ginks M, et al. Cardiac magnetic resonance-derived anatomy, scar, and dyssynchrony fused with fluoroscopy to guide LV lead placement in cardiac resynchronization therapy: a comparison with acute haemodynamic measures and echocardiographic reverse remodelling. Eur Heart J Cardiovasc Imaging. 2012;14(7):692–9.
2. Shetty A, Sohal M, Chen Z, et al. A comparison of left ventricular endocardial, multisite, and multipolar epicardial cardiac resynchronization: an acute haemodynamic and electroanatomical study. Europace. 2014; p. eut420.
3. Shin T, Lustig M, Nishimura D, et al. Rapid single-breath-hold 3D late gadolinium enhancement cardiac MRI using a stack-of-spirals acquisition. J Magn Reson Imaging. 2014;40(6):1496–502.
4. Kurzendorfer T, Brost A, Forman C, et al. Semi-automatic segmentation and scar quantification of the left ventricle in 3-D late gadolinium enhanced MRI. 32nd Annu Sci Meet ESMRMB. 2015; p. 318–9.
5. Unberath M, Maier A, Fleischmann D, et al. Comparative evaluation of two registration-based segmentation algorithms: application to whole heart segmentation in CT. Proc GRC. 2015; p. 5–8.
6. Klein S, Staring M, Murphy K, et al. elastix: a toolbox for intensity-based medical image registration. IEEE Trans Med Imaging. 2010;29(1):196–205.
7. Jolliffe I. Principal Component Analysis. Wiley Online Library; 2002.
8. Lorensen W, Cline H; ACM. Marching cubes: a high resolution 3D surface construction algorithm. ACM Siggraph Computer Graph. 1987;21:163–9.

Abstract: Clickstreamanalyse zur Qualitätssicherung in der crowdbasierten Bildsegmentierung

Eric Heim[1], Alexander Seitel[1], Christian Stock[2], Tobias Ross[1],
Lena Maier-Hein[1]

[1]Abteilung für Computer-assistierte medizinische Interventionen, Deutsches
Krebsforschungszentrum Heidelberg (DKFZ)
[2]Institut für Medizinische Biometrie und Informatik, Universitätsklinikum Heidelberg
e.heim@dkfz.de

Mit der vermehrten Verbreitung von Verfahren aus dem Bereich des Maschinellen
Lernens in der medizinische Bildverarbeitung wird eine große Menge von akkurat
annotierten medizinischen Bilddaten benötigt. Die begrenzten Ressourcen von
medizinischen Experten entwickeln sich dabei zum Flaschenhals für das gesamte
Forschungsgebiet. Eine neuartige Methode zum Annotieren von Daten im großen
Stil, die bereits Einzug in die medizinische Bildverarbeitung erhalten hat, ist
das sogenannte Crowdsourcing, welches auf dem Outsourcen kognitiver Aufgaben an anonyme Internetbenutzer basiert. Eine große Herausforderung in diesem
Zusammenhang ist die hohe Varianz der Annotationsqualität, die in der Regel
durch redundante Aufgabenverteilung gelöst wird. In diesem Beitrag stellen wir
einen neuartigen Ansatz zur Bewertung der Annotationsqualität auf Basis von
Clickstreams vor. Inspiriert von Verfahren zur Analyse von Benutzerverhalten in
sozialen Netzwerken [1] und biometrischen Benutzerauthentifizierung [2] konver-
tieren wir die Benutzereingaben in einen Vektor von Interaktionsmerkmalen und
trainieren einen Regressor, der die Annotationsqualität, repräsentiert durch den
DICE Koeffizienten, schätzt. Mehrere Annotationen können so konfidenzgewich-
tet zu einer finalen Objektsegmentierung fusioniert werden. Unter Verwendung
von 20.000 Crowdsegmentierungen auf öffentlich verfügbaren Datensätzen zeigen wir (1) dass unser Verfahren mit weniger als der Hälfte der Kosten dieselbe
Qualität im Vergleich zum verbreiteten Majority Voting erreicht und (2) her-
vorragend auf neue Domänen generalisiert, die nicht in den Trainingsbildern
enthalten sind. Durch die Kostenersparnis ist das Anwendungspotential für die
neue Methode hoch.

Literaturverzeichnis

1. Wang G, Konolige T, Wilson C, et al. You are how you click: Clickstream analysis
   for sybil detection. In: Proc. USENIX Security; 2013. p. 1–15.
2. Feher C, Elovici Y, Moskovitch R, et al. User Identity Verification via Mouse Dynamics. Information Sciences. 2012;201:19–36.

Model-Based 4D Segmentation of Cardiac Structures in Cine MRI Sequences

Nassim Bouteldja[1], Matthias Wilms[1], Heinz Handels[1], Dennis Säring[2],
Jan Ehrhardt[1]

[1]Institute of Medical Informatics, University of Lübeck
[2]University of Applied Sciences Wedel
wilms@imi.uni-luebeck.de

Abstract. A temporally consistent segmentation of cardiac structures in spatio-temporal cine MRI sequences is a prerequisite for in-depth analyses of the heart dynamics in clinical practice. Despite its great importance, automated cardiac segmentation is still an open problem, especially for spatio-temporal data due to challenging imaging characteristics, large anatomical heart variability, and diversity of cardiac dynamics. To cope with these challenges, an approach for model-based 4D segmentation of the left and right ventricle in clinical cine MRI sequences is presented in this paper. Central to our approach is a 4D statistical shape model that accounts for both inter- and intra-patient variability. It is fitted to the spatio-temporal image sequence by applying a computationally efficient MRF-based discrete optimization approach that uses BRIEF descriptors for image matching. The approach is evaluated on 15 cardiac cine MRI sequences of children and adults with different heart abnormalities. The segmentation results are compared with another effective 4D segmentation technique indicating similar segmentation accuracy but improved coherence and runtime performances.

1 Introduction

Cardiovascular diseases are reported to be the leading cause of death globally. Meaningful assessments of the cardiac function or myocardial viability are possible using spatio-temporal cine MRI sequences. For example, clinical parameters such as the ejection fraction or myocardial mass indicating heart abnormalities can be obtained based on segmentations. In clinical practice, automation plays a crucial role as manual segmentation is very time-consuming and prone to high inter-observer variability. Despite the advances in automatic cardiac segmentation in recent years ([1] for an overview), robust, accurate, and fast techniques for 4D biventricular segmentation in cardiac cine MRI sequences are still missing. In this context, it is important to note that segmentation of 4D image data should not be treated as multiple isolated 3D segmentation tasks, because advantages in terms of robustness and temporal consistency of real 4D segmentation approaches were shown, e.g., in [2, 3]. Existing approaches for 4D cardiac segmentation often utilize statistical shape models (SSMs) or spatio-temporal registration techniques. For example, Perperidis et al. built a 4D statistical shape model accounting for both inter- and intra-patient variability in [4], and Kepp et al. used atlas-based segmentation techniques based on time-consuming multichannel 3D registrations with trajectory constraints [3] for 4D cardiac image segmentation.

In this work, we present a fast spatio-temporal (4D) segmentation approach for cardiac structures in cine MRI data. Our approach is based on [4, 2] and compared to [3] on 15 cardiac cine MRI sequences.

2   Material and methods

We assume a training set of N_p different cine MRI sequences each consisting of N_j 3D images with segmentations (LV endocard, LV epicard, RV) to be given to build a 4D statistical shape model of both ventricles (Sec. 2.1), which can subsequently be fitted to an unseen sequence using a discrete optimization framework (Sec. 2.2).

2.1   Building the 4D statistical shape model

Our approach for establishing landmark correspondences for model building largely follows that of [2]. Briefly summarized, an atlas representing the average shape of the cardiac structures in the training set at a reference phase (here: end-diastolic) is constructed whose automatically generated M landmarks are propagated to the training shapes by atlas-patient and intra-patient non-linear diffeomorphic registration. Subsequently, all shapes are mapped to the atlas space via patient-specific similarity transforms. Now, we can build a model according to [4, 2] based on the set of aligned and corresponding training shapes $\{q_{p,j} \in \mathbb{R}^{3M} \,|\, p = 1, \ldots, N_p; j = 1, \ldots, N_j\}$ in atlas space with $\overline{q} \in \mathbb{R}^{3M}$ being the overall mean shape. Our spatio-temporal shape model is defined by

$$S_{4D}(b_{\text{inter}}, b_{\text{intra}}^j, \varphi) = \varphi(\overline{q} + P_{\text{inter}}b_{\text{inter}} + P_{\text{intra}}b_{\text{intra}}^j) . \qquad (1)$$

It is parameterized by a patient-specific subspace spanned by P_{inter} with weights b_{inter}, a phase-dependent subspace spanned by P_{intra} with weights b_{intra}^j, and an atlas-to-patient similarity transform φ. As the space of cardiac shapes is divided into two subspaces, the inter-patient covariance matrix

$$C_{\text{inter}} = \frac{1}{N_p} \sum_{p=1}^{N_p} (\overline{q}_p - \overline{q})(\overline{q}_p - \overline{q})^T \text{ with } \overline{q}_p = \frac{1}{N_j} \sum_{j=1}^{N_j} q_{p,j} \qquad (2)$$

represents shape variability appearing across the population, while the intra-patient covariance matrix

$$C_{\text{intra}} = \frac{1}{N_p N_j} \sum_{p=1}^{N_p} \sum_{j=1}^{N_j} (q_{p,j} - \overline{q}_p)(q_{p,j} - \overline{q}_p)^T \qquad (3)$$

holds information about shape variations occurring due to the cardiac cycle. Performing two separate PCAs on them yields the bases P_{inter} and P_{intra}.

2.2   Fitting the 4D statistical shape model

Fitting the 4D SSM to all N_j 3D images of an unseen sequence is done by estimating valid parameters $\{\tilde{b}_{\text{inter}}, \tilde{b}_{\text{intra}}^1, \ldots, \tilde{b}_{\text{intra}}^{N_j}, \tilde{\varphi}\}$ to optimally approximate the desired cardiac shape $r_j \in \mathbb{R}^{3M}$ by the model $S_{4D}(\tilde{b}_{\text{inter}}, \tilde{b}_{\text{intra}}^j, \varphi) \approx r_j$. Following [2], this is specified by the optimization problem

$$\sum_{j=1}^{N_j} \|r_j - S_{4D}(\tilde{b}_{\text{inter}}, b_{\text{intra}}^j, \varphi)\|^2 \longrightarrow \min \tag{4}$$

which is divided into the following two parts

$$(\tilde{b}_{\text{inter}}, \tilde{\varphi}) = \operatorname*{argmin}_{b_{\text{inter}}, \varphi} \|\frac{1}{N_j} \sum_{j=1}^{N_j} r_j - S_{4D}(b_{\text{inter}}, 0, \varphi)\|^2 \text{ and} \tag{5}$$

$$(\tilde{b}_{\text{intra}}^j) = \operatorname*{argmin}_{b_{\text{intra}}^j} \|r_j - S_{4D}(\tilde{b}_{\text{inter}}, b_{\text{intra}}^j, \tilde{\varphi})\|^2 \tag{6}$$

After initial placement of the model, these optimization problems can be solved iteratively by an alternating scheme largely similar to the classical active shape model algorithm. In each iteration a new candidate shape is generated by searching for new landmark positions along the surface normals, followed by a projection to the shape space(s) ([2] for details). In order to address the well-known limitations of this type of fitting, we look for candidates in an omnidirectional manner as proposed in [5]. We therefore denote a discrete set of uniformly distributed displacements within a sphere as S, and the triangulated surface mesh of the current model $S_{4D}(b_{\text{inter}}, b_{\text{intra}}^j, \varphi)$ as $R_j = (V_j, E_j)$ with vertex set V_j, edge set E_j and its displacement field $d_j : V_j \to S, d_j(v) =: d_{j,v}$. The optimization problem for 4D model adaptation

$$\sum_{j=1}^{N_j} \sum_{v \in V_j} \phi(v + d_{j,v}) + \sum_{j=1}^{N_j} \sum_{(v,w) \in E_j} \lambda \cdot \psi(d_{j,v}, d_{j,w}) \xrightarrow{\{d_j\}} \min \tag{7}$$

is encoded as an equally defined MRF despite of displacements being represented by MRF-states. Eq. 7 is about finding an optimal trade-off between image fit and local regularization, which is given by $\psi(d_{j,v}, d_{j,w}) = \|(d_{j,v} - d_{j,w})/\delta_s\|^3$ (according to [5]) to avoid topology inconsistencies. It also increases the robustness towards outliers. Here, δ_s denotes the sampling distance within the sphere. Additionally, edges between temporally corresponding vertices (analogy: 4D "ring-graph") and between landmarks on the LV epicard and their closest points on the LV endocard surface (within every phase j) are added to the MRF-edge set. Adding the former leads to maintaining temporal consistency, whereas the latter increases spatial consistencies by limiting the independence of their deformation. Finally, the MRF is efficiently optimized using primal dual strategies [6]. It yields the approximately optimal displacement field d summing up all d_j.

Furthermore, we need to specify the image fit function $\phi(v + d_{j,v})$. It is based on BRIEF-descriptors [7] which have shown their robustness in CV applications, and are extremely fast to compute and to compare due to the use of binarized pixel comparisons. During model training, for each landmark at each phase of all training images one BRIEF descriptor of length L is computed. As this leads to $N_p N_j$ extracted descriptors per landmark, K-medoids clustering is used to determine $K \ll N_p N_j$ representative descriptors. For model fitting, the unary potential function $\phi(v + d_{j,v})$ is defined as the minimal hamming distance between the binary descriptor at $v + d_{j,v}$ and the corresponding K representative descriptors.

It is also important to note that the segmentation process takes place in the atlas coordinate frame via the inverse of the model's initial transformation. This eliminates the problem of BRIEF not being rotation and scale invariant.

2.3 Experiments

Our evaluation is based on two different data sets. Data set A comprises 5 cardiac short-axis 4D cine MRI sequences of adults with acute myocardial infarction from our in-house database and data set C consists of 10 case subset of cardiac short-axis 4D cine MRI data of children with heart abnormalities provided by [8]. Data set C is also used in [3] allowing for the comparison of results reported below. Each 4D image sequence consists of 20 – 30 3D images volumes of size 256 – 320 $\times$ 256 – 320 $\times$ 8 – 15 with spacing of 0.93 – 1.64 mm $\times$ 0.93 – 1.64 mm $\times$ 6 – 13 mm covering the whole cardiac cycle. Manual ground-truth segmentations were available for 3 cardiac structures in all phases (LV endocard, LV epicard, RV). All images were preprocessed with a pipeline similar to [3] (bias correction and registration-based upsampling reducing the slice thickness to ≈ 1.5 mm) to account for intensity differences and large inter-slice distances.

Consequently, the model is built upon the complete training set of 15 cine MRI sequences and further consists of $M \approx 6000$ landmarks covering LV endocard, LV epicard and RV. As for evaluation, we apply leave-one-out tests and provide separate results for data set A and C. We also utilize the dice coefficient and the symmetric mean surface distance $d_{\mu_{\text{sym}}}$ as error metrics for ground-truth comparisons. Parameters were determined as the following: $K = 20$, $\lambda = 32$, $L = 256$, $\delta_s = 2, 6$ mm, sampling radius $r_s - 8$ mm.

3   Results

Tab. 1 shows separate results of our evaluation. Compared to the results of Kepp's et al. multichannel approach in [3], our approach shows similar segmentation accuracy but is substantially faster (ours: $\approx 7\,min$; [3, 9]: $\approx 18\,min$ on a quad-core Xeon CPU @ 2.67 GHz). Moreover, low standard deviations of $d_{\mu_{\text{sym}}}$ indicate the robustness of our approach and even more consistent results compared to [3]. Spatial and temporal consistencies are exemplary shown in Fig. 1 in which the model, especially in the first row, fits the data very well

Table 1. First/second coloum: Evaluation results of our approach based on data set A/C (hearts of adults/children). Third: Results of Kepp et al. [3] based on C. Both metric errors (dice, sym. mean surface distance) are averaged over patients and phases.

	Data set A Our approach		Data set C		Kepp et al. [3]	
	Dice	$d_{\mu_{\mathrm{sym}}}$	Dice	$d_{\mu_{\mathrm{sym}}}$	Dice	$d_{\mu_{\mathrm{sym}}}$
Endokard	0.76	3.38 ± 1.20	0.79	$2.47 \pm 0.95\,\mathrm{mm}$	0.82	$1.92 \pm 0.89\,\mathrm{mm}$
Epikard	0.82	$3.70 \pm 1.20\,\mathrm{mm}$	0.86	$2.37 \pm 0.73\,\mathrm{mm}$	0.86	$2.41 \pm 1.10\,\mathrm{mm}$
RV	0.77	$2.60 \pm 0.54\,\mathrm{mm}$	0.79	$2.27 \pm 0.69\,\mathrm{mm}$	0.77	$2.75 \pm 1.26\,\mathrm{mm}$
Mean	0.78	$3.23 \pm 1.12\,\mathrm{mm}$	0.81	$2.37 \pm 0.81\,\mathrm{mm}$	0.82	$2.36 \pm 1.14\,\mathrm{mm}$

being temporally smoothed. In contrast, adaptation difficulties at the outer side of the left ventricle are observed in the second row. Surprisingly, the model iteratively contracts its outer epicard contours onto the image's endocard due to widespread smooth intensity variations resulting from the smoothing processes. In fact, the model does not quantize the amplitude of local gradients due to the binary descriptor's strong quantization.

As our linear model can only adapt to variations seen in the training set, it has difficulties in expressing the true shape of some cardiac structures due to the small training set. Inaccurate reference data further badly affects the quality of the model and the descriptors. Nevertheless, it is able to cope with the challenges given by a small data set of hearts with huge differences in variation and scale.

4 Discussion

In this paper, we present a fast spatio-temporal cardiac segmentation approach that utilizes a 4D statistical shape model accounting for both inter- and intra-

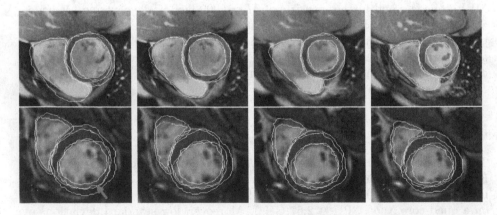

Fig. 1. Segmentation (yellow contours) on two patient's data compared to the ground trouth (green). First row: Uniformly depicted slices between ED and ES (temporal). Second row: Subsequently taken slices at ED (spatial).

patient variability to handle challenging image characteristics as well as large anatomical and physiological heart variabilities. Fitting the model is performed within a computationally efficient discrete MRF-based optimization framework that uses binary descriptors for image matching and ensures robustness as well as overall consistency through local and temporal regularization. The segmentation results showed that our approach leads to spatially and temporally consistent segmentations with a similar accuracy as the registration-based 4D segmentation approach used in [3]. However, our approach is substantially faster.

In future work, we plan to improve on the model's generalization ability by enlarging the training data set and by using new data augmentation approaches [10]. Moreover, we further intend to utilize other descriptors for model matching to reduce segmentation problems arising due to the BRIEF's strong quantization.

Acknowledgement. This work is supported by the DFG (EH 224/6-1).

References

1. Peng P, Lekadir K, Gooya A, et al. A review of heart chamber segmentation for structural and functional analysis using cardiac magnetic resonance imaging. Magn Reson Mater Phy. 2016;29(2):155–95.
2. Wilms M, Ehrhardt J, Handels H. A 4D statistical shape model for automated segmentation of lungs with large tumors. Proc MICCAI. 2012; p. 347–54.
3. Kepp T, Ehrhardt J, Handels H. Evaluation verschiedener Ansätze zur 4D-4D-Registrierung kardiologischer MR-Bilddaten. Proc BVM. 2015; p. 95–100.
4. Perperidis D, Mohiaddin R, Edwards P, et al. Segmentation of cardiac MR and CT image sequences using model-based registration of a 4D statistical model. Proc SPIE Medical Imaging. 2007;6512:65121D.
5. Kainmueller D, Lamecker H, Heller MO, et al. Omnidirectional displacements for deformable surfaces. Med Image Anal. 2013;17(4):429–41.
6. Komodakis N, Tziritas G, Paragios N. Performance vs computational efficiency for optimizing single and dynamic MRFs: setting the state of the art with primal-dual strategies. Comput Vis Image Underst. 2008;112(1):14–29.
7. Calonder M, Lepetit V, Strecha C, et al. BRIEF: binary robust independent elementary features. Proc ECCV. 2010; p. 778–92.
8. Andreopoulos A, Tsotsos JK. Efficient and generalizable statistical models of shape and appearance for analysis of cardiac MRI. Med Image Anal. 2008;12(3):335–57.
9. Kepp T. Atlasbasierte 4D-Segmentierung des Herzens durch Multichannel 3D-Registrierung. vol. 1. Infinite Science Publishing; 2014.
10. Ehrhardt J, Wilms M, Handels H. Patch-Based low-rank matrix completion for learning of shape and motion models from few training samples. Proc ECCV. 2016; p. 712–27.

Abstract: Kombination binärer Kontextfeatures mit Vantage Point Forests zur Multi-Organ-Segmentierung

Maximilian Blendowski, Mattias P. Heinrich

Institut für Medizinische Informatik, Stiftungsuniversität zu Lübeck
maximilian.blendowski@student.uni-luebeck.de

Verfahren zur automatischen Multi-Organ-Segmentierung in medizinischen Bildvolumina beruhen häufig auf annotierten Daten eines Patientenkollektivs (Atlas) und deren Anpassung z.b. durch zeitintensive nichtlineare Registrierung [1]. Bei der MICCAI 2016 Konferenz [2] stellten wir ein registrierungsfreies Framework für die Übertragung von Vorwissen in Form von segmentierten Trainingsdaten auf ungesehene Patienten mit Hilfe eines neuen starken Klassifizierer vor: die Vantage Point Forests (VPF). Ähnlich zu Random Decision Forests (RDF) werden schnelle Berechnungszeiten von wenigen Sekunden erreicht.

Unser Verfahren setzt nun am Schwachpunkt achsenparalleler Splitfunktionen der RDFs an, welche insbesondere für kleine Organstrukturen mit großer Formvariabilität an Grenzen stoßen. Der VPF-Klassifizierer ermöglicht das Finden von Zusammenhängen hochdimensionaler Eingabefeatures durch deren gemeinsame Betrachtung bei der Teilungsentscheidung in jedem Knoten. Als Baumstruktur wird die effiziente Datenpartitionierung in Hypersphären aus [3] eingesetzt, welche balancierte Bäume ergibt und auf aufwendige Optimierungen der Splits verzichtet (Quellcode siehe http://mpheinrich.de/research.html#vpf).

Wir verwenden eine Vielzahl einfacher Intensitätssvergleiche [4] zur Erzeugung von hochdimensionalen, binären Featurevektoren. Sie zeichnen sich durch eine sehr gute kontrastinvariante Kodierung der umgebenden Struktur aus und ermöglichen einen zusätzlichen Geschwindeskeits- und Speichervorteil durch Verwendung der effizienten Hammingdistanz zwischen Binärvektoren (POPCNT). Unsere Methode erreicht Stand-der-Technik Dice-Werte von 90% für Leber und Nieren in Abdominal-CTs (+10% im Vergleich zu RDF) und liefert gerade bei kleineren Strukturen eine große Verbesserung der Segmentierung.

Literaturverzeichnis

1. Xu Z, Lee CP, Heinrich MP, et al. Evaluation of six registration methods for the human abdomen on clinically acquired CT. IEEE Trans Biomed Eng. 2016;63(8):1563–72.
2. Heinrich MP, Blendowski M; Springer. Multi-organ segmentation using vantage point forests and binary context features. Proc MICCAI. 2016; p. 598–606.
3. Yianilos PN. Data structures and algorithms for nearest neighbor search in general metric spaces. Proc SODA. 1993;93(194):311–21.
4. Calonder M, Lepetit V, Strecha C, et al. BRIEF: Binary robust independent elementary features. Proc ECCV. 2010; p. 778–92.

Needle Detection in In-Plane-Acquired 3D Ultrasound Image Volumes Using Stick Filtering and a Heuristic

Heinrich M. Overhoff, Anke Poelstra, Sebastian Schmitt

Westfälische Hochschule, University of Applied Sciences,
Medical Engineering Laboratory, Gelsenkirchen, Germany
heinrich-martin.overhoff@w-hs.de

Abstract. We propose an image-based method to estimate the needle axis parameters in 3D ultrasound data although the needle is shown as flat, broad shape due to ultrasound elevation beam-width artifacts in ultrasound volumes. For this, ultrasound volumes are correlated with small 3D sticks of various azimuth and polar angles. The maximal correlation magnitude assigns the orientation of one of the sticks to each voxel position. Voxels of similar angles are clustered and modeled as lines by ℓ_2-norm minimization. The method was applied to 44 3D ultrasound volumes showing a 16 G needle which was pushed into pork liver. The estimated location and orientation of the needle axes coincide well with expert defined "reference" needles, as median (97%-quantile) estimation errors for orientation $\leq 1.24°$ ($\leq 5.16°$) and distance between needle tip and axis ≤ 0.53 mm (≤ 1.16 mm) indicate.

1 Introduction

Monitoring the position of surgical instruments in image guided, minimally invasive interventions is an important task to increase the success of the procedure. Ultrasound is a non-ionizing imaging modality with real-time capabilities. Therefore, it is the method of choice for monitoring instrument positions in minimally invasive interventions like core biopsies.

Various methods for detecting surgical instruments like biopsy needles in 3D ultrasound exist. They can be divided into external or position-sensor-based methods and internal or image-based methods. With position-sensor-based methods, additional position measuring systems are used for calculating the relative position between the intervention needle and the ultrasound probe. For reasons of a reduced measurement setup, the focus of this work lies on image-based methods. Commonly used image-based methods use the RANSAC (random sample consensus) algorithm to detect linear structures of high intensity in ultrasound volumes [1, 2, 3]. In [1] a needle localization accuracy of less than 1 mm is reported. However, this accuracy could only be reached in simulated ultrasound images with almost homogeneous background. For real images, the background is more inhomogeneous (tissue boundaries) and for a similar localization accuracy the number of iterations of the RANSAC algorithm has to be increased. In order to reduce calculation time, Zhao et al. developed a method for automatically reducing the ROI (region of interest) [3]. In [4] they present the validation of that method on real ultrasound data and achieve an accuracy (RMSE) for needle axis localization of $d^{\text{tip}} \leq 1.8\,\text{mm}$ and $\Delta\vartheta^\dagger \leq 8°$, $\Delta\varphi^\dagger \leq 5°$. With that method, the needle is assumed to be of a thin and cylindrical shape. However, one drawback of ultrasound imaging is the distortion of the image due to the insertion of highly echogenic objects, e.g. biopsy needles. Variations of needle-related ultrasound artifacts are discussed in [5]. For example, the elevation beam-width artifact leads to a broadened perception of the needle axis (band-shaped artifact). By image processing, this artifact must be reduced to the needle's linear shape. In [6], Czerwinski et al. describe an approach to enhance linear structures in medical images by filtering with "sticks". We adopted this idea for use in 3D data – called 3D stick filtering in the following. With the 3D stick filtering, the needle artifact is enhanced in such a way that it can be modeled by a straight line in the image volume coordinate system. This mathematical abstraction is then used for the evaluation of the presented image-based method for determining the location and orientation of the needle axis in 3D ultrasound volumes.

2   Materials and methods

2.1   Experimental setup

A total of 44 ultrasound volumes has been recorded via the Art.Lab interface of a MyLab 70 ultrasound system (Esaote Europe B.V., The Netherlands) connected to a mechanical 3D linear probe (BL433), which acquires the raw data image plane by image plane. These raw data – summed A-lines – contain the reflection signals of a $16\,\text{G}$ ($d^{\text{N}} = 1.29\text{mm}$) needle pushed into pork liver and have a sampling frequency of $f_s = 50\,\text{MHz}$. Image reconstruction of ultrasound raw data mainly consisted of Hilbert transform and logarithmic compression. Gray scaling is performed individually for each image. Each image volume G has size $N_X \times N_Y \times N_Z$, where N_X is the number of columns, N_Y the number of rows, and N_Z the number of image planes. The spatial resolution of G is $\Delta x = \Delta y = \Delta z = 0.245\,\text{mm/px}$ and the gray scale values at the coordinates (x, y, z) are denoted by $g(x, y, z)$. The needles are oriented to be visible in a minimal number of image planes (in-plane technique), i.e. $\vartheta \approx 90°$ (cf. (1)) such generating a line-like reflection in these planes.

2.2   Needle axis model

Mathematical formulation. In a 3D gray scale image volume, the needle refletion appears as a band-shaped structure. Fig. 1 shows two synthetic cross sectional views of a needle. The needle axis is part of this artifact. It can be represented in the image volume coordinate system in the bijective vector form of the equation of a line $\mathbf{p} - \mathbf{p}_0 - \lambda\mathbf{u} = \mathbf{0}$ s.t. $\mathbf{u}^T \cdot \mathbf{u} = 1$ (normalization) and

$\mathbf{u}^T \cdot \mathbf{p}_0 = 0$ (orthogonality). $\mathbf{p}$ denotes a point vector, λ a scalar parameter, $\mathbf{u} = [u_x \ u_y \ u_z]^T$, $u_y = \sqrt{1 - u_x^2 - u_z^2}$ a unit vector in the direction of the line, and $\mathbf{p}_0 = [p_{0_x} \ p_{0_y} \ p_{0_z}]^T$, $p_{0_z} = -\frac{1}{u_z}(p_{0_x} u_x + p_{0_y} u_y)$ the shortest point vector from the image volume coordinate system's origin to the line. $\mathbf{u}$ is derived from the direction vector in the needle coordinate system $\mathbf{u}^N = [0 \ 0 \ 1]^T$, which is first aligned to the image volume coordinate system and then consecutively rotated in polar ($0° \leq \vartheta < 180°$) and in azimuth ($0° \leq \varphi < 360°$) orientation

$$\begin{bmatrix} u_x \\ u_y \\ u_z \end{bmatrix} = \begin{bmatrix} \cos\varphi & -\sin\varphi & 0 \\ \sin\varphi & \cos\varphi & 0 \\ 0 & 0 & 1 \end{bmatrix} \begin{bmatrix} \cos\vartheta & 0 & \sin\vartheta \\ 0 & 1 & 0 \\ -\sin\vartheta & 0 & \cos\vartheta \end{bmatrix} \begin{bmatrix} 0 \\ 0 \\ 1 \end{bmatrix} = \begin{bmatrix} \sin\vartheta \cos\varphi \\ \sin\vartheta \sin\varphi \\ \cos\vartheta \end{bmatrix} = \mathbf{u}(\vartheta, \varphi) \tag{1}$$

Reference model of a needle axis. For each of the investigated ultrasound volumes, an expert determined a line $\mathbf{p} = \mathbf{p}_0^\dagger + \lambda\mathbf{u}(\vartheta^\dagger, \varphi^\dagger)$ as model of the needle. The parameter sets $\{p_{0x}^\dagger, p_{0y}^\dagger, \vartheta^\dagger, \varphi^\dagger\}$ thus define reference models of needle axes.

2.3 Automatic determination from image data

3D stick filtering. Given are three dimensional binary templates $H_{p,q}$ of size $N_{X'} \times N_{Y'} \times N_{Z'}$, with $N_{X'} = N_{Y'} = N_{Z'} = 2R + 1$. Straight lines pass the template's center $[x' \ y' \ z']^T = [0 \ 0 \ 0]^T$ in different discrete orientations

$$\vartheta'_p = (p-1)\Delta\vartheta', \ 1 \leq p \leq N_{\vartheta'}, \ N_{\vartheta'} = \left\lceil \frac{180°}{\Delta\vartheta'} \right\rceil,$$

$$\varphi'_q = (q-1)\Delta\varphi', \ 1 \leq q \leq N_{\varphi'}, \ N_{\varphi'} = \left\lceil \frac{180°}{\Delta\varphi'} \right\rceil \tag{2}$$

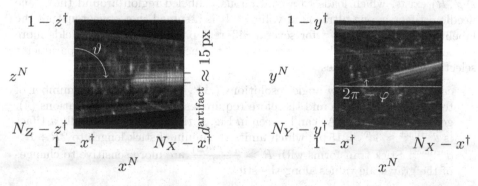

Fig. 1. Band-shaped cross section of the needle artifact with expert defined needle axis (red) and orientation angles (white, angles in reference coordinate system, (1)).

A gray scale volume G is filtered with each of the templates $H_{p,q}$, i.e. for each of the $N_{\vartheta'} \cdot N_{\varphi'}$ pairs (p,q) $g_{p,q}^{\mathrm{SF}}(x,y,z)$ is calculated

$$g_{p,q}^{\mathrm{SF}}(x,y,z) = \sum_{x',y',z'=-R}^{R} h_{p,q}(x',y',z') \cdot g(x+x',y+y',z+z') \qquad (3)$$

Labeling of 3D stick filtered image volumes. The best fitting stick (p^*,q^*) at each voxel position is found from $(p^*,q^*) = \underset{p,q}{\mathrm{argmax}}\, g_{p,q}^{\mathrm{SF}}(x,y,z)$. Each image volume G is such linked to a volume of stick orientations $G_{p,q}^{\mathrm{SF}}$ of size $N_X \times N_Y \times N_Z$. Sub-volumes with no obviously linearly distributed gray scale values usually result in randomly oriented sticks for neighboring voxels, i.e. the pairs (p^*,q^*) of neighboring voxels in $G_{p,q}^{\mathrm{SF}}$ differ. For needle axis detection only such sub-volumes shall be included, which fulfill the following heuristics:

- $3 \times 3 \times 3$ diamond-shaped sub-volumes with identical stick orientations are clustered to generate a label volume $\mathbf{L}_{\Delta\vartheta',\Delta\varphi',R}$ of size $N_X \times N_Y \times N_Z$. Labeled clusters represent sub-volumes with conjoint stick orientation.
- Clusters are omitted if they do not consist of more than $N^{\min}$ voxels.
- For each remaining cluster, its voxels are appoximated by a straight line (least squares approximation). This line has orientation angles (ϑ,φ). Labels are kept if the underlying cluster's stick and the line's orientation roughly coincide (cf. (1)): $(|\vartheta - (p^*-1)\Delta\vartheta'| < \Delta\vartheta') \wedge (|\varphi - (q^*-1)\Delta\varphi'| < \Delta\varphi')$. In this way, label volume $\mathbf{L}_{\Delta\vartheta',\Delta\varphi',R}^*$ is generated.

$\mathbf{L}_{\Delta\vartheta',\Delta\varphi',R}^*$ is linked to the voxels of image volume G and indicates sticks assumably belong to the needle axis. It has drastically less entries than $\mathbf{L}_{\Delta\vartheta',\Delta\varphi',R}$.

Estimating location and orientation of the needle axis. Because gray scaling is performed individually for each image, the gray scale contrast along the needle axis may vary. Therefore, no generally valid parameter setting $(\Delta\vartheta', \Delta\varphi', R)$ exists, which leads to a continuously labeled region around the whole needle artifact in one ultrasound volume. It is assumed that concatenating the labeling results $\mathbf{L}_{\Delta\vartheta',\Delta\varphi',R}^*$ for several different parameter settings yields more labeled voxels that match the geometry of the needle artifact. The parameter selection regards the issues

- calculation time: Low angle resolutions ($\Delta\vartheta'$, $\Delta\varphi'$) decrease the number of templates ($N_{\vartheta'} \cdot N_{\varphi'}$) and therefore require less correlation calculations (3).
- geometric relations: As can be seen in Fig. 1, the width of the needle artifact is $d^{\mathrm{artifact}} \approx 3d^{\mathrm{N}} \approx 15\,\mathrm{px}$, which limits the minimal stick length to $2R+1 > d^{\mathrm{artifact}}$. Stick transforms with $R \gg \frac{d^{\mathrm{artifact}}-1}{2}$ are more sensitive to changes of the gray scale values along the stick.

Therefore, for each volume, the stick transform is calculated for multiple parameter settings, which are characterized by different values for $\Delta\vartheta' \in \{10°,15°\}$, $\Delta\varphi' \in \{10°,15°\}$, and $R \in \{10,12,15\}$ px (Fig. 2).

All possible needle candidate voxels $(\mathbf{L}^*_{\Delta\vartheta',\Delta\varphi',R})$ for each parameter setting are merged for creating one combined label volume, which is clustered again in order to determine connected regions of possible needle candidates (Fig. 2). The cluster with the maximum number of voxels $N^{\max}$ is assumed to coincide with the "reference" needle axis (sec. 2.4). In order to reduce the band-shaped elevation beam-width artifact (Fig. 1) and by the way to overcome the poor angel resolutions, a line approximation of this cluster's voxels is calculated by ℓ_2-norm minimization. These line's parameters $\left\{\tilde{p}_{0x}, \tilde{p}_{0y}, \tilde{\vartheta}, \tilde{\varphi}\right\}$ are the estimates of location and orientation of the needle axis.

2.4   Evaluating the estimation of needle axis location and orientation

The estimated needle axis $\left\{\tilde{p}_{0x}, \tilde{p}_{0y}, \tilde{\vartheta}, \tilde{\varphi}\right\}$ differs from the "reference" needle axis $\left\{p^\dagger_{0x}, p^\dagger_{0y}, \vartheta^\dagger, \varphi^\dagger\right\}$ in location and orientation. The quality of the estimation is quantified by the difference in the axis orientation, $\Delta\vartheta^\dagger = \vartheta^\dagger - \tilde{\vartheta}$ and $\Delta\varphi^\dagger = \varphi^\dagger - \tilde{\varphi}$, and the minimal Euclidean distance between the needle tip and the estimated axis d^{tip}.

3   Results

For every volume, the stick transform has been calculated for multiple parameter combinations. The quality of the needle axis estimation slightly depends on the

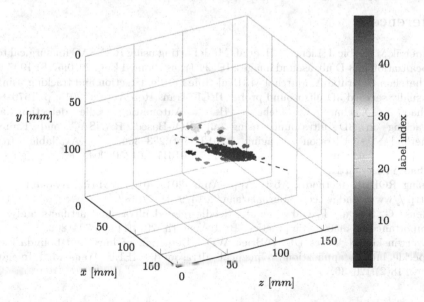

Fig. 2. Clusters of the combined label volumes. The linear regression of the cluster with the maximum number of voxels $N^{\max}$ is indicated by a black dashed line.

choice of the parameter settings for the stick transform. However, the errors of the needle axis location and orientation are almost the same for the different parameter settings. The 3%-, 50%-, and 97%-quantiles $(Q_{0.03}, Q_{0.50}, Q_{0.97})$ of the errors are $\Delta\vartheta^\dagger$: $(-5.16°, -0.20°, 3.78°)$, $\Delta\varphi^\dagger$: $(-4.71°, -0.20°, 2.38°)$, and d^{tip} : $(0.10\,\text{mm}, 0.53\,\text{mm}, 1.16\,\text{mm})$. For absolute differences, these errors become $\left|\Delta\vartheta^\dagger\right|$: $(0.07°, 1.24°, 5.16°)$ and $\left|\Delta\varphi^\dagger\right|$: $(0.05°, 0.56°, 4.71°)$.

4   Discussion

An image-based method for estimating needle axes in in-plane-acquired 3D ultrasound volumes has been derived. It was applied successfully to 44 volumes. Despite the needle's elevation beam-width artifact, a stick transform could be used to model the artifact by a straight line which coincides well with the "reference" needle axis, determined by an expert.

For the chosen parameter settings, the median errors of the estimated needle axis locations lie in the order of the needle's half diameter ($d^N/2 = 0.65\,\text{mm}$). The orientations of the estimated axes differ from the "reference" needle axes by $\left|\Delta\vartheta^\dagger\right| \approx 1.24°$ and $\left|\Delta\varphi^\dagger\right| \approx 0.56°$. The step of clustering regions with identical stick orientations, results in a resolution of the estimated axis orientation, which is much higher than the resolution of the stick orientations $(\Delta\vartheta', \Delta\varphi')$.

Acknowledgement. This work was funded by the Federal Ministry of Education and Research (BMBF) in the FHprofUnt program, grant no. 03FH041PX2.

References

1. Uhercik M, Kybic J, Liebgott H, et al. Model fitting using RANSAC for surgical tool localization in 3-D ultrasound images. IEEE Trans Biomed Eng. 2010;57(8):1907–16.
2. Chatelain P, Krupa A, Marchal M. Real-time needle detection and tracking using a visually servoed 3D ultrasound probe. IEEE Trans Rob Autom. 2013; p. 1676–81.
3. Zhao Y, Cachard C, Liebgott H. Automatic needle detection and tracking in 3D ultrasound using an ROI-Based RANSAC and Kalman method. Ultrason Imaging. 2013;35(4):283–306. Available from: http://uix.sagepub.com/lookup/doi/10.1177/0161734613502004.
4. Zhao Y, Bernard A, Cachard C, et al. Biopsy needle localization and tracking using ROI-RK method. Abstr Appl Anal. 2014;2014:e973147. Available from: http://www.hindawi.com/journals/aaa/2014/973147/abs/.
5. Reusz G, Sarkany P, Gal J, et al. Needle-related ultrasound artifacts and their importance in anaesthetic practice. Br J Anaesth. 2014;112(5):794–802.
6. Czerwinski RN, Jones DL, O'Brien WD. Detection of lines and boundaries in speckle images–application to medical ultrasound. IEEE Trans Med Imaging. 1999;18(2):126–36.

Extracting the Aorta Centerline in Contrast-Enhanced MRI

Marko Rak[1], Julian Alpers[1], Birger Mensel[2], Klaus-Dietz Tönnies[1]

[1]Department of Simulation and Graphics, University of Magdeburg
[2]Institute of Diagnostic Radiology and Neuroradiology, University of Greifswald
rak@isg.cs.ovgu.de

Abstract. We propose a semi-automatic approach for aorta centerline extraction in contrast-enhanced MRI, making aorta length analysis feasible on large scale. Starting from user-specified start and end regions, we extract the aorta path in between the regions automatically. The extraction is formulated as an optimization problem, seeking for the path that most likely runs central to the aorta. To this end, we exploit that the aorta distinguishes from the surrounding by strong image gradients that point inwards to the aorta's center due to contrast-enhanced imaging. We also include additional means of manual guidance to resolve erroneous cases. Experiments on data of 19 subjects yielded results that are close to the inter-reader variability. The average distance to the ground truth was 1.89 ± 1.54 mm, while aorta lengths deviated by only 0.66 ± 0.49 %.

1 Introduction

Arterial centerlines play a major role for indicators of arterial stiffness like the pulse wave velocity, which measures the speed of a pulse wave traveling between sections of the circulatory system. It may be calculated as quotient of the time delay of cardiac cycle, e.g., by assessing arterial diameters in cine sequences [1, 2], and the distance between the sections, i.e., the length of the arterial centerline. Epidemiological studies like the "Study of Health in Pomerania" [3] investigate arterial stiffness on a large scale, where manual lengths assessment is impractical due to the sheer number of subjects. Here, computerized concepts with a high degree of automation and adequate means of post-correction are necessary.

Related works are summarized in Tab. 1. The earliest approaches [4, 5, 6] apply threshold-based segmentation to identify the aorta and afterwards thin the result by skeletonization to extract the sought centerline. These works utilize morphological operations to cope with segmentation imperfections such as holes and disconnected segments. Later, [7, 8] formulate the extraction as an optimization task, trying to find the centerline path with highest likelihood w.r.t. the image. This avoids the issues of hard decision making by segmentation, but their approach introduces artifacts due to the heuristic spatial quantization that is used to simplify the optimization. Another heuristic approach was presented in [9], who grow a cylindrical model along the aorta. Their model is guided by

Table 1. Comparison with previous works on artery centerline extraction in MRI. '2d' implies long axis view; BB – black blood imaging; CE – contrast-enhanced imaging.

Works	Imaging	Arteries	Correction	Optimality	Length Error	Run Time
2d Gang '04 [4]		aorta	no	local	?	?
3d Giri '07 [6]		aorta	no	local	?	?
Babin '09 [5]	BB	aorta	no	local	1–4 %	> 5 m
Babin '12 [7]	BB	any	yes	local	1–3 %	> 1 m
Müller '12 [9]	CE	aorta	no	local	?	> 30 s
Babin '14 [8]	BB,CE	any	yes	local	?	> 1 m
Our Work	CE	any	yes	global	< 1 %	< 10 s

local intensity characteristics and rigidity is achieved by Kalman filtering of the model parameters. We do not apply heuristics, thereby guaranteeing global optimality of results, i.e., to find the centerline path with highest likelihood without getting stuck in local optima. At the same time, our approach is faster than those of the related works, making large scale investigations feasible in the first place.

2 Method

2.1 Maximum likelihood path

We interpret aorta centerline extraction as an optimization task, seeking the most likely aorta path between user-specified start and end regions. A region is placed by a mouse click and its radius may be adjusted by the mouse wheel if needed. The interaction does not need to be accurate, because the optimal start/end point inside the start/end region is estimated alongside the centerline extraction. The placement of regions is subject to the particular goal of investigation. For example, if the aortic arch is of interest then the user may use a single axial plane to specify a start region in the ascending and an end region in the descending aorta. If, on the other hand, the whole aorta is of interest, then the end region may be placed on the axial level where the aorta bifurcates into the common iliac arteries. We assume the latter setting, but the given arguments apply to other goals as well.

To formalize the problem, we think of the likelihood as a traveling speed, which allows to travel faster in regions of high likelihood and slower in regions of low likelihood. The extraction of the centerline with highest likelihood thus amounts to finding the fastest continuous path between the start and the end region as seen in Fig. 2.1. This problem is formalized by the Eikonal equation

$$|\nabla T(x)| \cdot L(x)^\alpha = 1 \tag{1}$$

where T is the sought arrival time at location x and L is an appropriate non-negative likelihood function. We introduced parameter α into the equation to amplify the influence of the likelihood, which is valuable for our task, because

Fig. 1. Exemplary stack of coronal slices (top) and the corresponding likelihood function (bottom). Overlayed centerlines were created manually (top) and calculated by our approach (bottom).

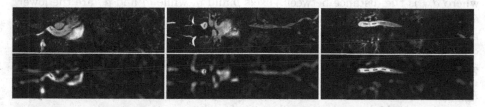

of the curved path through the aortic arch. The choice of α is discussed in the experiments. Solving Eq. (1) for any location can be done efficiently by fast marching methods. Afterwards, the globally optimal is extracted by backtracking the earliest arrival in the end region by streamline integration on $-\nabla T$.

2.2   Likelihood function

When tracing tubular structures it is most intuitive to utilize a so-called vesselness criterion. The most famous examples are based on scale space image representations like variants of Frangi's vesselness [10]. We cannot apply scale space concepts here, because significant smoothing is necessary to highlight rather thick structures like the aorta, which becomes problematic if other large hyperintense structures are close by, e.g., the heart. Thus smoothing will fuse both of these structures, skewing the vesselness estimate significantly.

We use a more application-specific criterion, which is based on two observations: (1) the aorta appears hyperintense with strong image gradients at its wall and (2) these gradients point inwards to the aorta's center. Combining both, we establish a voting scheme that favors locations which are pointed at by strong gradients. Our scheme utilizes soft votes to reflect that gradient strength may vary with the local concentration of the contrast agent and gradient direction may deviate depending on the local wall geometry. To be precise, we assign the likelihood $L(p)$ to any potential aorta center voxels p via the soft voting

$$L(p) = \max\left(0, \sum_{q \in \mathcal{N}(p)} w_{qp}(\boldsymbol{n}_{qp} \cdot \boldsymbol{g}_q)\right) \tag{2}$$

where q iterates all voxels inside a spatial neighborhood $\mathcal{N}$ of p. The unit vector $\boldsymbol{n}_{qp}$ points inwards from q to p, which results in larger votings whenever the image gradient $\boldsymbol{g}_q$ at neighborhood voxel q is strong and points into a similar direction. Weighting w_{qp} leverages centrality as discussed later. The $\max(0, \cdot)$ ensures the non-negativity of the likelihood function, i.e., non-negative speed.

As illustrated in Fig. 2.2, we define the neighborhood kernel $\mathcal{N}$ as all voxels within a pre-specified distance range to the voting center. The bounds of that range should capture the expected minimal and maximal aorta radii. To leverage centrality, the weighting in Eq. (2) should be a strictly concave, strictly monotonic decreasing function of the distance to the voting center. Accordingly, we use the first quadrant of the unit circle to weight votes via

$$w_{qp} = \sqrt{1 - ((d_{qp} - d_l)/(d_u - d_l))^2} \tag{3}$$

where d_{qp} is the distance between voxels p and q, while d_l and d_u are the lower and upper bound of the distance ranges, respectively. In particular, we use any radius inside $[5, 30]$ mm, which captures very thin and thick aortas alike.

2.3   Implementation

A naive implementation of the voting is not practicable for whole body images of medium or high resolution. To optimize the run time, we decompose the dot product in Eq. (2) into its three components (x, y and z), calculate the voting component-wise and aggregate the component results in the end. For each component, the voting resembles a convolution of a particular partial derivative of the image and the x, y or z component of the weighted unit vectors. Because the kernels are usually quite large, we use frequency domain filtering based on fast Fourier transformation to implement the convolutions.

2.4   Manual guidance

Adjacent hyperintense structures may still cause erroneous results if they touch the aorta at some point. In such cases our approach may take a short cut through this structure. For instance, a path through the heart may be preferred over one through the aortic arch if the heart and the descending aorta meet at some point. These cases can be addressed by manual interaction, letting the user specify one (or two) additional transition regions, e.g., inside the aortic arch, to constrain the centerline. Thus the maximum likelihood path splits into a number of sub-paths between the user-specified constraints.

2.5   Experiments

We carried out experiments on whole-body T_1-weighted fast low angle shot images of 19 subjects from the "Study of Health in Pomerania" [3]. Subjects were

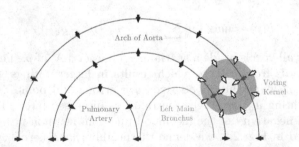

Fig. 2. Schematic illustration of the aortic arch and adjacent structures. When moved across the image, our voting kernel favors regions that are bounded by strong image gradients that point inwards to its center. Strong image gradients are visualized by filled arrows, while hollow arrows represent gradient directions favored by our voting.

Table 2. Number of erroneous cases as function of the likelihood amplifier α.

α	0.50	0.75	1.00	1.25	1.50	1.75	2.00	2.25	2.50	2.75	3.00	3.25	3.50	3.75	4.00
#	19	12	9	8	5	3	2	2	2	2	1	1	1	1	1

Table 3. Quantitative results of our approach for the aortic arch, the descending aorta and the aorta as a whole. AR – algorithmic results; IR – inter-reader variability.

	Length Error in %			Distance Error in mm		
	Arch	Desc.	Whole	Arch	Desc.	Whole
AR	1.56 ± 1.22	0.16 ± 0.12	0.66 ± 0.49	2.49 ± 1.87	1.47 ± 1.02	1.89 ± 1.54
IR	1.31 ± 0.92	0.11 ± 0.08	0.49 ± 0.37	2.29 ± 1.74	1.23 ± 0.80	1.64 ± 1.33

administered a contrast agent (Bayer Gadovist) to enhance aorta contrast. Images were acquired on a Siemens 1.5 Tesla Magnetom Avanto imager, whereby a field-of-view of about $1837 \times 366 \times 184$ mm was sliced coronally at a resolution of $0.98 \times 0.98 \times 1.5$ mm per voxel. To simplify processing, we downsampled all images to isotropical voxels of 1.5 mm. For each subject, annotations of the aorta centerline from two independent readers were given. We assess the centerline quality by the Euclidean distance to ground truth and the relative (unsigned) error in length compared to the reader's centerline.

3   Results and discussion

Firstly, we investigated how the likelihood amplifier α influences the number of cases that require additional manual guidance. As seen from results in Tab. 2, increasing α reduces the number of erroneous cases, until $\alpha = 3$ where only one data set is left. In this last case, we were unable to reconstruct the centerline even for higher α and additional manual guidance. We excluded this data set from further experiments, because the issue arose from image acquisition, where the contrast agent failed to fill the aortic arch during imaging. From the given results, we deduce that any α above two will be sufficient to minimize manual guidance. We use $\alpha = 3$ in what follows.

Secondly, we benchmarked result quality. From the results in Tab. 3, we observe that errors are significantly higher for the aortic arch compared to the descending part. This is true for our method and when comparing the two readers. This trend was expected, because selecting perpendicular view planes during ground truth creation likely produces inaccuracies at sections of high curvature. Overall, our results come close to the inter-reader variability for all listed sub-experiments. At the same time, our approach is fast, taking 5.39 ± 0.54 s per data set on a Intel Core i5 2500 @ 3.3 GHz. Most of the time was spent on likelihood function evaluation, which needs not be re-computed for manual guidance.

In conclusion, we proposed an approach to extract the aorta centerline and assess its length in contrast-enhance MRI. Our approach is semi-automatic, meaning that the user specifies start and end regions according to his/her goal. Subsequently, the aorta path in between is found automatically. Our approach integrates effective means of manual guidance, where the user specifies one (or two) additional transition regions to further constrain the centerline in case of erroneous results.

Experiments on data of 19 subjects yielded distances to ground truth center-lines of 1.89 ± 1.54 mm, while aorta lengths deviate by $0.66 \pm 0.49\,\%$. The results are close to the inter-reader variability. Our approach has limitations. One par-ticular case showed, that our approach will fail if large parts of the aorta cannot be distinguished from the surrounding due to missing contrast agent. In such rare cases, we would draw on manual extraction, since humans may compensate the missing information by knowledge about the general shape of the aorta.

Acknowledgement. We thank all parties of the Study of Health in Pomerania. This research was funded by the German Research Foundation (TO 166/13-2).

References

1. Rak M, Schnurr AK, Alpers J, et al. Measurement of the aortic diameter in plain axial cardiac cine MRI. Proc BVM. 2015; p. 293–8.
2. Rak M, Alpers J, Schnurr AK, et al. Aorta segmentation in axial cardiac cine MRI via graphical models. Proc BVM. 2016; p. 218–23.
3. Völzke H, Alte D, Schmidt CO, et al. Cohort profile: the study of health in Pomerania. Int J Epidemiol. 2011;40:294–307.
4. Gang G, Mark P, Cockshott P, et al. Measurement of pulse wave velocity using magnetic resonance imaging. In: Proc Int Conf IEEE Eng Med Biol Soc. IEEE; 2004. p. 3684–7.
5. Babin D, Vansteenkiste E, Pižurica A, et al. Segmentation and length measurement of the abdominal blood vessels in 3-D MRI images. In: Proc Int Conf IEEE Eng Med Biol Soc. IEEE; 2009. p. 4399–402.
6. Giri SS, Ding Y, Nishijima Y, et al. Automated and accurate measurement of aortic pulse wave velocity using magnetic resonance imaging. In: Comput Cardiol. IEEE; 2007. p. 661–4.
7. Babin D, Vansteenkiste E, Pižurica A, et al. Centerline calculation for extracting abdominal aorta in 3-D MRI images. In: Proc Int Conf IEEE Eng Med Biol Soc. IEEE; 2012. p. 3982–5.
8. Babin D, Devos D, Pižurica A, et al. Robust segmentation methods with an application to aortic pulse wave velocity calculation. Comput Med Imaging Graph. 2014;38:179–89.
9. Müller-Eschner M, Müller T, Biesdorf A, et al. 3D morphometry using automated aortic segmentation in native MR angiography: an alternative to contrast enhanced MRA? Cardiovasc Diagn Ther. 2014;4:80–7.
10. Frangi AF, Niessen WJ, Vincken KL, et al. Multiscale vessel enhancement filtering. In: Proc MICCAI. Springer; 1998. p. 130–7.

Noise Reduction in Low Dose DSA Imaging Using Pixel Adaptive SVD-Based Approach

Nikolas Menger[1], Thilo Elsässer[1], Guang-Hong Chen[2], Michael Manhart[1]

[1]Siemens Healthcare GmbH, Forchheim, Germany
[2]Department of Medical Physics, University of Wisconsin-Madison, WI 53705
studium@nmenger.de

Abstract. In this work, a new method for noise reduction in low dose DSA imaging is presented. The algorithm extends an existing approach using the low rank nature of DSA image series to enable considerable reduction of radiation dose while maintaining low image noise level and preserving spatial resolution and temporal dynamics of the DSA series. The algorithm is based on the singular value decomposition (SVD) using a pixel adaptive approach for the noise reduction. For validation of the method an in vivo animal study is examined.

1 Introduction

Digital subtraction angiography (DSA) is a standard technique for imaging of blood vessels. It has many applications in the diagnosis and treatment of vascular diseases in cardiology, neuroradiology and interventional radiology. Both patient and operators are exposed to ionizing radiation during the procedure [1]. This results in the necessity for robust and advanced algorithms which provide good reduction of image noise to enable dose reduction while retaining temporal dynamics and spatial resolution.

2 Materials and methods

2.1 SVD based DSA noise reduction method

Niu et. al. [2] proposed a novel algorithm for noise reduction in low dose DSA imaging using a low rank constraint. By creating a matrix X, which contains all images of the DSA series as column vectors, this matrix can be decomposed using the singular value decomposition (SVD) [3]

$$\mathbf{X}(\boldsymbol{x},t) = \sum_{i \in N} \boldsymbol{u}_i(\boldsymbol{x})\, \sigma_i\, \boldsymbol{v}_i^\top(t) \tag{1}$$

The result of the SVD are the spatial basis vectors $\boldsymbol{u}_i(\boldsymbol{x})$, the corresponding singular values σ_i and the temporal basis vectors $\boldsymbol{v}_i^T(t)$. By reshaping $\boldsymbol{u}_i$ to images, one gets the spatial bases images shown in Fig. 1. The first spatial basis contains the static structures of the time series (Fig. 1a). The following spatial bases contain the dynamic components of the time series, mainly induced by the contrast media injected into the vessels (Fig. 1b). With increasing index the noise level of the spatial basis rises. At first, the spatial basis images contain noise only in the image background outside of vessels (Fig. 1c). At even higher indices the spatial basis images only contain noise components (Fig. 1d). Niu et al. [2] reduced noise in the DSA series by weighting the spatial basis images. The weighting was done by setting the singular values with indices above a predefined threshold to zero. The denoised DSA series was then calculated from the remaining singular values, spatial basis and temporal basis using Eq. 1. With a low threshold the noise reduction is very effective. However, if the threshold

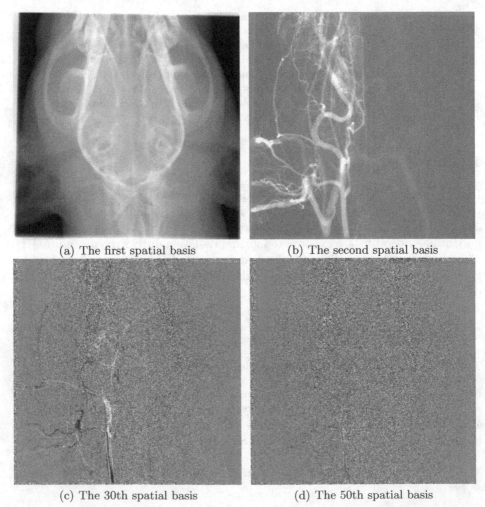

(a) The first spatial basis   (b) The second spatial basis

(c) The 30th spatial basis   (d) The 50th spatial basis

Fig. 1. Spatial basis images of a DSA series captured at 0.5 μGy/fr. With increasing index the noise level in the spatial basis rises.

is selected too low, the temporal resolution in image regions with high temporal dynamics, e.g. in aneurysms, might be lost. In DSA image series the temporal dynamics are highly spatially variant. For example, there is no dynamics in regions without contrast enhancement, medium dynamics in healthy vessels and very high dynamics in complex anatomical structures like aneurysms. Thus a denoising approach is desired, which incorporates the spatial variance to achieve the best noise reduction possible without loss of temporal information in all image regions.

2.2   Spatially adaptive SVD DSA noise reduction method

The new method calculates an individual cut off threshold $T_c(\boldsymbol{x})$ for each pixel of the DSA series. Every spatial basis pixel above this cut off threshold is set to zero. The image series is then reconstructed by multiplication of the remaining spatial basis pixels $\hat{\boldsymbol{u}}_i(\boldsymbol{x})$, the singular values σ_i and the temporal basis $\boldsymbol{v}_i^{\top}(t)$ using Eq. 1

$$\hat{\boldsymbol{u}}_i(\boldsymbol{x}) = \begin{cases} \boldsymbol{u}_i(\boldsymbol{x}), & \text{for } i \leq T_c(\boldsymbol{x}) \\ 0, & \text{for } i > T_c(\boldsymbol{x}) \end{cases} \tag{2}$$

The calculation of the threshold is based on the amplitude of the weighted spatial basis pixels $\boldsymbol{u}_{wi}(\boldsymbol{x}) = |\boldsymbol{u}_i(\boldsymbol{x})\,\sigma_i|$. Pixels in areas with low temporal dynamics (e.g. outside of vessels) have low amplitudes in the spatial basis pixels whereas the spatial basis pixels in areas with high temporal dynamics (e.g. vessels) have a high amplitude. Eq. 3 shows the calculation of $T_c(\boldsymbol{x})$. For each pixel all spatial basis pixels with an amplitude above the adaptive threshold T_A and the

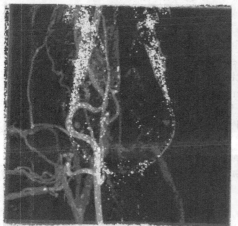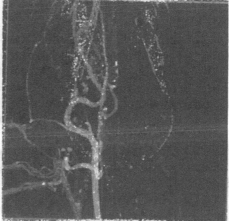

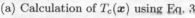

(a) Calculation of $T_c(\boldsymbol{x})$ using Eq. 3   (b) Improved calculation of $T_c(\boldsymbol{x})$ using Eq. 4

Fig. 2. Pixel wise cut off threshold $T_c(\boldsymbol{x})$. Dark colors represent a low $T_c(\boldsymbol{x})$, brighter colors a high $T_c(\boldsymbol{x})$. The improved calculation provides a lower $T_c(\boldsymbol{x})$ for bone structures and a higher $T_c(\boldsymbol{x})$ in the background area.

corresponding indices i are determined. The highest index is set as the cut off threshold $T_c(\boldsymbol{x})$

$$T_c(\boldsymbol{x}) = \max(i \,|\, \boldsymbol{u}_{wi}(\boldsymbol{x}) > T_A) \tag{3}$$

The result of this calculation is shown in Fig. 2a. While the cut off threshold is high in the areas containing vessels and bones, it is low in the background areas of the image. This leads to the needed denoising characteristics: Background areas are reconstructed from very few spatial bases, which results in a very low noise level, but also reduces the temporal dynamics. Vessel structures are reconstructed from more spatial bases, which preserves the temporal dynamics in these areas, but also results in a higher noise level. The limitations of decreased temporal dynamics or increased noise are only problematic if the cut off threshold calculation fails. Errors can be caused by thick bones, which are determined to be vessel structures with a very high cut off index. This error emerges from a high noise level inside bones in the original DSA-series, which produces high temporal dynamics. The resulting poor noise reduction is clearly visible compared to the low noise level in other background areas (see upper blue detailed view in Fig. 3b). Furthermore, errors occur in image areas with small vessels, which are determined to be image background. This results in blurring of these vessels due to the reconstruction from very few spatial bases (see lower red detailed view in Fig. 3b). These problems lead to an improved approach for the calculation of the cut off threshold $T_c(\boldsymbol{x})$

$$\hat{T}_c(\boldsymbol{x}) = \max(i < T_U \,|\, \boldsymbol{u}_{wi}(\boldsymbol{x}) > T_A)$$

$$T_c(\boldsymbol{x}) = \begin{cases} \hat{T}_c(\boldsymbol{x}), & \text{for } \hat{T}_c(\boldsymbol{x}) \geq T_L \\ T_L, & \text{for } \hat{T}_c(\boldsymbol{x}) < T_L \end{cases} \tag{4}$$

The upper threshold T_U is needed to avoid high cut off thresholds in bone areas. This threshold applies a weighting to the spatial bases like the original algorithm by Niu et al. [2]. Because of the additional calculation of $T_c(\boldsymbol{x})$, T_U can be chosen very high to avoid the loss of temporal dynamics. The lower threshold T_L guarantees that the cut off threshold is not too low in the background area. Fig. 2b shows the effect of the additional thresholds: While the threshold in the background area is higher compared to Fig. 2a, the bone structures have lower thresholds. This results in less noise in bone structures (upper blue detailed view in Fig. 3c) and avoidance of blurring of small vessels (lower red detailed view in Fig. 3c).

3   Results

Fig. 3 shows one image of the examined DSA series. The series contains 150 images which were recorded at a framerate of 30 fr/s and a radiation dose of 0.5 μGy/fr. The three thresholds were chosen as follows: $T_A = 20$, $T_L = 5$ and $T_U = 50$. The vessels in the unprocessed image (Fig. 3a) are superposed by strong image noise. This results in diffuse edges of large vessels and poor visibility of small vessels. The new algorithm produces an image (Fig. 3c) which contains very low noise. Therefore the visibility of all vessels, especially of small ones, is improved. Because of the sharp edges vessels and image background can be differentiated very well. Fig. 3d shows the difference between the unprocessed image and the result of the new method. The image consists only of image noise and does not contain any visible vessel structures implying that the algorithm just removes the image noise while preserving spatial resolution and temporal

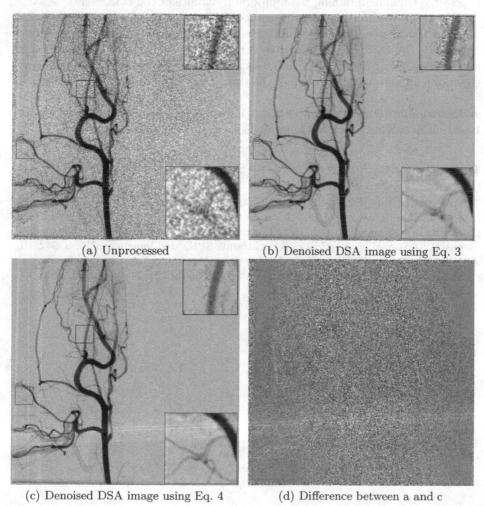

(a) Unprocessed   (b) Denoised DSA image using Eq. 3

(c) Denoised DSA image using Eq. 4   (d) Difference between a and c

Fig. 3. Original DSA-image and results of the denoising methods. Both methods show a reduction of the image noise. The improved method supresses the blurring of small vessels and reduces the noise in bones further. The difference image indicates, that only image noise is reduced while vessel structures are preserved.

Menger et al.

dynamics. Comparing time attenuation curves of highly dynamic pixels (Fig. 3a vs. Fig. 3c) showed an average difference approaching zero.

4 Discussion

This paper introduced a new approach for the noise reduction in DSA imaging. By spatially adaptive SVD threshold a considerable reduction of radiation dose is possible while maintaining the temporal dynamics of the DSA series.

For future research the algorithm should be tested on clinical datasets with different framerates, dose levels and injection protocols to validate the results. Especially, the choice of the adaptive threshold T_A resulting in the best image quality, depending on the acquisition setting, should be further examined. Furthermore, an automatic selection of the three thresholds should be investigated.

Acknowledgement. The concepts and information presented in this paper are based on research and are not commercially available.

References

1. Wagner LK, Eifel PJ, Geise RA. Potential biological effects following high X-ray dose interventional procedures. J Vasc Interv Radiol. 1994;5(1):71–84.
2. Niu K, Li Y, Schafer S, et al. Ultra low radiation dose digital subtraction angiography (DSA) imaging using low rank constraint. SPIE Med Imaging. 2015; p. 941210.
3. Golub G, Kahan W. Calculating the singular values and pseudo-inverse of a matrix. SIAM Rev Soc Ind Appl Math Numer Anal. 1965;2(2):205–24.

Skin Detection and Tracking for Camera-Based Photoplethysmography Using a Bayesian Classifier and Level Set Segmentation

Alexander Trumpp[1], Stefan Rasche[2], Daniel Wedekind[1], Martin Schmidt[1],
Thomas Waldow[3], Frederik Gaetjen[2], Katrin Plötze[2], Hagen Malberg[1],
Klaus Matschke[2], Sebastian Zaunseder[1]

[1]Institute of Biomedical Engineering, TU Dresden
[2]Department of Cardiac Surgery, Herzzentrum Dresden
[3]Center for Wound Therapy in Medical Rehabilitation, Klinik Bavaria Kreischa
alexander.trumpp@tu-dresden.de

Abstract. Camera-Based Photoplethysmography is a measuring technique that permits the remote assessment of vital signs by using cameras. The face is the preferred area of measurement (region of interest: ROI) that has to be selected automatically for convenient application. Most works use common face detection algorithm for this purpose. However, these approaches often fail if the face is partly occluded or distorted. In this work, we propose an automatic method for ROI detection and tracking that does not rely on facial features. First, a Bayesian skin classifier was applied. Second, the detected areas were refined and tracked by level set segmentation. We tested our method on videos of 70 patients. The determined ROIs were used for signal extraction and heart rate (HR) estimation. The results showed that our method can detect and track suitable skin regions. We achieved a median HR detection rate of 80 % which was only 6 % lower than when applying manually defined ROIs.

1 Introduction

Camera-based photoplethysmography (cbPPG) is an optical measuring technique that permits the contactless derivation of cardiorespiratory signals by using normal video cameras [1]. Similar to the common reflective photoplethysmography, backscattered light from superficial skin layers is captured over time and converted into a signal which relates to the cardiac cycle. In addition to the advantage of a remote application, cbPPG can be operated with only ambient light and can allow a spatial assessment of the recorded area [2].

For a variety of reasons, the face is the preferred region of measurement for cbPPG. Therefore, the automatic detection and tracking of suitable facial areas are essential for a convenient use of this technique. Existing approaches mostly rely on detection algorithms for the whole face or facial landmarks and subsequently involve a tracking based on either re-detection or by using determined image features [3, 4, 5]. However, faces that are partially occluded, rotated or not in a frontal position towards the camera might hinder any valid detection. To our knowledge, there are only few works related to cbPPG which propose an automatic detection and tracking method that does not require the initial registration of facial areas.

In this paper, we present a fully automated approach for the detection and tracking of face regions that are most suitable for cbPPG. For this approach, no prior knowledge about the image content is needed. We tested our method for camera recordings of 70 patients in an intensive care unit. The evaluation was performed using cbPPG's detection rate of the heart rate (HR). We compared the results of our method to results obtained by applying manually annotated regions of interest (ROIs).

2 Material and methods

2.1 Data and technical setup

For our tests, we analyzed measurements of a study that featured 70 patients (50 male, 20 female, ages 70.3 ± 11.4 years) after cardiac surgery [6]. All participants were recorded for about 30 min using a two-camera system. In this work, we only considered the RGB camera (IDS UI-3370CP-C-HQ) which was set to a resolution of 420x320 pixels, a frame rate of 100 fps and a color depth of 12 bit. During the recording, the patients were usually not conscious but sometimes woke up and moved their head. The illumination conditions were mainly defined by the indoor light source and outdoor sunlight. Synchronously to the videos, we captured reference signals from the clinical monitor system. The study was approved by the Institutional Review Board of the TU Dresden (IRB00001473, EK168052013) and each patient gave written consent.

2.2 Image processing

To verify our assumption, we tested common face detection algorithms like the Viola-Jones method on the videos. These algorithms mostly failed due to patients' head position and occlusion caused by fixation tapes as well as intubation tubes. Therefore, we applied a Naive Bayes classifier to detect suitable skin areas instead of faces. Following the description of Jones and Rehg [7], we built two RGB histograms, one for skin color, and one for non-skin color. We used labeled skin and non-skin images for this purpose that were made available by this group. The normalization of the histograms on the total number of entries provided the probability density functions (PDFs) for the classes skin and ¬skin: $p(\mathbf{c}|\text{skin})$, $p(\mathbf{c}|\neg\text{skin})$. The classifier could then be formulated using the Bayesian decision rule [8]. An RGB pixel $\mathbf{c}$ was set as skin if

$$\frac{p(\mathbf{c}|\text{skin})}{p(\mathbf{c}|\neg\text{skin})} \geq \theta \qquad (1)$$

We applied the classifier on the first image of each RGB video. For every patient, the threshold θ was automatically adapted between 0.1 and 10 based on the number of detected skin pixels. This adaption allowed us to compensate varying conditions among the patients. The classifier is generally a good choice due to its simplicity, the free access of the training data, and because it was often validated. However, in our case, the results did usually not represent the skin regions well enough (Fig. 2). Therefore, we applied a segmentation algorithm based on level set methods to refine the outcome.

Level set methods are able to describe the propagation of a segmentation contour using an implicit representation [9]. This representation is accomplished by the level set function $\Phi(x, y, t)$, where $\Phi = 0$ defines the contour, $\Phi > 0$ the inside region Ω_1 and $\Phi < 0$ the outside region Ω_2. For each segmentation procedure, the contour propagates from an initialization point to an optimal state that minimizes an appropriate energy function. The minimization is performed by a gradient descent. We applied a region-based approach by Brox et al. [10] in which the gradient descent reads to

$$\frac{\partial \Phi}{\partial t} = H'(\Phi) \left[\sum_{j=1}^{3} \log \frac{p_{1j}(I_j)}{p_{2j}(I_j)} + \nu \cdot \operatorname{div} \frac{\nabla \Phi}{|\nabla \Phi|} \right] \tag{2}$$

For the considered image I (j: color channels) in our study, the segmentation was initialized by setting Ω_1 to the skin classification result. During the segmentation, the first sum term allows to separate Ω_1 and Ω_2 due to their local intensities. The PDFs p_{1j} and p_{2j} are modeled using Gaussian distributions and describe the probabilities that an regional image pixel belongs to Ω_1 or Ω_2, respectively. For an optimal outcome, p_{1j} is maximal in Ω_1 and p_{2j} is maximal in Ω_2. The latter term in the equation is the curvature term which allows to control the smoothness of the contour (ν is a weighting factor). $H(\Phi)$ is a Heaviside function. We used 300 iteration steps to achieve the final segmentation result which was defined by Ω_1 and represents our ROI (Fig. 2).

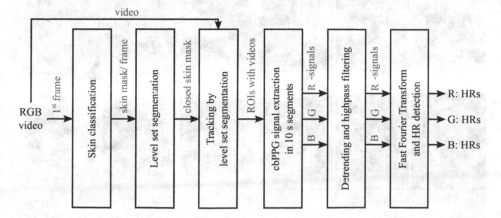

Fig. 1. Program sequence of the proposed procedure (ROI: region of interest, HR: heart rate, R: red, G: green, B: blue). They gray terms represent the transferred data.

The segmented skin regions in the first RGB images were further tracked in order to obtain ROIs for the whole videos. We also applied level set segmentation for this purpose and always used the last segmentation result as initialization point for the next image. Consequently, the contour quickly stabilized even in the case of motion or light variations. If the result changed at all between two images, a maximum of only 50 iteration steps was necessary. The chosen level set method (combined with the classifier) allowed us to track skin regions with similar intensity distributions instead of certain anatomical areas. We hypothesize that the consideration of these distributions provides a benefit for ROI selection.

2.3   Signal processing and evaluation

In order to extract cbPPG signals, the pixel values within the determined ROIs were averaged frame by frame. Due to the three color channels (R,G,B), we obtained three different signals for each patient. All signals were divided into 10 s segments and then detrended and highpass filtered (FIR filter, a cutoff frequency of 30 bpm, an order of 250). Afterward, a Fast Fourier Transform was applied and an amplitude spectrum was built for each segment. We detected the HR in this spectrum by searching for the maximum peak between 30 and 200 bpm. Fig. 1 summarizes the signal and image processing steps.

The detected HRs were compared to reference HRs that were determined from the electrocardiogram. A camera-based HR was considered correct if it differed less than 5 bpm. Using this outcome, we could calculate a mean HR detection rate (HRDR) for each patient and color channel. In a previous work [6], we worked with the same video data but manually annotated ROIs and only calculated HRDR values for the green channel. We used these results as the gold standard to validate our method.

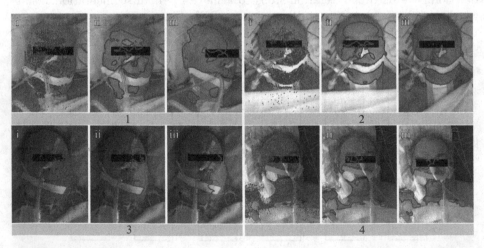

Fig. 2. Skin detection and tracking results for four patients (only contours are shown): i) skin classification, ii) initial segmentation, iii) tracking to a later point in the video.

3   Results

The proposed method proved to be applicable to detect and track suitable skin regions in RGB videos. Besides the face, also regions from the upper body part were occasionally included. Fig. 2 shows four patients where the skin detection, segmentation and one tracking result are visualized. The combination of the classifier and level set segmentation leads to the separation of skin areas (ROIs) with similarly distributed intensities. We can argue that this distribution plays a role for the quality of the extracted cbPPG signals when averaging the ROI pixel values. Patient 3 and 4 in Fig. 2 serve as examples. The light conditions caused the face to be illuminated differently. Our method only selected the appropriate part as ROI and therefore caused a better outcome than using the whole face. We also tested the processing time of our algorithm. Except for the initial detection and segmentation, it can be operated in real-time (MATLAB).

Fig. 3 shows the results for HRDR of the 70 patients (depicted in boxplots). When our ROI selection method was applied, the green channel provided the best rates with a median of 80 %. This median is remarkably high considering that the gold standard, where ROIs were selected manually, yielded 86 %. However, low HRDR values cause a large variance for our method. In comparison to the green channel, the red and blue channel provided a generally poor outcome with a median HRDR of 17 % and 14 %, respectively.

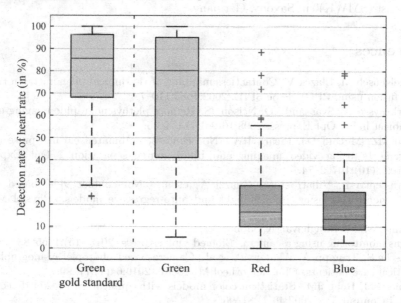

Fig. 3. Results for the detection rate of the heart rate. The first box shows the results using manually annotated ROI. The other boxes show the results for each color channel using our method.

4   Discussion

To some extent, the low HRDR values in the green channel can be explained by a group of patients where the ROI selection process was unsuccessful. Reasons are: (i) insufficient skin classification, (ii) inclusion of non-skin regions in the segmentation, (iii) failed tracking because contour did not stabilize enough. Moreover, the inclusion of non-facial skin regions can also affect the HRDR. Such regions might hold pulse signals with different characteristics and could degrade the outcome if they are combined with facial regions. Although we used the same ROIs for the red and blue channel as we used for the green one, the results differed significantly. This effect can be partly attributed to generally low cbPPG signal amplitudes for red and blue and coincides with the fact that the green channel provides the strongest plethysmographic signal [2]. Nevertheless, signals from the red and blue channel still offer valuable information which should be exploited in future analyses. For example, Poh et al. [3] applied an independent component analysis to the signals of all three channels and, therefore, could achieve a better HR detection than just considering the green channel.

In conclusion, our method allows to automatically determine facial ROIs in videos without using any prior knowledge about the image content. Furthermore, these regions proved to be suitable for cbPPG signal extraction and HR estimation. This work was funded by the "Staatsministerium für Wissenschaft und Kunst (SMWK)" in Saxony, Germany.

References

1. Huelsbusch M, Blazek V. Contactless mapping of rhythmical phenomena in tissue perfusion using PPGI. Proc SPIE. 2002;4683:110–7.
2. Verkruysse W, Svaasand LO, Nelson JS. Remote plethysmographic imaging using ambient light. Opt Express. 2008;16(26):21434–45.
3. Poh MZ, McDuff DJ, Picard RW. Non-contact, automated cardiac pulse measurements using video imaging and blind source separation. Opt Express. 2010;18(10):10762–74.
4. Tarassenko L, Villarroel M, Guazzi A, et al. Non-contact video-based vital sign monitoring using ambient light and auto-regressive models. Physiol Meas. 2014;35(5):807–31.
5. Kumar M, Veeraraghavan A, Sabharwal A. DistancePPG: robust non-contact vital signs monitoring using a camera. Biomed Opt Express. 2015;6(5):1565–88.
6. Rasche S, Trumpp A, Waldow T, et al. Camera based photoplethysmography in critical care patients. Clin Hemorheol Microcirc. 2016;64(1):77–90.
7. Jones MJ, Rehg JM. Statistical color models with application to skin detection. Int J Comput Vis. 2002;46(1):81–96.
8. Duda RO, Hart PE, Stork DG. Pattern Classification. John Wiley & Sons; 2001.
9. Osher S, Fedkiw R. Level Set Methods and Dynamic Implicit Surfaces. New York: Springer; 2003.
10. Brox T, Rousson M, Deriche R, et al. Colour, texture, and motion in level set based segmentation and tracking. Image Vis Comput. 2010;28(3):376–90.

Abstract: Können wir Rankings vertrauen?

Eine systematische Analyse biomedizinischer Challenges hinsichtlich Reporting und Design

Matthias Eisenmann[1], Patrick Scholz[1], Marko Stankovic[1], Pierre Jannin[2], Christian Stock[3], Lena Maier-Hein[1]

[1]Computer-assistierte medizinische Interventionen, DKFZ Heidelberg
[2]MediCIS, UMR 1099 LTSI, INSERM, Fakultät für Medizin, Universität Rennes 1
[3]Institut für Medizinische Biometrie und Informatik, Universitätsklinikum Heidelberg
m.eisenmann@dkfz-heidelberg.de

Im Bereich der biomedizinischen Bildanalyse werden vermehrt öffentliche Wettbewerbe (*Challenges*) durchgeführt, die den Vergleich von Methoden unter denselben Bedingungen ermöglichen. Ergebnisse aus solchen Challenges gewinnen zur Bewertung von Forschungsresultaten – z.B. im Reviewprozess von Publikationen – immer mehr an Bedeutung. Demgegenüber steht eine mangelnde Qualitätskontrolle im Challengedesign. Dieser Beitrag beruht auf der Hypothese, dass eine unzureichende Qualitätskontrolle zu einer geringen Aussagekraft der Challengeergebnisse führen kann. Basierend auf dem Validierungsprotokoll von Jannin et al. [1] wurden sämtliche biomedizinischen Challenges des Kollektivs „Grand Challenges in Biomedical Image Analysis" [2] bis zum Jahr 2016 erfasst und systematisch analysiert. Wir präsentieren die Analyseergebnisse hinsichtlich der Vollständigkeit des Reportings und des Einflusses verschiedener Entscheidungen im Challengedesign auf das finale Ranking der Teilnehmer. Unsere Analyse demonstriert die Notwendigkeit einer Qualitätskontrolle, welche dazu beitragen sollte, dass Rankings nachvollziehbar sowie reproduzierbar sind und die Aussagefähigkeit erhöht wird.

Literaturverzeichnis

1. Jannin P, Grova C, Maurer CR. Model for defining and reporting reference-based validation protocols in medical image processing. Int J Comput Assist Radiol Surg. 2006;1(2):63–73.
2. Grand Challenges in Biomedical Image Analysis; 2016. Available from: https://grand-challenge.org/All_Challenges/ [cited 18.10.2016].

Overexposure Correction by Mixed One-Bit Compressive Sensing for C-Arm CT

Xiaolin Huang[1,3], Yan Xia[2], Yixing Huang[1], Joachim Hornegger[1], Andreas Maier[1]

[1]Pattern Recognition Lab, Friedrich-Alexander-University Erlangen-Nürnberg
[2]Department of Radiology, Stanford University
[3]Institute of Image Processing and Pattern Recognition,
Shanghai Jiao Tong University
xiaolinhuang@sjtu.edu.cn

Abstract. This paper proposes a novel method to deal with overexposure for C-arm CT reconstruction. The proposed method is based on recent progress of one bit compressive sensing (1bit-CS), which is to recover sparse signals from sign measurements. Overexposure could be regarded as a kind of sign information, thus the application of 1bit-CS to overexposure correction in CT reconstruction is expected. This method is evaluated on a phantom and its promising performance implies potential application on clinical data.

1 Introduction

In the Angiographic C-arm Computed Tomography (C-arm CT), due to the limited dynamic range of C-arm flat detectors and the high contrast variation of different imaged object components, the problem of overexposure arises in the acquired projections during a 3D acquisition. Consequently, the reconstructed image, especially the low contrast structures, will be severely degraded by streak artifacts and capping artifacts due to the overexposed projection values. Thus, it is important to establish overexposure correction methods to reduce these artifacts.

The overexposure problem is similar to the truncation problem [1] in the sense of the resulting discontinuity between measured and unmeasured data and hence the truncation correction methods [2, 3, 4, 5] are potentially feasible for overexposure correction. Generally, these methods heavily rely on the prior-knowledge about the object structure. As a specific example, [6] is to correct the overexposure for knee images based on cylinder shapes that are fitted in the sinogram domain. But such methods are no longer accurate if there is little prior-knowledge or the shapes are too complicated to be modeled.

The essence of overexposure artifacts is the lack of measurements, which inspires us to think about compressive sensing (CS). Based on sparsity, CS can recover signals/images with a relatively small number of observations. The related theory and algorithms can be found in, e.g., [7, 8, 9]. When overexposure occurs, the observed projection value is zero. The value itself is useless, but it implies that the true projection is less than the threshold. Thus, in over-exposure correction, it is still possible to acquire some information from those projections, which is closely linked with so-called one-bit compressive sensing (1bit-CS) [10, 11, 12]. Our task is between CS and 1bit-CS: we have both anal-ogy observations (un-overexposed part) and one-bit information (overexposed part). Therefore, we call our correction method as mixed one-bit compressive sensing (M1bit-CS).

In the rest of this paper, we first mathematically formulate the overexpo-sure correction problem and give M1bit-CS method for this problem. Then the proposed method is evaluated on the Shepp-Logan phantom and the paper is concluded with some discussions.

2   Materials and methods

2.1   Overexposure on CT projection

The X-ray transform of an object $\mathbf{f}$ is denoted by $\mathbf{R}$. Then the ideal acquired projection is

$$\mathbf{p} = \mathbf{Rf} \tag{1}$$

However, due to the dynamic range of the detector, projections could be over-exposed such that our observations $\mathbf{y}$ is a truncation of $\mathbf{p}$. Mathematically

$$y_i = \begin{cases} p_i, & \text{if } p_i > s \\ 0, & \text{if } p_i \leq s \end{cases} \tag{2}$$

where s is the threshold of overexposure determined by the highest X-ray in-tensity that can be measured by the detector. In this paper we assume that we know which projection is overexposured, which could be modeled as a boolean indicator vector Φ

$$\Phi_i = 1 \iff p_i > 0 \text{ and } y_i = 0 \tag{3}$$

Our aim in this paper is to reconstruct $\mathbf{f}$ from the truncated projection $\mathbf{y}$ with the above prior assumption.

2.2   Mixed one bit compressive sensing

Compared to the regular CT construction, the major problem of overexposure is that we do not have the exact values for the overexposed projections. Instead, we only know that $(\mathbf{Rf})_i < s$ if $\Phi_i = 1$. This inequality inspires us to consider 1bit-CS, which is to recover sparse signals from sign measurements. As afore-mentioned, we have both un-overexposed projections and one-bit information. Therefore the following M1bit-CS model is proposed

$$\min_{\mathbf{f}} \ \mu\|\mathbf{f}\|_{\text{TV}} + \frac{1}{2}\sum_{i:\Phi_i=0} ((\mathbf{Rf})_i - y_i)^2 + \lambda \sum_{i:\Phi_i=1} \max\{0, (\mathbf{Rf})_i - s\} \tag{4}$$

Table 1. Root of mean square error (RMSE) of reconstruction results.

method	FBP	SART	TV	M1bit-CS
RMSE	0.3148	0.0242	quad 0.0147	0.0098

where μ and λ are relaxation parameters, $\| \cdot \|_{TV}$ is the total variation term that pursues sparsity, $(\cdot)^2$ is the least squares loss to penalize the inconsistency on analogy measurers, and $\max\{0, \cdot\}$ is the hinge loss for the inequality consistency. Obviously, (4) is a convex model and can be solved by standard convex optimization methods, such as interior-point method, coordinate descent algorithm, alternating direction method of multipliers, and so on. The parameter μ is to adjust the sparsity on the gradient of the image. In our experiment, we set $\mu = 10^{-3}$ and in practice it could be tuned based on prior-knowledge or by cross-validation. The parameter λ is the trade-off between the regular measurements and the overexposed ones. Heuristically, when there are more overexposes, we prefer a smaller λ. In this paper, we set $\lambda = 10$.

3 Results

3.1 Simulated phantom design

To demonstrate the performance of M1bit-CS method on overexposure correction, the standard high contrast Shepp-Logan phantom is employed; see, Fig. 2(a). The image size is 256×256 with an isotropic pixel length of 1 mm. We simulate a fan-beam scan to acquire the overexposed sinogram. The source-to-isocenter distance is 750 mm and isocenter-to-detector distance is 450 mm. The angular step is $1°$ and the total scan range is $360°$. The equal-spaced detector length $s_{\max}$ is 620 mm with pixel element length $\Delta s = 1$ mm.

The ideal sinogram of the Shepp-Logan phantom is shown in Fig. 1(a). Without overexposure, the classical reconstruction algorithms such as FBP [13] and

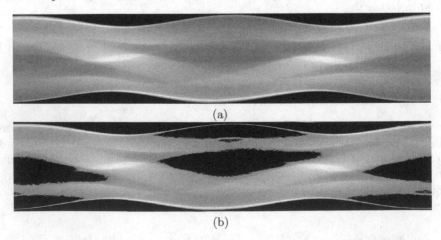

(a)

(b)

Fig. 1. (a) Projection of the Shepp-Logan; (b) Projection with overexposure.

SART [14] can be applied for reconstruction. However, overexposure that leads to severe information loss makes these reconstruction algorithms not applicable. To simulate the overexposure, we take the threshold $s = 0.55p_{max}$, where p_{max} is the maximum value in the projection domain. The sinogram with overexposure is shown in Fig. 1(b) and our task is to accurately reconstruct the image from this overexposed sinogram.

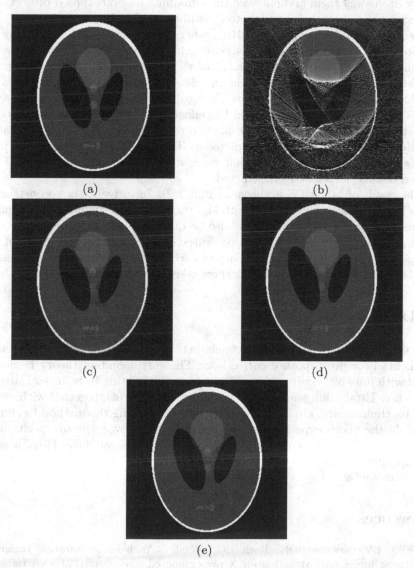

Fig. 2. Image reconstructed from the overexposed sinogram with different algorithms: (a) Shepp-Logan phantom; (b) FBP; (c) SART; (d) TV minimization; (d) M1bit-CS.

3.2   Reconstructed image

We first show the reconstructed results of FBP and SART in Fig. 2(b) and 2(c), respectively. FBP utilizes all the "fake" zeros, i.e., the overexposure projections that correspond to non-zero real values but zero observations. For SART, if we use those fake projection data, the performance will be similar to FBP. If we simply drop away them and only use the remaining un-overexposed projections, the reconstructed result is much better, as illustrated in Fig. 2(c).

Recall the projections in Fig. 1(b), where the overexposed part is not in the boundary. Thus, SART yields good image quality on the boundaries of the Shepp-Logan phantom. However, in the center, the performance is not satisfactory: there are streaks inside and detailed structures are blurred. One possible improvement comes from the TV regularization, which can help recovery from a relatively less measurements. The effect of TV regularization is rooted in compressive sensing theory and can also be regarded as a smoothing operator. Fig. 2(c) displays the image reconstructed by TV minimization. Comparing with the result of pure SART, we find that some streaks are suppressed but still the blurred details cannot be reconstructed.

The result of M1bit-CS is shown in Fig. 2(e). Intuitively, the reconstructed image is very close to the ground truth and the streaks are significantly reduced. The reconstruction performance can also be quantitatively measured by the the root-mean-square errors, which are presented in Tab. 1. The gray value of the Shepp-Logan is between 0 and 1. One can see that the reconstructed image of M1bit-CS is quite accurate, although there is serious overexposure in projections.

4   Discussion

From the evaluation results, we can conclude that the proposed M1bit-CS method is beneficial for overexposure correction. The corresponding theory is closely linked with (one-bit) compressive sensing and is interesting to be investigated in the future. Establishing an efficient algorithm to solve (4), together with evaluation on clinical data, are both necessary before applying the method to clinical trials. In the above experiment, we assume that the overexposure positions is known. But in clinical applications, this may not be available. Thus, a good overexposure detection method is required for practical use and is interesting in the future study.

References

1. Sidky EY, Kraemer DN, Roth EG, et al. Analysis of iterative region-of-interest image reconstruction for X-ray computed tomography. J Med Imaging. 2014;1(3):031007.
2. Ohnesorge B, Flohr T, Schwarz K, et al. Efficient correction for CT image artifacts caused by objects extending outside the scan field of view. Med Phys. 2000;27(1):39–46.

3. Hsieh J, Chao E, Thibault J, et al. A novel reconstruction algorithm to extend the CT scan field-of-view. Med Phys. 2004;31(9):2385–91.
4. Maier A, Scholz B, Dennerlein F. Optimization-based extrapolation for truncation correction. 2nd CT Meet. 2012; p. 390–4.
5. Xia Y, Hofmann H, Dennerlein F, et al. Towards clinical application of a Laplace operator-based region of interest reconstruction algorithm in C-arm CT. IEEE Trans Med Imaging. 2014;33(3):593–606.
6. Preuhs A, Berger M, Xia Y, et al. Over-exposure correction in CT using optimization-based multiple cylinder fitting. Proc BVM. 2015; p. 35–40.
7. Donoho DL. Compressed sensing. IEEE Trans Inf Theory. 2006;52(4):1289–306.
8. Candès EJ. The restricted isometry property and its implications for compressed sensing. Comptes Rendus Mathematique. 2008;346(9):589–92.
9. Eldar YC, Kutyniok G. Compressed Sensing: Theory and Applications. Cambridge University Press; 2012.
10. Boufounos PT, Baraniuk RG; IEEE. 1-bit compressive sensing. 42nd Annu Conf Inf Sci Syst. 2008; p. 16–21.
11. Yan M, Yang Y, Osher S. Robust 1-bit compressive sensing using adaptive outlier pursuit. IEEE Trans Signal Process. 2012;60(7):3868–75.
12. Jacques L, Laska JN, Boufounos PT, et al. Robust 1-bit compressive sensing via binary stable embeddings of sparse vectors. IEEE Trans Inf Theory. 2013;59(4):2082–102.
13. Feldkamp L, Davis L, Kress J. Practical cone-beam algorithm. J Opt Soc Am A. 1984;1(6):612–9.
14. Andersen AH, Kak AC. Simultaneous algebraic reconstruction technique (SART): a superior implementation of the ART algorithm. Ultrason Imaging. 1984;6(1):81–94.

Self-Calibration and Simultaneous Motion Estimation for C-Arm CT Using Fiducial Markers

Christopher Syben[1], Bastian Bier[1], Martin Berger[1], André Aichert[1]
Rebecca Fahrig[2], Garry Gold[2], Marc Levenston[2] and Andreas Maier[1]

[1]Pattern Recognition Lab, Friedrich-Alexander-University Erlangen-Nuremberg
[2]Radiological Sciences Lab, Stanford University, Stanford, USA
christopher.syben@fau.de

Abstract. C-arm cone-beam CT systems have an increasing popularity in the clinical environment due to their highly flexible scan trajectories. Recent work used these systems to acquire images of the knee joint under weight-bearing conditions. During the scan, the patient is in a standing or in a squatting position and is likely to show involuntary motion, which corrupts image reconstruction. The state-of-the-art fully automatic motion compensation relies on fiducial markers for motion estimation. Due to the not reproducible horizontal trajectory, the system has to be calibrated with a calibration phantom before or after each scan. In this work we present a method to incorporate a self-calibration into the existing motion compensation framework without the need of prior geometric calibration. Quantitative and qualitative evaluations on a numerical phantom as well as clinical data, show superior results compared to the current state-of-the-art method. Moreover, the clinical workflow is improved, as a dedicated system calibration for weight-bearing acquisitions is no longer required.

1 Introduction

The high flexibility of C-arm cone-beam CT (CBCT) systems allow their usage in a wide range of new applications. Recently, these systems have been used to acquire data from knee joints under weight-bearing conditions [1, 2, 3]. For this purpose, the C-arm has to move on a horizontal trajectory around the standing patient. During the scan, involuntary patient motion can occur, which causes blurring, double edges and streaks in the 3D image reconstruction. Estimation and compensation of patient motion improves the quality of the reconstructed images. The state-of-the-art method estimates motion based on fiducial markers, which are attached to the patients knee [4].

However, the method requires a time consuming calibration with a calibration phantom for each scan, since the horizontal trajectory is not supported and thus, not reliably reproducible with the used C-arm system [5]. A self-calibration approach would be beneficial in such a setting. Current approaches can be divided into methods, which use external tools, like calibration markers or tracking systems [6], or rely only on the acquired data [7, 8].

The proposed approach in this work uses fiducial markers to calibrate the system, while simultaneously compensating for the patient's motion. Hence, dedicated time consuming calibration scans are dispensable.

2 Materials and methods

2.1 State-of-the-art motion compensation framework

The state-of-the-art motion estimation framework is introduced in the following [4, 3]. First, a reference 3D marker position is estimated for each marker by backprojecting the detected 2D marker positions into the volume. Then, the 3D reference positions are registered with the detected 2D positions [9]. Afterwards, the rigid motion consisting of three translation and three rotation parameter is estimated, such that the reprojection error (RPE) of the projected 3D reference marker positions on the 2D detected marker is minimized

$$\arg\min_{\boldsymbol{\alpha}} f(\boldsymbol{\alpha}) = \arg\min_{\boldsymbol{\alpha}} \frac{1}{2} \sum_{j=1}^{J} \sum_{i=1}^{M} ||h(\boldsymbol{n}) - \boldsymbol{u}_{ij}||_2^2$$

$$\boldsymbol{n} = \begin{pmatrix} n_1 & n_2 & n_3 \end{pmatrix}^\top = \mathbf{P}_j \cdot \mathbf{M}_j(\boldsymbol{\alpha}) \cdot (\boldsymbol{v}_i \quad 1)^\top \qquad (1)$$

where vector $\boldsymbol{\alpha} \in \mathbb{R}^{6J}$ contains three rotation and translation parameters for each projection. The matrix $\mathbf{M}_j(\alpha)$ applies the rigid motion to the calibrated projection matrix $\mathbf{P}_j \in \mathbb{R}^{3\times4}$ for projection j. The estimated i-th 3D marker position is given by $\boldsymbol{v}_i$ and the corresponding detected 2D position on the j-th projection is given by $\boldsymbol{u}_{ij}$. The function $h : \mathbb{R}^3 \mapsto \mathbb{R}^2$ describes the mapping from 3D homogeneous coordinates to 2D coordinates, i.e., a division by the third component $h(\boldsymbol{n}) = \begin{pmatrix} \frac{n_1}{n_3} & \frac{n_2}{n_3} \end{pmatrix}^\top$. In a last step, motion is compensated by incorporating the estimated motion into the projection matrices and using these updated projection matrices for the reconstruction [3, 4].

2.2 Joint motion estimation and system calibration

We face two problems if no calibration scan is performed and thus no initial estimation of the projection matrices is available. Valid system matrices are needed for the backprojection in the marker detection and for the forward projection to evaluate the objective function. To overcome the missing calibration, we propose to initialize with an ideal circular trajectory and to decompose the projection matrices into an extrinsic and intrinsic matrix, such that the intrinsic parameter estimation can be incorporated in the estimation process.

Initialization. The projection matrices $\mathbf{P}_j$ are initialized with the ideal horizontal circular trajectory based on the systems properties. The 3D marker detection and the evaluation of the objective function can be performed sufficiently well.

Intrinsic camera model. For the self-calibration of the system, the projection matrices need to be estimated. The decomposed projection matrix is $\mathbf{P} = \mathbf{K}[\mathbf{R}|\mathbf{t}]$, where $\mathbf{K} \in \mathbb{R}^{3 \times 3}$ is the intrinsic camera matrix and $\mathbf{R} \in \mathbb{R}^{4 \times 3}$ and $\mathbf{t} \in \mathbb{R}^{4 \times 1}$ contain the extrinsic parameters. For the extrinsic matrix, three rotation and three translation parameters are needed. For the projection matrices, it is not distinguishable whether the patient or the CT system itself is moving. These parameters are able to cover both rigid scanner and patient motion. The intrinsic camera matrix has five degree of freedom. Assuming isotropic detector pixels it can be further reduced to three parameters, i.e., the focal length f and the location of the principal point c_x and c_y. These parameters are estimated using an extended model by Wein et al. [7], which is well suited to the source detector geometry. The model is given by

$$f_x = \frac{p_x}{s_x} \cdot d, \qquad f_y = \frac{p_y}{s_y} \cdot d$$

$$c_x = \frac{p_x}{2} + \frac{p_x}{s_x} \cdot \tan \eta \cdot d, \qquad c_y = \frac{p_y}{2} + \frac{p_y}{s_y} \cdot \tan \theta \cdot d \qquad (2)$$

where d is the source detector distance (SDD) in mm. The width and height of the detector is given by s_x and s_y in mm and p_x and p_y are the width and height of the projection image in pixels. Further, η is the angle to which the detector is tilted with respect to the plane orthogonal to the principal axis around the vertical detector axis $\boldsymbol{v}$. Similarly angle θ describes the rotation around the horizontal detector axis $\boldsymbol{u}$.

Joint motion and system estimation. To achieve a simultaneous motion and system calibration, the calibrated projection matrices in Eq. 1 are replaced with the decomposition of $\mathbf{P}_j$. The cost function for the joint estimation is given by

$$\underset{\boldsymbol{\alpha}, \boldsymbol{\beta}}{\arg \min} \, f(\boldsymbol{\alpha}, \boldsymbol{\beta}) = \underset{\boldsymbol{\alpha}, \boldsymbol{\beta}}{\arg \min} \, \frac{1}{2} \sum_{j=1}^{J} \sum_{i=1}^{M} \|h(\boldsymbol{n}) - \boldsymbol{u}_{ij}\|_2^2$$

$$\boldsymbol{n} = \boldsymbol{P}_j(\boldsymbol{\alpha}, \boldsymbol{\beta}) \cdot (\boldsymbol{v}_i \quad 1)^\top = \mathbf{K}_j(\boldsymbol{\beta}) \cdot \left[\mathbf{R}_j | \boldsymbol{t}_j\right] \cdot \mathbf{M}_j(\boldsymbol{\alpha}) \cdot (\boldsymbol{v}_i \quad 1)^\top \qquad (3)$$

where vector $\boldsymbol{\beta} \in \mathbb{R}^{3J}$ contains the three intrinsic parameters of presented model, for each projection. Hence, $\mathbf{K}_\beta$ describes the intrinsic matrix for the j-th projection. The patient motion and the mechanical deviations from the system are applied by multiplying with $\mathbf{M}_\alpha$, which describes the deviation from the ideal circular trajectory. Further $[\mathbf{R}_j | \boldsymbol{t}_j]$ describes the initial circular trajectory and is fixed during optimization.

The function is solved using a gradient-based optimizer. An analytical derivative of the objective function is computed, which achieves a remarkable speedup. The optimization is carried out in two steps. First, the cost function is minimized with respect to $\boldsymbol{\beta}$ and afterwards $\mathbf{K}_\beta$ is fixed and the function is optimized w.r.t. $\boldsymbol{\alpha}$. Additionally, an iterative scheme is applied, where the new projection

matrices are used to obtain new, more precise 3D marker positions. In the next
iteration the updated 3D marker positions are used for the optimization. After
two iterations the resulting projection matrices contain the patient motion as
well as the system matrices for the scan.

2.3 Data and experiments

For the evaluation a numerical phantom and clinical data from three healthy
patients are used. The phantom models a simplified leg, that consists of three
encapsulated cylinders with a radii of 36, 40, and 100 mm and attenuations of
bone marrow, femur and water, respectively. Beads, with an attenuation of
stainless steel, are included into the phantom on a helical trajectory on the
surface of the outer cylinder. Additionally, a wire with a diameter of 0.2 mm
and with material set to bone is placed in the isocenter, pointing in direction
$(1\ 1\ 1)^T$ [8]. The projections are generated with the CONRAD framework [10]
using calibrated projection matrices with additional estimated patient motion
from clinical scans. Additionally, clinical datasets were acquired with a Siemens
Artis zeego system (Siemens Healthcare GmbH, Forchheim, Germany). The scan
range of the acquisition is 200° acquiring 248 projections in 10 s. Each projection
image has 1240 × 960 pixels with isotropic pixel spacing of 0.308 mm.

For evaluation we use quantitative metrics and visual inspection. The first
metric is the RPE, which is the result of the cost function. The second is the Full-
width at Half-Maximum (FWHM) obtained averaging 720 line profiles through
the cross-section of the wire in case of the numerical phantom and the metallic
beads in case of the clinical datasets. Note for visual inspection that row one is
rotated due to different initialized trajectories.

3 Results

We compared the proposed method with the results of the state-of-the-art method
and the results if no correction is applied. The first column in Fig. 3 shows reconstructions of the phantom dataset with the wire in the ROI. Without correction,
motion artifacts are clearly visible: streaks are present and the shape of the wire
cannot be identified. The state-of-the-art method and the proposed approach
were able to reconstruct the elliptical cross-section of the wire. However, our
method could reconstruct the shape more clear.

The RPE's for the phantom dataset are shown in Tab. 1. Both correction
methods could improve registration accuracy, where we obtained the best results
for the proposed method. The FWHM results are shown in Tab. 2. Without
application of motion correction, the FWHM value could not be measured, due
to strong artifacts. The state-of-the-art and the proposed method achieve comparable FWHM results.

Columns two to four in Fig. 3 show reconstructions of clinical datasets.
Without any correction the reconstructions of all three datasets are affected
by streaking artifacts and the bone outline can not be restored properly. Both

Table 1. RPE in pixel for the described methods and datasets.

Dataset	No Correction	Berger et al.	Proposed Method
Phantom	84.85	1.36	0.07
Clinical 1	96.70	6.07	0.25
Clinical 2	71.29	0.72	0.19
Clinical 3	38.20	0.59	0.43

the state-of-the-art method and the proposed method are able to improve image quality at the bone structures for the clinical datasets. However, the proposed method could further eliminate residual streaking artifacts that could not be fully corrected by the state-of-the-art approach.

Without correction, the highest RPE values for the clinical datasets can be obtained (Tab. 1). The state-of-the-art method achieves for all three clinical datasets good RPE values. However, the RPE values of the proposed method are the best for all three clinical datasets. The FWHM results in Tab. 2 for the clinical dataset 1 are similar for the state-of-the-art method and the proposed method. For clinical datasets 2 and 3 the median FWHM and the standard deviation (std) of the proposed method are lower compared to the state-of-the-art-method.

4   Discussion

Incorporating a self-calibration component into the state-of-the-art method shows promising results. The proposed method is able to achieve reconstruction results, which are superior to the results of the state-of-the-art method, yet, it does not

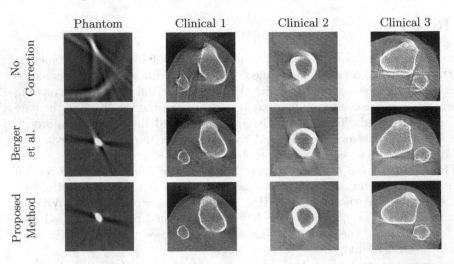

Fig. 1. ROI reconstruction for the described methods and datasets.

Dataset	Berger et al. (median ± std)	Proposed Method (median ± std)
Phantom	0.36 ± 1.80	0.35 ± 1.21
Clinical 1	0.62 ± 3.32	0.63 ± 3.11
Clinical 2	0.84 ± 2.68	0.81 ± 1.31
Clinical 3	0.88 ± 3.22	0.81 ± 1.57

Table 2. FWHM (median ± std) for the described methods and datasets.

require a separate calibration scan. The proposed method consists of two improvements: an self-calibration component and the iterative scheme for updated 3D marker positions. These improvements leads to the superior performance of the proposed method and to a less time consuming procedure. Future work will extend the state-of-the-art method with the iterative scheme using updated 3D reference marker positions to improve the estimation results.

References

1. Choi JH, Fahrig R, Keil A, et al. Fiducial marker-based correction for involuntary motion in weight-bearing C-arm CT scanning of knees - Part I - Numerical model-based optimization. Med Phys. 2013;40(9):091905–n/a.
2. Choi JH, Maier A, Keil A, et al. Fiducial marker-based correction for involuntary motion in weight-bearing C-arm CT scanning of knees - II - Experiment. Med Phys. 2014;41(6):061902–n/a.
3. Müller K, Berger M, Choi JH, et al. Automatic motion estimation and compensation framework for weight-bearing C-arm CT scans using fiducial markers. IFMBE Proc. 2015; p. 58–61.
4. Berger M, Müller K, Aichert A, et al. Marker-free motion correction in weight-bearing cone-beam CT of the knee joint. Med Phys. 2016;43(3):1235–48.
5. Maier A, Choi JH, Keil A, et al. Analysis of vertical and horizontal circular C-arm trajectories. Proc SPIE. 2011;7961:7961231–8.
6. Mitschke M, Navab N. Recovering the X-ray projection geometry for three-dimensional tomographic reconstruction with additional sensors: attached camera versus external navigation system. Med Image Anal. 2003;7(1):65–78.
7. Wein W, Ladikos A, Baumgartner A. Self-Calibration of geometric and radiometric parameters for cone-beam computed tomography. Fully3D Proc. 2011; p. 327–30.
8. Ouadah S, Stayman JW, Gang GJ, et al. Self-Calibration of cone-beam CT geometry using 3D–2D image registration. Phys Med Biol. 2016;61(7):2613.
9. Berger M, Forman C, Schwemmer C, et al. Automatic removal of externally attached fiducial markers in cone beam C-arm CT. Proc BVM. 2014; p. 168–73.
10. Maier A, Hofmann HG, Berger M, et al. CONRAD–A software framework for cone-beam imaging in radiology. Med Phys. 2013;40(11):111914.

Robust Groupwise Affine Registration of Medical Images with Stochastic Optimization

Hristina Uzunova, Heinz Handels, Jan Ehrhardt

Institute of Medical Informatics, University of Lübeck, Germany
ehrhardt@imi.uni-luebeck.de

Abstract. Robust registration of medical images with missing correspondences caused by pathological structures or anatomical variations is still a challenging problem. This paper presents a robust method for groupwise affine registration based on the RASL algorithm [1] that formulates the registration problem as a sparse and low-rank decomposition. We adapt the RASL algorithm for the alignment of 3D image data and introduce a stochastic optimization scheme to enable the computational tractability. Further, a normalization scheme generates more plausible and unique transformations. In our experiments, the algorithm has been applied to various medical images, and proves its suitability for medical image registration. Especially, the approach shows advantages in the presence of pathologies and outperforms iterative groupwise registration based on ITK. The stochastic optimization scheme generates a significant acceleration allowing for a groupwise affine registration of ten 3D CT images in $\sim$ 5 minutes on CPU without elaborate optimization.

1 Introduction

Image registration is a crucial part of various applications in medical image analysis and processing. The robust registration of medical images is particularly challenging if pathologies hinder correspondence detection. The usual definition of image registration uses a template image, which is then aligned to a chosen reference image by finding proper transformations. However, it is often necessary to be able to align multiple images at the same time – a *groupwise* registration. This is e.g. needed for atlas construction.

In this work we present an efficient and robust algorithm for groupwise affine registration of medical images in the presence of pathological structures. Our algorithm bases on robust alignment by sparse and low-rank decomposition for linearly correlated images (RASL), which has been used in previous work to align non-medical 2D images [1]. The authors of [1] have shown the efficacy of the robust alignment algorithm RASL over a wide range of realistic misalignments and image corruptions. A drawback of RASL is the high computational demand required to solve the underlying optimization problem which prevents the application to 3D (medical) data. The contribution of our paper is threefold: first, the algorithm has been expanded for aligning 3D images and a stochastic sampling scheme was integrated leading to a significant speedup allowing for efficient 3D registration, second, we introduce a normalization scheme that results in more plausible transformations, and further, the algorithm has been applied in various medical settings, to prove its suitability for medical image registration and to show its advantage in the presence of pathologies.

2   Methods and experiments

2.1   Robust image alignment by sparse and low-rank decomposition

Suppose we are given n grayscale images $I_1, \ldots, I_n \in \mathbb{R}^{w \times h}$ and vec : $\mathbb{R}^{w \times h} \to \mathbb{R}^m$ is an operator which stacks the pixels of an image as a vector. Under the assumption that aligned images are linearly correlated, the data matrix

$$D = [\text{vec}(I_1)| \ldots |\text{vec}(I_n)] \in \mathbb{R}^{m \times n} \tag{1}$$

should be approximately *low-rank* if the images are well-aligned. However, even small misalignments will lead to an increased rank of the matrix D. The misalignment of the input images is modeled by transformations τ_i, such that $I_1 \circ \tau_1, \ldots, I_n \circ \tau_n$ are aligned. In practice images are often corrupted or happen to have differing pixels to each other – in medical images, those can be differing pathologies, artifacts or anatomical variations not modeled by the transformation class. Thus, it is practical to assume that each image I_j has a corresponding additive error e_j. These observations are formulated as optimization problem

$$\min_{A,E,\tau} \text{rank}(A) + \gamma ||E||_0 \quad \text{s.t.} \ D \circ \tau = A + E \tag{2}$$

where $\gamma > 0$, A represents a low-rank matrix, $E = [\text{vec}(e_1)| \ldots |\text{vec}(e_n)]$ is assumed to be a *sparse matrix*, because errors usually affect only a fraction of the image, and under abuse of notation we write $D \circ \tau = [\text{vec}(I_1 \circ \tau_1)| \ldots |\text{vec}(I_n \circ \tau_n)]$. While Eq. (2) follows naturally from the problem definition, this problem cannot be directly solved [2]. Therefore, a relaxed convex optimization problem is formulated using nuclear norm $|| \cdot ||_*$ and $\mathcal{L}^1$ norm

$$\min_{A,E,\tau} ||A||_* + \lambda ||E||_1 \quad \text{s.t.} \ D \circ \tau = A + E \tag{3}$$

To solve Eq. (3) w.r.t. the transformations τ, the constraint $D \circ \tau = A + E$ is linearised using Taylor's formula: $D \circ (\tau + \Delta \tau) \approx D \circ \tau + \sum_{i=1}^{n} J_i \Delta \tau \epsilon_i^T$, where $J_i = \frac{\partial}{\partial \xi} \text{vec}(I_i \circ \xi)|_{\xi = \tau_i}$ is the Jacobian of the i-th image with respect to the transformation parameters and ϵ_i denotes the standard basis for $\mathbb{R}^n$. Based on this linearization the authors of [1] propose the iterative RASL algorithm to solve the given optimization problem. The algorithm uses an outer loop to update the transformations $\tau_1, \ldots, \tau_n$ and an inner loop to minimize Eq. (3) with respect to A, E and $\Delta \tau$ using the alternating direction method of multipliers (ADMM) [3].

2.2   Restriction to plausible transformations

A significant problem in the existing algorithm is the fact, that the calculated transformations $\tau_1, \ldots, \tau_n$ are not restricted and computed independently. This can lead to implausible results such as zooming all images in or out up to a certain area of one colour. Such transformations are, indeed, solutions of the minimization problem, but are not desirable in practice. The authors propose an intensity rescaling step in each iteration to avoid this problem, however, in our observations the resulting transformations do not correspond to the intuition (Fig. 1). Therefore, we propose the following additional constrain

$$\tau_1 \circ \tau_2 \circ \cdots \circ \tau_n = Id \qquad (4)$$

where $\circ$ denotes the concatenation of affine transformations. Note, that Eq. (4) implicitly registers all images to the average shape (Fig. 1).

2.3   Solving RASL efficiently by stochastic optimization

In previous work, RASL is particularly used for the rigid, affine and projective alignment of 2D photographic images [1]. The extension of the algorithm to 3D image data is straight forward by using a vectorization operator vec : $\mathbb{R}^{w \times h \times d} \rightarrow \mathbb{R}^m$. The RASL registration of images with $200 \times 200 \times 100$ voxels then requires multiple times the ADMM optimization of Eq. (3) for matrices with 4 million rows. One possible solution is to reduce the image size in a multi-resolution mode, however, this might contradict the sparsity assumption. Instead, we propose to use stochastic sampling in the outer loop of the RASL algorithm to reduce the matrix size in Eq. (3) to be solved in the inner loop. Therefore, we select randomly a percentage $p \in (0, 1]$ of pixel positions in each iteration to compute the transformation updates $\Delta\tau$. Because only a small number of transformation parameters needs to be computed (e.g. 12 per image for affine transformations), we assume that a robust registration is possible even for small values p. The stochastic RASL optimization is shown in Alg. 1. Note, that the matrices A and E are not needed within the outer while loop, and have only $p \cdot m$ rows.

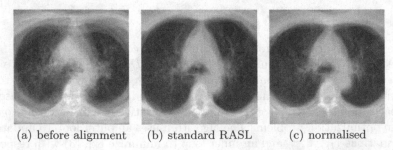

(a) before alignment   (b) standard RASL   (c) normalised

Fig. 1. Mean of ten lung CT images (a) before alignment, (b) after RASL alignment and (c) after RASL alignment using the transformation constrain in Eq. (4).

Algorithm 1 Stochastic RASL optimization

INPUT: Images $I_1,\ldots,I_n \in \mathbb{R}^{w \times h \times d}$, initial transformations $\tau_1,\ldots,\tau_n$, weights $\lambda > 0$, percentage of used rows $p \in (0,1]$.

Step 0: Vectorize and stack the images:

$$D \leftarrow [vec(I_1)|\ldots|vec(I_n)]$$

while not converged **do**

    Step 1: Select $p \cdot m$ rows of D and save them in $\hat{D}$ corresponding to the reduced images $\hat{I}_i$

    Step 2: Compute Jacobian matrices w.r.t. transformation:

$$J_i \leftarrow \frac{\partial}{\partial \xi}\left(vec(\hat{I}_i \circ \xi)\right)\Big|_{\xi = \tau_i}, i = 1,\ldots,n$$

    Step 3: Transform the images:

$$\hat{D} \circ \tau \leftarrow \left[vec(\hat{I}_1 \circ \tau_1)|\ldots|vec(\hat{I}_n \circ \tau_n)\right]$$

    Step 4: Solve the linearized convex optimization with ADMM (inner loop):

$$(A^*, E^*, \Delta\tau^*) \leftarrow \arg\min_{A,E,\Delta\tau} ||A||_* + \lambda ||E||_1,$$

$$\text{s.t. } \hat{D} \circ \tau + \sum_{i=1}^{n} J_i \Delta\tau \epsilon_i \epsilon_i^T = A + E$$

    Step 5: Update and normalize transformations:

$$\tau \leftarrow \tau + \Delta\tau^* \qquad\qquad \text{(linearized update)}$$

$$\tau_i \leftarrow \tau_i \circ \bar{\tau}^{-1} \text{ with } \bar{\tau} = exp(\tfrac{1}{n}\textstyle\sum_i log(\tau_i)) \text{ (normalization, Eq.(4))}$$

end while

Step 6 (optional): Compute $D \circ \tau$ and solve (for fixed τ):

$$(A^*, E^*) \leftarrow \arg\min_{A,E} ||A||_* + \lambda ||E||_1, \text{ s.t. } D \circ \tau = A + E$$

OUTPUT: Transformations $\tau_1,\ldots,\tau_n$ (optional A^* and E^*) as solution of Eq. (3)

The stochastic optimization leads to a necessary adaption of the weighting parameter λ depending on the parameter p. According to the suggestion in [1], we use the following adaptation rule: $\lambda = \frac{\lambda_0}{\sqrt{p}}$, where λ_0 is the weighting parameter for the full resolution images ($p = 1$). Note, that the Log-Euclidean formula in [4] is used for the normalization in step 5.

3 Experiments and results

The first experiment evaluates the influence of the percentage p of the used image pixels on the registration accuracy and run-time. Tab. 1 shows the results for an affine registration of ten 3D CT images of the thorax without visible pathologies ($200 \times 200 \times 180$ voxels). Registration accuracy is measured by average pair-wise Dice overlaps of the lung masks. Computation time is measured for the complete groupwise registration process on a quad core 2.67GHz Xeon(R) CPU W3520. A speed-up of ≈ 35 can be achieved by using only 1% of the voxels in each iteration without degrading registration accuracy significantly.

The following experiments assess the registration accuracy of the stochastic 3D RASL algorithm in the presence of pathologies using four different data sets:

$p =$	Time (min.)	Dice
100%	202:14	0.7815
50%	91:51	0.7815
10%	21:29	0.7818
1%	05:43	0.7805
initial		0.7175

		Groupwise stochastic	
data set	Initial	ITK-Reg	3D RASL
Lung CT Tumor	0.7175	0.7915	0.8135
Lung CT diverse	0.6397	0.6692	0.7586
Brain MRI Tumor	0.9502	0.8966	0.9741
Brain MRI Lesion	0.9017	0.9568	0.9576

Table 1. Sample size and its effect on speed and quality of alignment, measured using Dice-coefficient.

Table 2. Registration accuracy measured in Dice coefficients for four different 3D data sets. Compared are the initial alignment, the results of the groupwise ITK-based registration and the proposed stochastic RASL algorithm.

- *Lung CT Tumor:* Ten 3D CT images of the thorax with large lung tumors, $200 \times 200 \times 180$ voxels.
- *Lung CT diverse:* Ten 3D CT images of the thorax with diverse lung pathologies like fibrosis or lung edema, $210 \times 210 \times 190$ voxels.
- *Brain MRI Tumor:* 10 MRI images with brain tumors, $200 \times 200 \times 80$ voxels.
- *Brain MRI Lesion:* 10 MRI images of the head with artificially generated stroke lesions, $140 \times 180 \times 140$ voxels.

In all experiments an affine transformation model with $p = 0.01$ and $\lambda_0 = \frac{1}{\sqrt{m}}$ is used, where $m = w \cdot h \cdot d$ is the number of voxels. Registration accuracy is measured in terms of average pair-wise Dice overlaps of lung or brain masks, and compared to the iterative groupwise registration approach proposed in [5].This approach was implemented using the intensity-based affine registration method implemented in ITK. Here we use 3-level multiresolution, regular gradient descent optimizer and SSD as distance measurement. The quantitative results are summarized in Tab. 2. As shown in Fig. 2 and 3 the sparse component contains predominantly pathological structures beside the residual alignment errors, except for the Brain MRI Lesion data set. Here, the lesions do not affect the registration accuracy due to slight intensity differences to healthy brain tissue and they are consequently not present in the sparse component. In contrast, RASL strongly improves the registration accuracy for data sets with prominent space-consuming pathologies like Lung CT diverse.

4   Discussion and conclusions

We presented a stochastic groupwise robust registration method and applied this method to 3D medical images. The algorithm is run-time efficient and outperforms standard intensity-based registration methods, particularly for images with missing correspondences caused by space-consuming pathologies.

The RASL algorithm can be applied to 3D images because of a significant acceleration generated by a stochastic optimization scheme. The normalization of the transformations shown in Sec. 2.2 results in a registration to the group

Fig. 2. Results of the groupwise stochastic 3D RASL registration for the Lung CT Tumor (top row) and Lung CT diverse (bottom row) data sets. Shown are the transformed images (left) as well as sparse (middle) and low-rank components (right).

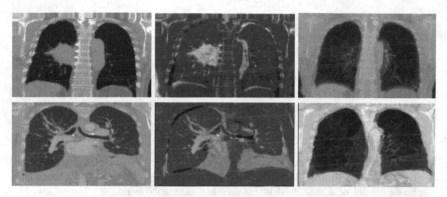

Fig. 3. Results of the groupwise stochastic 3D RASL registration for the Brain MRI Tumor (left) and Brain MRI Lesion (right) data sets. Shown are the transformed images and the sparse components.

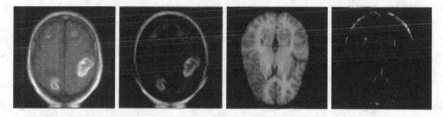

average shape and therefore increases the plausibility of the resulting transformations.

References

1. Peng Y, Ganesch A, Wright J, et al. RASL:robust alignment by sparse and low-rank decomposition for linearly correlated images. IEEE Trans Pattern Anal Mach Intell. 2012;34(11):2233–46.
2. Wright J, Ganesh A, Rao S, et al. Robust principal component analysis: exact recovery of corrupted low-rank matrices via convex optimization. Adv Neural Inf Process Syst. 2009; p. 2080–8.
3. Boyd S, Parikh N, Chu E, et al. Distributed optimization and statistical learning via the alternating direction method of multipliers. Foundations Trends® Mach Learn. 2011;3(1):1–122.
4. Arsigny V, Commowick O, Ayache N, et al. A fast and log-euclidean polyaffine framework for locally linear registration. J Math Imaging Vis. 2009;33(2):222–38.
5. Guimond A, Meunier J, Thirion JP. Average brain models: a convergence study. Comput Vis Image Underst. 2000;77(2):192–210.

GPU-Based Image Geodesics for Optical Coherence Tomography

Benjamin Berkels[1], Michael Buchner[2], Alexander Effland[2], Martin Rumpf[2], Steffen Schmitz-Valckenberg[3]

[1] AICES Graduate School, RWTH Aachen University
[2] Institute for Numerical Simulation, University of Bonn
[3] Department of Ophthalmology, University of Bonn
`michael.buchner@uni-bonn.de`

Abstract. Within a manifold framework, the interpolation of tomographic image time series is investigated. To this end, the metamorphosis model of a manifold of images is taken into account. Based on a variational time discretization, discrete geodesic paths in this space of images are computed. The space discretization is based on finite elements spanned by tensor product cubic B-splines. An efficient implementation is obtained by utilizing graphics hardware and a proper combination of GPU and CPU computation. First results for time series of optical coherence tomography images of a macular degeneration demonstrate the applicability of this geometric concept.

1 Introduction

This paper deals with the interpolation of images considered as objects in a Riemannian manifold $\mathcal{M}$ of images. In this context, image interpolation can naturally be phrased as computing a geodesic path between the input images. Geodesics on Riemannian manifolds are minimizers of the path energy, which in particular implies that they also minimize the path length and are arclength parametrized. The path energy of a path $u : [0,1] \to \mathcal{M}$, $t \mapsto u(t)$, is given by $\mathcal{E}[u] = \int_0^1 g_u(\dot{u}, \dot{u}) \, dt$, where $\dot{u}$ is the time derivative of the curve. In our case, $t \mapsto u(t)$ is a curve of images and the metric $g_u(v,v)$ is a bilinear form measuring the cost of an infinitesimal variation $u + \delta v$ of an image u. To define the metric, we follow the *metamorphosis* model, which was analyzed by Trouvé and Younes [1]. The associated metric is defined as an integral over the image domain $\Omega \subset \mathbb{R}^2$ and reflects

- the cost caused by viscous Newtonian and multipolar dissipation $|Dv|^2 + \gamma|D^2v|^2$ due to friction, where Dv, D^2v are the Jacobian and Hessian of v,
- the cost of the intensity modulation $(\dot{u} + v \cdot \nabla u)^2$ along transport paths described via the so-called material derivative $\dot{u} + v \cdot \nabla u$.

To evaluate the metric, we take into account the flow field v, which causes the minimal cost. Altogether, we obtain for a fixed $\delta > 0$ the path energy

$$\mathcal{E}[u] = \int_0^1 \min_{\text{flow fields } v} \int_\Omega |Dv|^2 + \gamma|D^2v|^2 + \frac{1}{\delta}(\dot{u} + v \cdot \nabla u)^2 \, dx \, dt \qquad (1)$$

Geodesic paths in the space of images, i.e. minimizers of this path energy, provide smooth interpolations between the input images. In [2], Berkels et al. introduced a variational time discretization of the path energy and proved Γ-convergence to the time continuous path energy under slightly stronger assumptions. This in particular implies the convergence of the minimizers of the discrete path energy to (time continuous) geodesics. Furthermore, they proposed an algorithm to numerically compute time discrete geodesics, for which a spatial discretization of the underlying deformations and image intensities by piecewise affine finite elements is employed.

Here, we improve the robustness and approximation quality taking into account cubic spline spaces. The algorithm is based on an alternating descent scheme, during which multiple images are updated. To speed up these registration subproblems, which are the computational bottleneck, a GPU implementation [3] significantly improves the performance of the proposed method.

In this paper, we demonstrate the applicability of this approach to optical coherence tomography (OCT) images in age-related macular degeneration, the most common cause of irreversible visual loss in industrial countries. In this retinal disease, in-vivo imaging by OCT allows to detect and monitor progressive microstructural changes of the outer retina that lead to photoreceptor cell degeneration and thus functional loss [4]. As shown below, the approach generates suitable interpolations equipped with explicitly computed pointwise motion fields and intensity modulations. Furthermore, we compare a piecewise geodesic path between images recorded annually against geodesic paths spanning a four year period to test the prediction quality of the geodesic interpolation.

2   Materials and methods

2.1   Time discrete geodesics in the metamorphosis model

This section summarizes the time discrete metamorphosis model from [2], which builds on a variational time discretization. To approximate the path energy (1), we consider a time discrete curve $\mathbf{u} = (u_0, \ldots, u_K)$ in the space of images (with $u_k : \Omega \to \mathbb{R}$ being a gray valued intensity map) and define a dissimilarity

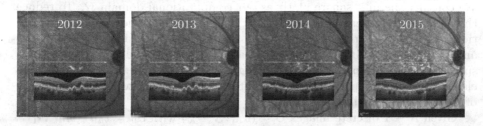

Fig. 1. Ophthalmoscopy (background) and a slice (perpendicular to the green line) from an optical coherence tomography of a human eye (foreground) show an age-related macular degeneration in four consecutive years.

measure

$$\mathcal{W}^D[u, \tilde{u}, \phi] := \int_\Omega |D(\phi - \mathrm{Id})|^2 + \gamma |D^2\phi|^2 + \frac{1}{\delta} |\tilde{u} \circ \phi - u|^2 \, \mathrm{d}x \qquad (2)$$

for two images u, $\tilde{u}$, and a deformation $\phi : \Omega \to \Omega$. By minimizing w.r.t. all deformations ϕ with $\phi(x) = x$ for all $x \in \partial\Omega$, we actually solve a very simple (elastic) matching problem between the template image $\tilde{u}$ and the reference image u. Now, we define $\mathcal{W}[u, \tilde{u}] := \min_\phi \mathcal{W}^D[u, \tilde{u}, \phi]$ as the optimal matching cost and use this to introduce a discrete path energy $\mathbf{E}^K[\mathbf{u}] = K \sum_{k=1}^K \mathcal{W}[u_{k-1}, u_k]$ summing over the (minimal) dissimilarity measure of consecutive image pairs. Indeed, [2] shows that the first two terms in $\mathcal{W}^D$ approximate the viscous friction reflected in the first two terms of the path energy (1), whereas the last term approximates the squared material derivative term appearing in (1). Here, the associated time step is $\tau = \frac{1}{K}$.

Now, a *discrete geodesic* connecting two images u_A and u_B is a discrete curve in the space of images that minimizes $\mathbf{E}^K$ over all discrete curves $\mathbf{u}$ with $u_0 = u_A$ and $u_K = u_B$. For a curve $\mathbf{u}$ and deformations $\phi = (\phi_1, \ldots, \phi_K)$, we set

$$\mathbf{E}^{K,D}[\mathbf{u}, \phi] = K \sum_{k=1}^K \mathcal{W}^D[u_{k-1}, u_k, \phi_k] \qquad (3)$$

Thus, a discrete geodesic from u_A to u_B is obtained by minimizing $\mathbf{E}^{K,D}[\mathbf{u}, \phi]$ with respect to $\mathbf{u}$ and ϕ while fixing $u_0 = u_A$ and $u_K = u_B$. Minimizing with respect to ϕ for fixed images $\mathbf{u}$ results in K independent image registration problems (registering u_{k-1} to u_k), while minimizing with respect to $\mathbf{u}$ for fixed deformations ϕ leads to a linear system of equations for $\mathbf{u}$, i.e. for $k = 1, \ldots, K - 1$

$$\left(1 + (\det D\phi_k)^{-1} \circ \phi_k^{-1}\right) u_k = u_{k+1} \circ \phi_{k+1} + (u_{k-1} \circ \phi_k^{-1}) \left((\det D\phi_k)^{-1} \circ \phi_k^{-1}\right) \qquad (4)$$

2.2   Spatial discretization and computation of geodesics

We consider the unit square $[0, 1]^2$ as our computational domain Ω. To reduce the complexity, we take into account a fine grid $\mathcal{G}_h$ for the image discretization and a coarse grid $\mathcal{G}_H$ for the deformation discretization – both regular and quadrilateral. Grid elements of $\mathcal{G}_h$ and $\mathcal{G}_H$ are denoted by e_h and e_H, respectively. For the space of discrete images, we use the piecewise bilinear finite element space. The space of discrete deformations is the Cartesian product space of (vector valued) cubic splines.

Given $K + 1$ discrete images $\mathbf{U} = (U_0, \ldots, U_K)$ with $U_0 = \mathcal{I}_h u_A$ and $U_K = \mathcal{I}_h u_B$ ($\mathcal{I}_h$ is the nodal interpolation operator onto the discrete image space), and K discrete deformations $\Phi = (\Phi_1, \ldots, \Phi_K)$, we use a numerical quadrature scheme to compute the discrete path energy

$$\mathbf{E}_{h,H}^{K,D}[\mathbf{U}, \mathbf{\Phi}] = K \sum_{k=1}^{K} \left(\sum_{e_H \in \mathcal{G}_H} \sum_{Q=0}^{3} \omega_Q^{e_H} \left(|D\Phi_k - \mathrm{Id}|^2(x_Q^{e_H}) + \gamma |D^2\Phi_k|^2(x_Q^{e_H}) \right) \right.$$
$$\left. + \frac{1}{\delta} \sum_{e_h \in \mathcal{G}_h} \sum_{q=0}^{8} \omega_q^{e_h} \left(U_k \circ \Phi_k(x_q^{e_h}) - U_{k-1}(x_q^{e_h}) \right)^2 \right)$$

Here, we use Gauss-Legendre quadrature of order 3 in 2D on elements of $\mathcal{G}_H$ to compute the prior with quadrature points $x_Q^{e_H}$ and weights $\omega_Q^{e_H}$. The fidelity term is computed using a tensor product Simpson quadrature on $\mathcal{G}_h$ with quadrature points $x_q^{e_h}$ and weights $\omega_q^{e_h}$. Alternatively, we also use cubic splines for the image intensity discretization on $\mathcal{G}_h$ and adapted the quadrature accordingly.

2.3 GPU-accelerated computation of geodesics

In the numerical applications, it became apparent that the time-critical step in the computation of geodesics was the solution of the registration subproblem. The assembly of the discrete energy as well as the gradient exhibit data parallelism as the same integrand has to be evaluated on all elements during the numerical integration. As GPUs are particularly well suited for the computation of the data parallel parts of the program, the energy and gradient assembly are implemented on the graphics card. Elements in the mesh are identified with a thread on the GPU. For the assembly of the discrete energy, a reduction scheme is employed to perform the integration on each element embedded into streams to overlap computation on the GPU. As the assembly of the energy and the gradient involves the evaluation of deformed images, the assembly can be further accelerated by a pre-computing of deformed images via existing GPU image warping tools (Fig. 2 for some speed up results).

3 Results

We applied the proposed method to two OCT image sequences, each consisting of four images taken in consecutive years (Fig. 1 for one of the sequences) and computed a piecewise geodesic curve interpolating these input images consisting of $3 \cdot K + 1$ images ($K = 27$). Fig. 3 shows the input images in red boxes and the

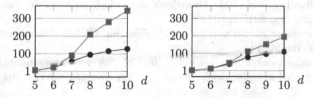

Fig. 2. Left: speedup for assembly of the energy without (blue) and with (red) image warping at image size $(2^d+1) \times (2^d+1)$. Right: Same data shown for gradient assembly.

interpolated intermediate time steps u_9 and u_{18} in between. Furthermore, the corresponding velocity fields $\frac{1}{\tau}(\phi_k-\mathrm{Id})$ and the intensity modulation given by the discrete material derivative $\frac{1}{\tau}(u_k \circ \phi_k - u_{k-1})$ are shown. Finally, selected images from a direct geodesic connection ($K = 27$) between the 2012 and 2015 images are shown together with the associated velocity fields and intensity modulations. This in particular enables a comparison of this wide span temporal geodesic interpolation with the images recorded for the years in between.

4   Discussion

Based on the tool of discrete geodesics, we are able to compute interpolation paths for a given time series of images. The method also provides information on a probable motion field reflecting the actual deformation process of tissue structures in tomographic images. In our application, a detailed analysis of dynamic disease evolution in age-related macular degeneration may serve for a better understanding of the underlying pathogenetic processes, an identification of prognostic biomarkers for progression and for the evaluation of new therapeutical strategies. In addition, we compared the piecewise geodesic interpolation with key frames for every year with the geodesic interpolation of a four year span. A qualitative comparison of recorded and interpolated images allows a validation of the physical model underlying the image manifold. Indeed, the obtained interpolation properly shows the progressive thinning of the outer retinal layers, while subtle dynamic hyperreflective dots–presumably reflecting migration of retinal pigment epithelium cells–are less accurately detectable by the long range interpolation. For the assessment of velocity fields, an accurate alignment of images at different visits using the hyperreflective outer band of the retinal pigment epithelium as a reference should be incorporated. Motivated by the quality of the obtained interpolation–even over wider time spans–we aim for the computation of image extrapolation to predict the progression of the decease based on in-vivo imaging. This might be of particular importance for future interventional clinical trials that aim to prevent blinding retinal diseases.

References

1. Trouvé A, Younes L. Local geometry of deformable templates. SIAM J Math Anal. 2005;37(1):17–59.
2. Berkels B, Effland A, Rumpf M. Time discrete geodesic paths in the space of images. SIAM J Imaging Sci. 2015;8(3):1457–88.
3. Cheng J, Grossmann M, McKercher T. Professional CUDA C Programming. John Wiley & Sons, Inc.; 2014.
4. Holz FG, Schmitz-Valckenberg S, Fleckenstein M. Recent developments in the treatment of age-related macular degeneration. J Clin Invest. 2014;124(4):1430–8.

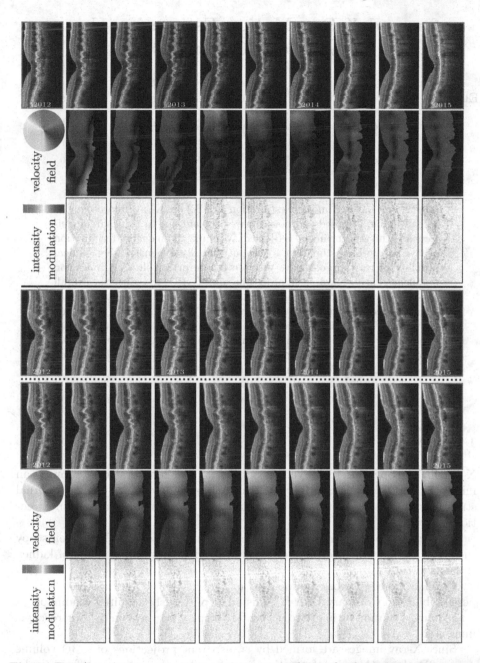

Fig. 3. First/fourth row: piecewise geodesic interpolation for four consecutive years of human eyes for two patients (input data in red boxes). Second/third row: the associated discrete velocity field (the hue refers to the direction and the intensity is proportional to the norm) and the intensity modulation of the first patient. Fifth to seventh row: geodesic interpolation between the years 2012 and 2015 of the second patient and the associated discrete velocity field and intensity modulation, respectively.

Layered X-Ray Motion Estimation Using Primal-Dual Optimization

Ehsan Mehmood[1], Peter Fischer[1,2], Thomas Pohl[2], Tim Horz[2], Andreas Maier[1]

[1]Pattern Recognition Lab, FAU Erlangen-Nürnberg, Erlangen, Germany
[2]Siemens Healthineers, Forchheim, Germany
esn.mehmood@gmail.com

Abstract. Layered motion estimation (LME) in X-ray fluoroscopy is a challenging, ill-posed and non-convex problem due to transparency effects and the way the image is defined. Minimizing an energy formulation of layered motion estimation is computationally expensive. For clinical usability of this approach, we propose to use primal-dual optimization parallelized using a graphical processing unit (GPU) to reduce the overall run-time of this algorithm. Experimentally this method is able to substantially reduce target registration error by 70% on manually annotated landmarks on five distinct image sequences compared to the static baseline, similar to prior work on this domain. However, the overall runtime of our method on a conventional GPU is less than 3.3 seconds compared to several minutes for the state of the art. Considering typical frame-rates of X-ray fluoroscopy devices, this runtime makes the application of layered motion estimation feasible for many clinical workflows.

1   Introduction

X-ray fluoroscopy, due to its very good spatial and temporal resolution, is an important modality for clearly visualizing human body functions and internal structures, and is commonly used for guidance in minimally invasive interventions.

Motion estimation is useful for many clinical applications in X-ray fluoroscopy such as blood flow monitoring, detection of dead tissues and tracking of kidney stones and tumors.

Cardiac and respiratory motion can be compensated to improve visibility and perceptibility in Coronary DSA [1]. Fusion of previously acquired roadmaps requires a motion estimate to accurately display overlays on live fluoroscopic images [2].

Since X-ray images are formed by transparent projections of a 3D volume onto a 2D plane, there is information loss as well as transparency effects in the images. To solve the transparency problem in X-ray image registration, motion layers are introduced with a goal to calculate a 2-D motion field for each layer. This approach involves estimation of both layers and motions with information on neither available initially. Their dependency on each other causes a chicken-and-egg problem since computation of layers requires motion estimated and vice versa. Szeliski et al. assume parametric motion to simplify the problem and describe two methods to compute layers, using max and min composites for sequential initialization and using constrained least squares optimization for iterative refinement [3]. Preston et al. introduce a method to jointly estimate layers and motions by using a total-variation layer gradient penalty and a smoothness prior for motions [4]. To generate physiologically plausible motions, Fischer et al. proposed to use surrogate signals to define a model of the layer motions [5] and an alternating minimization scheme to calculate motions and layers.

The existing work by Fischer et al. [5] is able to plausibly estimate layers and motions. However, the runtime is several minutes and thus not feasible for time-critical clinical applications. We propose to solve the layered motion estimation problem using primal-dual optimization. Compared to other optimizers, primal-dual methods are simple, easily parallelizeable, and can handle non-smooth problems naturally. They involve splitting of the main problem into simpler sub-problems that can be solved efficiently using computationally efficient proximity operators. Thus, we implement layered motion estimation on the graphical processing unit (GPU) to achieve a clinically acceptable time. In the experiments, we demonstrate that a similar accuracy of motion estimation as in [5] is achieved. Additionally, we analyze and compare the runtimes of the different algorithms.

2   Methods

2.1   Layered motion estimation

We are interested in separating transparent X-ray images, denoted in this paper as i (with dimensions $N_t \times H \times W$) into multiple layers l_n (with dimensions $N_l \times H \times W$) and motions v_n (with dimensions $N_l \times H \times W \times 2$) that each layer n undergoes, where N_t, N_l, W, H are number of images in the sequence, number of layers, width of an image and height of an image respectively. In mathematical terms, we can define our image as

$$I = \mathbf{a}\,(l, v) + \eta \tag{1}$$

where $\mathbf{a}\,(l, v)$ is a function that creates an image sequence estimate using bilinear remapping of layers and motions and η is introduced to account for model errors and observation noise in the log-transformed X-ray model [4].

Moreover, to make motions physiologically plausible, calculated base motions ν_n are scaled using surrogate signals to obtain motions according to [5]

$$v_n\,(\boldsymbol{x}, t) = s_n\,(t) \cdot \nu_n\,(\boldsymbol{x}) \tag{2}$$

In discretized form, the energy equation of the layered motion estimation (LME) problem can be written as

$$\min_{l,v} \underbrace{\|\mathbf{a}\,(l, v) - I\|_1}_{\text{Data term}} + \underbrace{\lambda_l \,\|\nabla l\|_{2,1}}_{\text{Layer regularizer}} + \underbrace{\lambda_v \,\|\nabla v\|_{2,1}}_{\text{Motion regularizer}} \tag{3}$$

where ∇ is the gradient operator and λ_l and λ_v are the regularizer weights. The layer and motion regularization terms in this setup are to ensure layer and motion smoothness. As proposed by Fischer et al. we solve this energy minimization problem through alternate minimization by keeping one variable (layers or motions) constant and minimizing energy function with respect to the other [5].

2.2   Primal-dual minimization

Primal-dual minimization minimizes a given problem with respect to its primal and dual form. For the given general problem, its primal form

$$x^* \in \mathrm{argmin}\,2453_x G(x) + H(Lx) \tag{4}$$

and dual form

$$y^* \in \mathrm{argmin}\,2453_y G^*(-L^T y) + H^*(y) \tag{5}$$

can be solved using Chambolle-Pock algorithm as proposed by Chambolle et al. [6], where $x \in \mathbb{R}^N$ and $y \in \mathbb{R}^K$ are vectors (primal and dual solutions) in real Hilbert spaces, G and H are proper, convex and simple functions, and $L : \mathbb{R}^N \to \mathbb{R}^K$ is a bounded linear operator.

Layer minimization. For layer minimization we can develop an algorithm using appropriate proximity operators for our functions similar to Sidky et al. [7]. Algorithm 1 shows layer minimization algorithm which involves solving with respect to three variables, the primal variable l and the dual variables p and q. A_l is a matrix encoding the application of the function $a\,(l, v)$ from Eq. (3) to l, which is linear in l assuming constant motion.

Algorithmus 1 : Pseudo-code for N-steps $l_1 - $ TV Chambolle-Pock algorithm for layers. The constant K is the $l_2 - $ norm of the matrix defining L, τ and σ are non-negative step-size parameters, θ is the update coefficient for primal variable, j is the iteration index and J are the total predefined number of iterations.

$K \leftarrow \|(\mathbf{A}_l, \nabla)\|_2\,; \tau \leftarrow 1/K; \sigma \leftarrow 1/K; n \leftarrow 0; \theta \leftarrow 1; j \leftarrow 0$
$l_0 \leftarrow 0, \bar{l}_0 \leftarrow l_0, p_0 \leftarrow 0, q_0 \leftarrow 0$
while $j \leq J$ **do**

    $p_{j+1} \leftarrow (p_j + \sigma\,(\mathbf{A}_l \bar{l}_j - i))\,/ \max(1_D, |p_j + \sigma\,(\mathbf{A}_l \bar{l}_n - i)|)$
    $q_{j+1} \leftarrow \lambda\,(q_j + \sigma \nabla \bar{l}_j)\,/ \max(\lambda 1_D, |q_j + \sigma\,(\nabla \bar{l}_j)|)$
    $l_{j+1} \leftarrow l_j - \tau \mathbf{A}_l^T p_{j+1} - \tau \nabla^T q_{j+1}$
    $\bar{l}_{j+1} \leftarrow l_{j+1} + \theta\,(l_{j+1} - l_j)$
    $j \leftarrow j + 1$

end
return l_J

Motion minimization. Similarly, Algorithm 1 can be modified to develop a minimization algorithm for motions with change of primal variable, $l_n \rightarrow v_n$ and remapping function $A_l \rightarrow A_v$, where A_v is approximating the application of $a\,(l, v)$ to v. A_v is not linear in v, but the algorithm still converges empirically.

2.3   Implementation

The implementation for the layered motion estimation algorithm is based on a coarse-to-fine method and a two-layer model, a static layer and a respiratory layer. The surrogate signal for the static layer is $s_1\,(t) = 0$ to describe static components in the images. For the respiratory layer, the surrogate signal $s_2\,(t)$ is extracted from the intensities of the entire X-ray image sequence using manifold learning. The regularisation term weights for layer and motion smoothness are empirically calculated and set to $\lambda_L = 0.05$ and $\lambda_x = 0.025$. Similarly the step sizes for layer and motion minimization problems are also empirically calculated. For all the results obtained during the experiments, an Nvidia Quadro K5000 GPU and an Intel Xeon E5-1650 processor were used. The code was optimized with respect to minimum data transfer between CPU and GPU and data spread over maximum number of threads on the GPU.

3   Experiments and results

The experiments were calculated on 5 clinical data sets containing 50 frames each at a maximum resolution of 128×128 pixels. As a measure of error, target registration error (TRE) was calculated using differences between each point on a manually annotated curve on landmark regions and the computed curve [5]. To obtain a benchmark for comparison, layered motion estimation was implemented using a L-BFGS-B minimizer with tolerance level of 10^{-6}, similar to [5]. Fig. 1 shows results of the proposed algorithm on an image sequence. Fig. 1(a)-(d) show four frames from the image sequence while Fig. 1(e)-(h) show respective calculate motions on those frames. Fig. 1(i) shows the calculated static layer and Fig. 1(j) the respiratory layer while Fig. 1(k) shows TRE over time in comparison to the dotted line which represents the case when there is no motion in the sequence.

The aim of this work was to bring the overall runtime into a clinically feasible range. Fig. 2(a) shows the improvements in overall runtime between the different implementations of this algorithm, primal-dual (PD) and L-BFGS-B (QN) executed on CPU and GPU. Moreover, the decrease in time should not compromise on the quality of results. To study the performance of our primal-dual algorithm relative to L-BFGS-B, we tested the two versions on 5 distinct image sequences and calculated TRE error means and standard deviations. When compared to TRE on a stationary sequence, 4.98 ± 3.14 mm, L-BFGS-B reduced the TRE to 1.45 ± 0.50 mm and primal-dual also showed similar results, 1.46 ± 0.47 mm for empirically tuned step-sizes with respect to each image sequence.

Fig. 1. Layered motion estimation results on an image sequence.

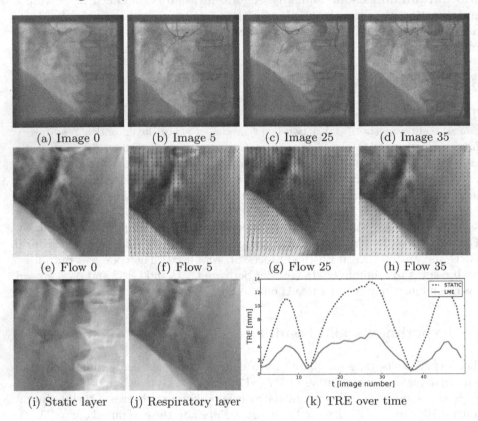

(a) Image 0   (b) Image 5   (c) Image 25   (d) Image 35

(e) Flow 0   (f) Flow 5   (g) Flow 25   (h) Flow 35

(i) Static layer   (j) Respiratory layer   (k) TRE over time

To compare the performance of the two methods in more detail, we look at the convergence of both algorithm versions for same data set. Fig. 2(b) shows the energy convergence with respect to number of iterations while Fig. 2(c) shows the convergence of both algorithm versions with respect to time.

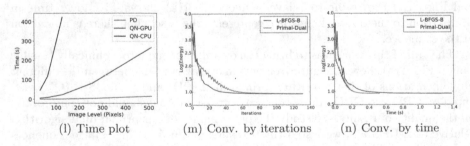

(l) Time plot   (m) Conv. by iterations   (n) Conv. by time

Fig. 2. Comparison: Primal-Dual vs. L-BFGS-B.

4   Conclusion and outlook

Use of a faster and easily parallelizeable primal-dual method instead of L-BFGS-B minimization together with implementation on the GPU helped us to reduce the overall runtime of the algorithm from 642 seconds to less than 3.3 seconds for an image sequence containing 50 frames while maintaining the quality of results. This algorithm can handle a rate of 15 frames per second which is usually quite high for an x-ray fluoroscopy machine. Moreover, it was able to reduce the overall TRE by 70% for step-size parameters tuned with respect to each image sequence, which means primal-dual method performed on par with L-BFGS-B method.

In future work, more layers can be incorporated into this model especially to cater for cardiac motion. Automatic step-size calculation for primal-dual optimizer is an important improvement that can be worked on in order to rely less on empirically calculated values. Although this algorithm has been tested on clinical data, it still needs to be incorporated into a clinical prototype and tested on live subjects.

Acknowledgement. The authors gratefully acknowledge funding of the Erlangen Graduate School in Advanced Optical Technologies (SAOT), by the German Research Foundation (DFG) in the framework of the German excellence initiative and by Siemens Healthineers. The concepts and information presented in this paper are based on research and are not commercially available.

References

1. Zhu Y, Prummer S, Wang P, et al.; Springer. Dynamic layer separation for coronary DSA and enhancement in fluoroscopic sequences. Int Conf Med Image Comput Comput Assist Interv. 2009; p. 877–84.
2. Brost A, Liao R, Strobel N, et al. Respiratory motion compensation by model-based catheter tracking during EP procedures. Med Image Anal. 2010;14(5):695–706.
3. Szeliski R, Avidan S, Anandan P; IEEE. Layer extraction from multiple images containing reflections and transparency. Proc IEEE Comput Soc Conf Comput Vis Pattern Recognit. 2000;1:246–53.
4. Preston JS, Rottman C, Cheryauka A, et al.; Springer. Multi-layer deformation estimation for fluoroscopic imaging. Inf Process Med Imaging. 2013; p. 123–34.
5. Fischer P, Pohl T, Maier A, et al.; Springer. Surrogate-driven estimation of respiratory motion and layers in x-ray fluoroscopy. Int Conf Med Image Comput Comput Assist Interv. 2015; p. 282–9.
6. Chambolle A, Pock T. A first-order primal-dual algorithm for convex problems with applications to imaging. J Math Imaging Vis. 2011;40(1):120–45.
7. Sidky EY, Jakob H, Pan X. Convex optimization problem prototyping for image reconstruction in computed tomography with the Chambolle-Pock algorithm. Phys Med Biol. 2012;57(10):3065.

Barrett's Esophagus Analysis Using Convolutional Neural Networks

Robert Mendel[1], Alanna Ebigbo[2], Andreas Probst[2], Helmut Messmann[2], Christoph Palm[1,3]

[1]Regensburg Medical Image Computing (ReMIC)
Ostbayerische Technische Hochschule Regensburg (OTH Regensburg)
[2]III. Medizinische Klinik, Klinikum Augsburg
[3]Regensburg Center of Biomedical Engineering (RCBE)
OTH Regensburg and Regensburg University
robert.mendel@st.oth-regensburg.de

Abstract. We propose an automatic approach for early detection of adenocarcinoma in the esophagus. High-definition endoscopic images (50 cancer, 50 Barrett) are partitioned into a dataset containing approximately equal amounts of patches showing cancerous and non-cancerous regions. A deep convolutional neural network is adapted to the data using a transfer learning approach. The final classification of an image is determined by at least one patch, for which the probability being a cancer patch exceeds a given threshold. The model was evaluated with leave one patient out cross-validation. With sensitivity and specificity of 0.94 and 0.88, respectively, our findings improve recently published results on the same image data base considerably. Furthermore, the visualization of the class probabilities of each individual patch indicates, that our approach might be extensible to the segmentation domain.

1 Introduction

Barrett's esophagus (BE) is a precancerous condition with a high risk of developing high-grade dysplasia and adenocarcinoma (AD). Early neoplasia can even be cured by endoscopic treatment [1]. However, despite of endoscopic surveillance and random biopsies, many AD remain undetected in the first instance. A study of leading experts achieved sensitivity and specificity of 80% and 89%, respectively, in diagnosis of high grade neoplasia and mucosal cancer. This might give evidence of the difficulty to differentiate BE and early stage AD [2]. In this paper, we introduce a method for their automatic classification based on endoscopic white light images. Having remarkable breakthroughs of deep neural networks in mind [3], we propose the learning of features with the help of a pretrained deep residual network instead of handcrafted texture features [4].

2 Material and method

To enable automatic classification, convolutional neural networks (CNNs) need a large number of training data. Here, we describe the available image data and the preprocessing steps, which result in a reasonably large and balanced data set. Then, a brief overview of deep learning and the architecture used in this work is provided, followed by a description of the evaluation method.

2.1   Image database

Our work is based on an image data set provided by the Endoscopic Vision Challenge MICCAI 2015. It contains 100 high-definition (1600×1200 pixels) endoscopic images from 39 patients. While 22 patients show cancerous lesions, 17 were diagnosed as non-cancerous Barrett. Each patient contributes between one and eight images to the database yielding 50 images of class non-cancerous (C0, Fig. 1 (a)) and class cancerous (C1, (Fig. 1 (b))), respectively. The images were annotated independently by five experts. Since these manual segmentations vary significantly, their intersection was defined as cancerous region (C1-region) within each C1-image (Fig. 1 (c)). Please note, that not only C0-images contain non-cancerous regions (C0-regions), but C1-images as well.

2.2   Preprocessing and training data generation

Each image was split into patches of size 224×224 pixels with the label depending on the extent of the C0- and C1-regions present in the patch. Since the union of all C1-regions in the image database is much smaller than the union of C0-regions, equidistant sampling of both regions for patch generation results in imbalanced number of training data. Therefore, C0-regions were sampled differently from C1-regions.

C0 and C1 sampling. The full image was sampled equidistantly with an offset of 120 pixels. The resulting patches were labeled with C0, if at least 75% of the pixels are part of the C0-region. Additionally, 30% of the labeled patches were randomly selected and rotated by 90°, 180° or 270°. The rotated versions were added to the C0-region samples, resulting in 4157 C0-patches.

Proportionally to the size of the C1-region of a full C1-image, random pixels of the C1-region were chosen. Each pixel defined the upper left corner of a C1-patch candidate. The patch was labeled as C1, if at least 75% of its pixels are

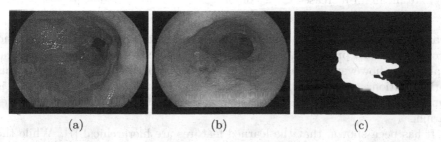

(a)   (b)   (c)

Fig. 1. Examples of C0 (a) and C1 (b) images. The cancerous region of (b) is marked by the intersection of 5 manual expert segmentations (c).

part of the C1-region. Augmentation of the data due to rotation was performed in the same fashion as for the C0-region samples resulting in 3666 C1-patches.

2.3   Deep learning with ResNets

CNNs are multilevel architectures organized into layers. The input of the first layer consists of the raw color pixel values followed by several hidden layers. For each hidden layer the output of the previous layer serves as input of the current layer. Historically three types of layers, convolution, activation and pooling, are grouped together and repeated to build the complete network.

A convolution layer computes a feature map calculating the discrete convolution between a convolutional kernel or filter and the input of the layer. The elements of a convolutional kernel are the parameters learned by the CNN. The activation modifies the input values with the help of a nonlinear function. Pooling layers are used to decrease the spatial dimension of the input by computing for example the average of a square window of the input. The extend of the reduction is dependent on the window size and the stride, which is the step size of the moving window. Further details can be found e.g. in [5].

ResNets. For our work, we choose the ResNet architecture of Kaiming He et al. [6]. Their contribution was the introduction of a shortcut connection within a Residual Unit (RU). An RU $\mathcal{F}(x^{(l)}, W)$ consists of two or three stacked convolutions and activations. In the case of two convolutions, $\mathcal{F}$ computes $W_2 * \sigma(W_1 * x^{(l)})$ where $x^{(l)}$ is the input at layer l, W_1 and W_2 contain the parameters to be learned and σ is the ReLU activation: $\sigma(x) = \max(0, x)$. The shortcut connection results from the elementwise addition of the input

$$x^{(l+1)} = x^{(l)} + \mathcal{F}(x^{(l)}, W) \tag{1}$$

In the case of an identity mapping $x^{(l+1)} = x^{(l)}$ being optimal, shortcut connections alleviate learning of this mapping. Additionally, this might have an effect like depth shrinkage of the network if the output of $\mathcal{F}(\cdot)$ vanishes. He et al. showed that a model augmented by shortcut connections could be extended to over 1000 layers. Without this effect, architectures with a depth greater than 18 layers result in an increased error compared to shallower models [6].

Transfer learning. CNNs achieve impressive results for object detection and recognition tasks, provided a large dataset is available. In the area of medical applications however, the amount of data is usually limited. As applied in this work, rotations e.g. can artificially increase the amount of data, but this is commonly not sufficient. This problem can in part be bypassed by transfer learning.

It has been shown, that the learned features are hierarchical [7]. While the first few layers are quite abstract and low level like corners, edges, etc., the further layers are more and more application specific. Transfer learning makes

Table 1. Classification performance measures for varying thresholds t with best results for $t = 0.8$.

threshold t	0.70	0.75	0.80	0.85	0.90	0.95	0.99
specificity	0.78	0.82	0.88	0.90	0.92	0.98	0.98
sensitivity	0.96	0.96	0.94	0.90	0.78	0.68	0.46
F1-score	0.86	0.88	**0.91**	0.90	0.84	0.80	0.63

use of this characteristic by initializing the CNN with parameters learned from images of a completely different domain. Subsequently, the CNN is adapted to the medical domain introducing the medical training images during a further learning process. Commonly, during this learning process the learning rate updating the parameters of the abstract layers is small, whereas the learning rate at the more domain specific higher levels is larger.

2.4 Training and evaluation process

The training data (Sec. 2.2) were generated following a class specific sampling protocol of the full images. Only clean patches were considered where more than 75% of the pixel were labeled with the respective class. For evaluation, however, the full images were sampled equidistantly in patches of size 224×224 with an offset of 50 pixel. This resulted in 768 patches for each image. The models were trained and evaluated with leave one patient out cross-validation (LOPO-CV).

Our experiments result in a probability value for each class and each patch of an image, given a model based on the training samples of all other patients. To come to a class decision (C0 or C1) for the full images on the basis of these patch results, a threshold t was applied. If only one patch probability for C1 exceeds t, the whole image is classified as C1. Variation of t yields to a Receiver-Operator-Characteric (ROC) analysis. To evaluate the results further, a probability map was created. It visualizes the spatial distribution of probabilities of class C1. For this, the images are divided into 50×50 regions and the C1-probability of that patch is assigned which is centered at the region.

3 Results

One hundred full images were sampled into 7823 patches (Sec. 2.2) according to C0- and C1-regions. Then, the models were trained with the ResNet approach and a 50-layer architecture. The ResNet was initialized with the parameters learned on the ImageNet dataset [8]. For transfer learning, a base learning rate of 0.00025 across all layers were chosen, which was halved every 1500 iterations. Further hyperparameters of the ResNet were a batch size of eight, a weight decay of 0.0008 and a momentum of 0.9. For details to these parameters we refer e.g. to [5]. With this initial configuration, the models were trained for at least 1000 iterations. The median iteration count until convergence was 2750.

A LOPO-CV approach resulted in probabilities for C0 and C1 for each patch, respectively. Transferring these patch probabilities to a full image classification decision via threshold t (Sec. 2.4) we achieved different results for sensitivity (SE), specificity (SP) and F1 for every t. TN and FP being the number of true negative and false positives, respectively, FN and TP analogously. Then, these standard measures are defined as

$$ \mathrm{SE} = \frac{\mathrm{TP}}{\mathrm{TP} + \mathrm{FN}}, \quad \mathrm{SP} = \frac{\mathrm{TN}}{\mathrm{TN} + \mathrm{FP}}, \quad F1 = 2 \cdot \frac{\mathrm{SE} \cdot \mathrm{SP}}{\mathrm{SE} + \mathrm{SP}} \tag{2} $$

The ROC like evaluation of the results for varying t yields the best result for $t = 0.8$ with SE $= 0.94$, SP $= 0.88$ and $F1 = 0.91$ (Tab. 1).

The evaluation of the probability maps show a strong consensus between the location of high C1 probabilities and the intersection of all expert annotations in most of the cases (Fig. 2, (a, b)). In only two images, the region of C1 classification did not overlap the expert ground truth. In false negative cases, the patch probabilities of C1 did not exceed t (Fig. 2, (c)).

4 Discussion

We have shown that features learned by CNNs are appropriate for early detection of adenocarcinoma in case of Barrett's esophagus. Although the data base has limited size, a model initialized with weights learned from data of a different domain was able to generalize for the medical task. Our results with $F1 = 0.91$ improved recently published results of $F1 = 0.83$ [4] on the same data.

Even though the final classification of an image depends only on the threshold exceeding probability of at least one patch, this straightforward approach still led to high values for sensitivity and specificity. Additionally, the regions with high probability for C1 overlap in almost all cases to a significant amount with the expert annotations. Therefore, our approach seems to be extensible to a segmentation approach.

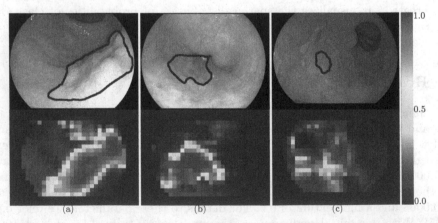

Fig. 2. Visualization of the original images, the annotations, and probability maps for three patients. Both (a) and (b) highlight correct classification and localisation, when choosing $t = 0.8$, whereas (c) is an example of a false negative classification.

In two images the threshold exceeding region did not overlap the expert annotations. We count this systematically as true positive classification. On the other hand, a segmentation on this basis would have failed completely here. In this respect, these two can be seen as fluke. Taking this into account, our F1 score would decrease to 0.89, which is still a very promising result. Nevertheless, accurate localisation is an important part of Barrett's analysis, so further work is needed to strengthen this aspect of our model.

In literature, adapting an already trained model via transfer learning is either done by treating the model as fixed feature extractor or by decreasing the learning rate for the abstract first layers in comparison to the domain specific higher layers. In our case, however, we achieved our best results with an equal learning rate for all layers. Up to now, we have no explanation for that behaviour of our net. In terms of convergence, a median iteration count of 2750 is quite low, but justified due to transfer learning approach, which is initialized with a pretrained model. Further experiments revealed that the models converge to equal results for increased iteration count to 50000.

Further research will be done to extend our approach to the segmentation domain. Additionally, minimizing the need of expert annotations by unsupervised deep learning would enable a computer assisted diagnosis system.

References

1. Probst A, Aust D, Märkl B, et al. Early esophageal cancer in europe: endoscopic treatment by endoscopic submucosal dissection. Endosc. 2015;47(02):113–21.
2. Sharma P, Bergman JJ, Goda K, et al. Development and validation of a classification system to identify high-grade dysplasia and esophageal adenocarcinoma in barrett's esophagus using narrow-band imaging. Gastroenterol. 2016;150(3):591–8.
3. He K, Zhang X, Ren S, et al. Delving deep into rectifiers: surpassing human-level performance on imagenet classification. Proc IEEE Int Conf Comput Vis. 2015; p. 1026–34.
4. van der Sommen F, Zinger S, Curvers WL, et al. Computer-aided detection of early neoplastic lesions in barrett's esophagus. Endosc. 2016;48(7):617–24.
5. LeCun Y, Kavukcuoglu K, Farabet C. Convolutional networks and applications in vision. ISCAS. 2010; p. 253–6.
6. He K, Zhang X, Ren S, et al. Deep residual learning for image recognition. ArxivOrg. 2015;7(3):171–80.
7. Farabet C, Couprie C, Najman L, et al. Learning hierarchical features for scence labeling. IEEE Trans Pattern Anal Mach Intell. 2013; p. 1–15.
8. Russakovsky O, Deng J, Su H, et al. Imagenet large scale visual recognition challenge. Int J Comput Vis. 2015;115(3):211–52.

Brain Tumor Segmentation Using Large Receptive Field Deep Convolutional Neural Networks

Fabian Isensee[1], Philipp Kickingereder[2], David Bonekamp[3], Martin Bendszus[2], Wolfgang Wick[4], Heinz-Peter Schlemmer[3], Klaus Maier-Hein[1]

[1]Junior Group Medical Image Computing, German Cancer Research Center (DKFZ)
[2]Department of Neuroradiology, University of Heidelberg
[3]Department of Radiology, German Cancer Research Center
[4]Neurology Clinic, University of Heidelberg Medical Center
f.isensee@dkfz-heidelberg.de

Abstract. Glioblastoma segmentation is an important challenge in medical image processing. State of the art methods make use of convolutional neural networks, but generally employ only few layers and small receptive fields, which limits the amount and quality of contextual information available for segmentation. In this publication we use the well known U-Net architecture to alleviate these shortcomings. We furthermore show that a sophisticated training scheme that uses dynamic sampling of training data, data augmentation and a class sensitive loss allows training such a complex architecture on relatively few data. A qualitative comparison with the state of the art shows favorable performance of our approach.

1 Introduction

Tumor detection and more importantly tumor segmentation are difficult challenges in medical image processing. Automated solutions can aid diagnosis, and assist in therapy planning and radiotherapy. Over the years efforts have been made to develop algorithms that are capable of automatically segmenting glioblastomas in MRI images, most of which are presented in the Brain Tumor Segmentation Challenge (BraTS) [1]. While BraTS submissions in 2012 and 2013 were almost exclusively based on conventional machine learning approaches, deep learning became popular in the recent years and is now the state of the art.

1.1 Contributions

In this paper we present our most recent efforts for brain tumor segmentation. Our network is based U-Net [2]. It is trained using a sophisticated scheme that reduces overfitting and allows the training of such a deep network for glioblastoma segmentation. Our key contributions are:

86

1. Application of the U-Net architecture for glioblastoma segmentation, allowing multi-level integration of context information over a large receptive field.
2. Development of a sophisticated training scheme that combines excessive data augmentation and dynamic sampling of training data.

1.2   Related work

Many deep learning approaches for brain tumor segmentation exist, and we can only give a short overview in the scope of this article. For a more complete list, see [3].

We denote a training set of N images by $\chi = \{(X_n, Y_n), n = 1, ...N\}$ with X_n being the nth image in the set with corresponding label map Y_n. x_n^i denotes the ith voxel in X_n with $i \in \mathbb{R}^3$ and its corresponding label is given by y_n^i.

Early deep learning approaches used pixel-wise classification. A classification network is trained to predict the class label y_n^i of a pixel x_n^i using the information available in a patch $p_{x_n^i}$ surrounding it. Such an approach is for instance applied by Zikic et al. [4] who use three convolutional layers followed by one dense layer for the classification. Pereira et al. [5] use a deeper model by stacking layers with smaller (3×3) convolutional filters. Later approaches make use of fully convolutional neural networks. Havaei et al. [6] apply a cascaded model where the first network (2D convolutions) outputs a dense prediction map which is then fed into a second network that classifies y_n^i by also considering the class of neighboring pixels. Kamnitsas et al. [7] use 3D convolutions in their network. The network has 11 convolutional layers and is 7 layers deep. Kamnitsas et al. as well as Havaei et al. incorporate features of different scales by using two feature extraction pathways. Milletari et al. [8] extend the 3D U-Net [9] with residual connections and solve the class imbalance problem using a robust dice loss layer.

2   Materials and methods

Although the above mentioned methods all achieve good results in the BraTS challenge data, we believe that these architectures lack two key features that could enable us to get even better prediction. For once, the receptive fields of the networks are rather small, thereby limiting the amount of contextual information that can be incorporated into the features. Second, integration of features derived from several levels of abstraction is lackluster, if present at all, and hindered by the rather shallow nature of the networks. We use the U-Net architecture that alleviates the above mentioned issues. It possesses a large receptive field (180×180) as well as multi-level integration of abstract features (combines *what* with *where*).

2.1   Data

We use an in-house dataset (used in [10]) for our experiments. In comparison to BraTS, our dataset possesses a higher resolution in the axial direction, which is especially useful for our 2D convolutional neural network. The majority of the BraTS data ($\geq$ 2014) was annotated automatically by a consensus vote of the top ranking methods submitted in earlier challenges. In contrast, our dataset has been annotated semi-automatically using ITK-SNAP by an expert.

Our dataset comprises 98 MRI scans of different patients each diagnosed with glioblastoma. The following modalities a: T1, contrast-enhanced T1 (T1c), Flair, ADC and CBV. Brain extraction was performed using FSL. Bias field correction on T1, T1c and Flair was performed, followed by white-stripe normalization [11] on T1, T1c and Flair. The tumor was segmented into edema, necrosis and contrast enhancing tumor. All datasets are resampled to a spacing of $0.5 \times 0.5 \times 1.0[mm]$. We use 80 patients for training, 9 for validation and 9 for testing.

2.2 Architecture

We use the U-Net architecture [2] which is significantly deeper (18 convolutional layers) and has a much larger receptive field (180×180) than previously employed architectures. More importantly it uses skip connections which allows it to fast forward features from shallow layers very deep into the network. They allow the network to combine semantic information (from the encoding layers at the bottom) with location information encoded in shallower layers. U-Net is fully convolutional and makes use of unpadded convolutions, which results in a segmentation that is smaller than the network input.

The U-Net model we use in this publication has some minor modifications. We replace the rectified linear unit nonlinearities with exponential linear units to combat the vanishing gradient problem and speed up the training. Furthermore, we replace the deconvolution layers with simple up-scaling layers which we found to perform equally well while being less computationally intensive. The number

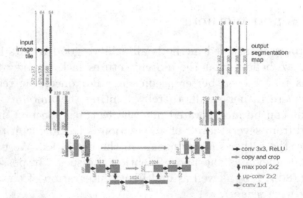

Fig. 1. U-Net architecture as proposed by Ronneberger et al. [2]. Skip connections at various stages of the network allow the combination of precise localization information from the contracting pathway with more coarse semantic information from the expanding pathway.

of feature channels is reduced to 16 in the first convolutional layer and doubled whenever the network increases in depth.

2.3   Training procedure

We exploit the fully convolutional nature of U-Net to train with whole axial slices instead of small patches. This allows maximum re-use of computations and speeds up the training substantially. The kth slice of training image X_n is denoted $S_{X_n}^k$. To allow for spatial smoothing over the third dimension, the input channel of the network is overloaded with 2 slices above and below the slice of interest for each modality, resulting in a total of 25 input channels. We make extensive use of data augmentation. The images are rotated $\pm 180°$ around the axial axis, mirrored randomly in x- and y-direction and we apply elastic deformations. The latter are created by randomly sampling a 2D displacement vector field which is subsequently smoothed using a Gaussian filter.

The training is done using a pixel-wise categorical cross-entropy loss. The loss for a training slice $\mathcal{L}(S_{X_n}^k)$ is computed as the average over all pixels in that slice. We use adam for stochastic optimization with learning rate 0.001, $\beta_1 = 0.9$, $\beta_2 = 0.999$ and $\epsilon = 10^{-8}$

$$L_{\text{corr}}(x_n^i) = L(x_n^i)\sqrt{\frac{1}{f(y_n^i)}} \tag{1}$$

$$d^{\text{new}}(S_{X_n}^k) = \frac{d^{\text{old}}(S_{X_n}^k) + 2 * \mathcal{L}(S_{X_n}^k)}{3} \tag{2}$$

The loss of each pixel is weighted by the inverse of the square root of the corresponding class frequency $f(y_n^i)$ (Eq. 1). Additionally, we dynamically sample training slices based on their difficulty $d(S_{X_n}^k)$, an idea that originates in reinforcement learning. Thereby, slices with more tumor pixels are sampled more often than non-tumor slices since they are more difficult to segment. The difficulty $d(S_{X_n}^k)$ of all slices is initialized to an arbitrary number (here 100) and subsequently modified using the training loss and an exponential moving average. The difficulty update is shown in Eq. 2. Our network is trained for 70 epochs (batch size 20, 600 batches per epoch). We then fine tune 2 epochs using neither dynamic sampling nor class sensitive loss.

3   Results

We evaluate our predictions on the test set qualitatively as well as quantitatively using the standard metrics that are also commonly applied in the BraTS challenge: precision, recall and the DICE coefficient.

Qualitative results are shown in Fig. 2. Similarly to BraTS, we group the segmentations into the categories whole tumor (edema + necrosis + contrast enh. tumor), tumor core (necrosis + contrast enh. tumor) and enh. tumor (contrast enh. tumor). Visual inspection confirmed high overall segmentation

Table 1. Comparison of our approach with state of the art algorithms from the BraTS challenge.

	DICE			Precision			Recall		
	Whole	Core	Enh.	Whole	Core	Enh.	Whole	Core	Enh
Pererira et al. [5]	87	73	68	89	74	72	86	77	70
Havaei et al. [6]	88	79	73	89	79	68	87	79	80
Kamnitsas et al. [7]	**90.1**	75.4	72.8	**91.9**	85.7	75.5	89.1	71.7	74.4
ours	85.0	**90.0**	**84.5**	83.1	**89.2**	**83.6**	90.2	**91.9**	**87.3**

quality, exemplarily shown in Fig. 2. Furthermore, although each pixel is classified independently, the generated segmentation map is surprisingly smooth. This hints that using a fully connected CRF on top would not improve the performance by a large margin. Due to the overloading of the input channels (2.3) the predictions are also consistent between slices.

Quantitative evaluation criteria were computed using the MedPy package and are shown in Tab. 1. Naturally, a direct comparison with results from the BraTS challenge is not possible because we here use a different dataset. We nonetheless show results of BraTS as a general guideline of what numbers can be achieved with other state of the art algorithms. Overall, our results are promising, especially considering that our architecture employs 2D convolutions as opposed to the best performing competing method [7].

4   Discussion

In this paper we demonstrated that using a large receptive field combined with multi-level semantic cue integration provided via skip connections can be ben-

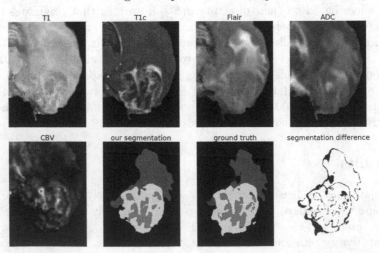

Fig. 2. Qualitative results of our approach. Edema is shown in blue, contrast enhancing tumor in green and necrosis in red.

eficial for glioma segmentation. We tackled the class imbalance implicitly by presenting training examples with a high loss more frequently to the network. Our segmentations, although pixels are classified independently, are smooth, which we explain by the combination of location and semantic information via skip layers in the U-Net architecture. Our training scheme allowed us to train the large U-Net on a relatively small dataset without considerable overfitting. Data augmentation and loss sampling were the key methods to make this possible. Segmentation of a 3D volume ($350 \times 265 \times 142$ voxels) took less than 10s on a Pascal Titan X GPU. Although some spatial information is integrated into the architecture via overloading the input channels, our approach doe not tap the potential of 3D convolutions. Considering that human annotators regularly move between slices during annotation, we believe that there is potential in switching to 3D convolutions. It should be noted that there may be a bias in our training data due to their semi-automatically generated segmentations.

In future work, we plan to validate our approach on the BraTS challenge data. Furthermore, we will switch to 3D convolutions and investigate the interplay between a robust loss layer [8] and our loss sampling strategy.

References

1. Menze BH, Jakab A, Bauer S, et al. The multimodal brain tumor image segmentation benchmark (BRATS). IEEE TMI. 2015;34(10):1993–2024.
2. Ronneberger O, Fischer P, Brox T. U-Net: Convolutional networks for biomedical image segmentation. Proc MICCAI. 2015; p. 234–41.
3. Havaei M, Guizard N, Larochelle H, et al. Deep learning trends for focal brain pathology segmentation in MRI. ArXiv. 2016; p. 1607.05258.
4. Zikic D, Ioannou Y, Brown M, et al. Segmentation of brain tumor tissues with convolutional neural networks. MICCAI BraTS Challenge. 2014; p. 36–9.
5. Pereira S, Pinto A, Alves V, et al. Brain tumor segmentation using convolutional neural networks in MRI images. IEEE TMI. 2016;35(5):1240–51.
6. Havaei M, Davy A, Warde-Farley D, et al. Brain tumor segmentation with deep neural networks. Med Image Anal. 2017;35:18–31.
7. Kamnitsas K, Ledig C, Newcombe VFJ, et al. Efficient multi-scale 3D CNN with fully connected CRF for accurate nrain lesion segmentation. ArXiv. 2016; p. 1603.05959.
8. Milletari F, Navab N, Ahmadi SA. V-Net: Fully convolutional neural networks for volumetric medical image segmentation. ArXiv. 2016; p. 1606.04797.
9. Cicek O, Abdulkadir A, Lienkamp SS, et al. 3D U-Net: Learning dense volumetric segmentation from sparse annotation. Proc MICCAI. 2016;9901:1–9.
10. Kickingereder P, Bonekamp D, Nowosielski M, et al. Radiogenomics of glioblastoma: machine learning-based classification of molecular characteristics by using multiparametric and multiregional MR imaging features. Radiology. 2016; p. 101382.
11. Shinohara RT, Sweeney EM, Goldsmith J, et al. Statistical normalization techniques for magnetic resonance imaging. Neuroimage Clin. 2014;6:9–19.

A Deep Learning Architecture for Limited-Angle Computed Tomography Reconstruction

Kerstin Hammernik[1], Tobias Würfl[2], Thomas Pock[1,3], Andreas Maier[2]

[1]Institute of Computer Graphics and Vision, Graz University of Technology
[2]Pattern Recognition Lab, Friedrich-Alexander-University
[3]Digital Safety and Security Department, AIT Austrian Institute of Technology
hammernik@icg.tugraz.at

Abstract. Limited-angle computed tomography suffers from missing data in the projection domain, which results in intensity inhomogeneities and streaking artifacts in the image domain. We address both challenges by a two-step deep learning architecture: First, we learn compensation weights that account for the missing data in the projection domain and correct for intensity changes. Second, we formulate an image restoration problem as a variational network to eliminate coherent streaking artifacts. We perform our experiments on realistic data and we achieve superior results for destreaking compared to state-of-the-art non-linear filtering methods in literature. We show that our approach eliminates the need for manual tuning and enables joint optimization of both correction schemes.

1 Introduction

Computed Tomography (CT) is a clinical routine imaging modality that is used to diagnose certain diseases and trauma. In some applications, CT data cannot be acquired over the full angular range which is known as limited-angle CT. Examples for such setups are robot assisted scanners in medicine or scanning of very large objects in industrial CT. As limited-angle CT does not acquire data over the full angular range, the projection data is incomplete which results in intensity inhomogeneities as well as streaking artifacts in the image domain. Further sources for streaking artifacts are the non-linear attenuation of polychromatic X-rays or inelastic scattering of photons. All these artifacts are corrected with specialized heuristic compensation procedures that tune each step independently.

Many specialized iterative algorithms exist which clearly improve the image quality [1, 2]. A disadvantage of iterative techniques is their high runtime requirement. In contrast, analytical algorithms are less demanding, but typically suffer from intensity inhomogeneities and streaking artifacts in the image domain due to missing projections. To correct for intensity inhomogeneities, Riess et al. [3] use a heuristic scheme to estimate compensation weights. Würfl et al. [4] reformulate filtered back-projection as a neural network and learn compensation weights for limited-angle CT reconstruction. However, their approach cannot account for the remaining streaking artifacts due to the missing non-linear filtering step.

To correct for remaining streaking artifacts, Riess et al. [3] apply a bilateral filter [5] after the compensation of missing projection data. Although there exists a number of other non-linear filtering methods such as BM3D [6] and Total (Generalized) Variation (T(G)V) [7, 8], they can mainly correct for unstructured Gaussian noise. These models cannot describe the complex image content as they make assumptions on the image statistics such as piece-wise constancy in the case of TV. This motivates the use of deep learning approaches that learn the statistics of images [9], and thus can account for coherent noise artifacts. Recently, Hammernik et al. [10] proposed a deep learning approach to remove coherent backfolding artifacts in accelerated magnetic resonance image reconstruction.

In this paper, we propose a deep learning architecture for limited-angle CT reconstruction. In a first step, we estimate compensation weights in the projection domain [4]. The focus of our work is the second step: We propose to learn a non-linear filtering method inspired by variational image restoration problems [9] to remove streaking artifacts in the image domain.

2   Materials and methods

The basic network architecture for artifact compensation in limited-angle CT is illustrated in Fig. 1. To account for missing projection data due to the limited-angle CT acquisition, a neural network architecture is used to estimate the compensation weights in the first step. In a second step, we eliminate streaking artifacts using a variational network architecture.

2.1   Step 1: A neural network to learn compensation weights

To correct for intensity inhomogeneities in limited-angle CT, we use the network architecture of Würfl et al. [4]. The input of the neural network is a sinogram

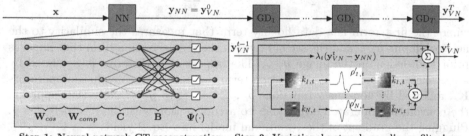

Step 1: Neural network CT reconstruction   Step 2: Variational network non-linear filtering

Fig. 1. Deep learning architecture for limited-angle CT reconstruction. The first neural network (blue) models filtered backprojection and corrects the intensity inhomogeneities in the image domain by learning compensation weights $\mathbf{W}_{comp}$ in the projection domain. The second variational network (red) formulates non-linear filtering as T unrolled gradient descent steps (GD). In each step t, the filters $k_{i,t}$, derivative of potential functions $\rho'_{i,t}$ and the regularization parameter λ_t are learned to remove the remaining streaking artifacts.

with missing angular data, denoted by x. The network reformulates the fan-beam reconstruction as

$$y_{NN} = \Psi\left(\mathbf{BCW}_{\text{comp}}\mathbf{W}_{\cos}x\right) \tag{1}$$

where $\mathbf{B}$ denotes the backprojection operator, $\mathbf{C}$ implements filtering with a one-dimensional convolution kernel and the weighting operators $\mathbf{W}_{\cos}$, $\mathbf{W}_{\text{comp}}$ implement elementwise multiplications with cosine weights and compensation weights, respectively. The non-negativity constraint is realized via the operator Ψ. While the operators $\mathbf{B}, \mathbf{C}$ and $\mathbf{W}_{\cos}$ are fixed, the compensation weights in $\mathbf{W}_{\text{comp}}$ are learned. After training, the network can be applied to a new sinogram and yields the intensity corrected reconstruction y_{NN}. This output defines the input for the following variational network that focuses on destreaking.

2.2   Step 2: A variational network to remove streaking artifacts

To remove streaking artifacts in the neural network reconstruction y_{NN}, we learn a non-linear filtering method. We seek an optimal image with eliminated streaking artifacts y_{VN}. Based on the theory of [9], we formulate a network for non-linear filtering as a fixed number of T unrolled gradient descent steps

$$y_{VN}^t = y_{VN}^{t-1} - g^t(y_{VN}^{t-1}) \tag{2}$$

The gradient of these steps is set to the gradient of a variational model

$$g^t(y_{VN}^{t-1}) = \nabla_y E(y)\big|_{y=y_{VN}^{t-1}} \tag{3}$$

The variational image restoration problem is given as

$$E(y) = \frac{\lambda}{2}\|y_{VN} - y_{NN}\|_2^2 + \sum_{i=1}^{N_k} \rho_i(\mathbf{K}_i y_{VN}) \tag{4}$$

where the first term is a data fidelity term that measures the similarity to the network input y_{NN} and the second term is the regularization term that imposes prior knowledge on the image y_{VN}. The impact of both terms is regulated by a parameter λ. For the regularization term, we apply N_k convolution operators $\mathbf{K}_i$, followed by non-linear functions $\rho_i : \mathbb{R}^N \mapsto \mathbb{R}$ to y_{VN}. Note that applying the convolution operator $\mathbf{K}_i y$ equals to a convolution with filter kernels $k_i * y$. Plugging the gradient of the variational model into Eq. 2 yields

$$y_{VN}^t = y_{VN}^{t-1} - \sum_{i=1}^{N_k} \mathbf{K}_{i,t}^T \rho_{i,t}'(\mathbf{K}_{i,t} y_{VN}^{t-1}) - \lambda_t(y_{VN}^{t-1} - y_{NN}) \tag{5}$$

This allows the parameters to adapt in every gradient descent step. In the gradient calculation, we additionally introduce the derivative of potential functions $\rho_{i,t}' : \mathbb{R}^N \mapsto \mathbb{R}^N$ and transpose convolution operators $\mathbf{K}_{i,t}^T$. The vector $\rho_{i,t}'$ is understood in a point-wise manner. After a training procedure, we obtain the convolution kernels $k_{i,t}$, non-linear derivatives of potential functions $\rho'_{i,t}$ and the regularization parameter λ_t for each of the T gradient steps by minimizing the the mean-squared error (MSE)

$$L_{MSE} = \frac{1}{2S} \sum_{s=1}^{S} \| \boldsymbol{y}_{VN,s}^{T} - \boldsymbol{z}_s \|_2^2 \tag{6}$$

where S is the number of training samples and $\boldsymbol{z}$ defines the full scan reference.

2.3   Experimental setup

To obtain training data, we simulated 450 fan-beam projections of size 512×512 from volumetric datasets of ten different patients. For evaluation, we performed a 5-fold cross validation and split the dataset into 80% training data and 20% validation data. As we focused on the evaluation of destreaking, we refer the interested reader to [4] for more details on the estimation of compensation weights. For our variational network architecture, we report results for different kernel sizes $k \in \{5, 7, 9, 11, 13\}$ and fixed the number of filter kernels $N_k = 24$ and gradient steps $T = 5$ empirically. For training, we used the L-BFGS-B optimizer and run 1200 iterations in total, i.e. 5×100 iterations pre-training of each gradient step and 700 iterations joint training of all gradient steps [9].

3   Results

We compared our variational network results to bilateral filtering, BM3D, TV and TGV quantitatively and to BM3D qualitatively. Tab. 1 shows the mean values and standard deviations for Peak Signal-to-Noise Ratio (PSNR) and Structured Similarity Index (SSIM). In order to perform a fair comparison, the parameters for all methods were estimated by grid search such that the PSNR of the validation data was maximized. Fig. 2 shows the qualitative comparison of different methods and illustrates that the variational network result has less streaking artifacts and appears more natural compared to BM3D, which is like T(G)V and bilateral filtering not well suited for structured noise. Our deep learning architecture outperforms all methods qualitatively and quantitatively. The best results were achieved for a filter kernel size of 13.

4   Discussion

We propose a two-step deep learning architecture to correct for imperfections in limited-angle CT reconstruction due to missing projection data. In a first step, we correct intensity inhomogeneities in the image domain by learning compensation weights in the projection domain. In a second step, we train a variational network to learn regularization to remove structured streaking artifacts. Our results reduce streaking artifacts significantly and outperform current state-of-the-art non-linear filtering approaches that can mainly deal with unstructured noise.

Table 1. Quantitative comparison of non-linear filtering methods along with the used parameter settings. The comparison is performed in terms of PSNR and SSIM (mean ± standard deviation) in the field-of-view. The intensity corrected neural network reconstruction defines the input to all methods. Our variational network results outperform all reference methods significantly.

Method	PSNR	SSIM
Neural Network	34.66 ± 2.07	0.908 ± 0.015
Bilateral Filtering ($\sigma_s = 0.5, \sigma_c = 0.1$)	29.93 ± 3.61	0.907 ± 0.021
BM3D ($\sigma = 1.5$)	34.75 ± 2.09	0.911 ± 0.015
TV ($\lambda = 300$)	34.82 ± 2.10	0.914 ± 0.014
TGV ($\lambda = 2, \alpha_0 = 0.01, \alpha_1 = 0.02$)	34.80 ± 2.09	0.914 ± 0.014
Variational Network ($k = 5$)	36.16 ± 2.13	0.930 ± 0.010
Variational Network ($k = 7$)	36.86 ± 2.01	0.938 ± 0.010
Variational Network ($k = 9$)	38.14 ± 2.27	0.947 ± 0.009
Variational Network ($k = 11$)	37.87 ± 1.98	0.949 ± 0.009
Variational Network ($k = 13$)	*38.23 ± 2.06*	*0.952 ± 0.010*

The strength of our proposed model is that it eliminates the need for manual

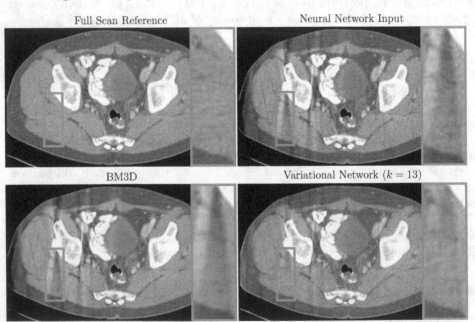

Full Scan Reference   Neural Network Input

BM3D   Variational Network ($k = 13$)

Fig. 2. Qualitative comparison of different non-linear filtering methods to the full scan reference. The neural network result is the intensity corrected output of a first correction step and defines the input to all methods. The variational network reconstruction with kernel size $k = 13$ shows significantly reduced streaking artifacts compared to BM3D.

tuning and replaces heuristic compensation steps by data-driven optimization. In the future, we want to explore further extensions to our network architecture that account for more physical effects and train both networks jointly.

Acknowledgement. We acknowledge grant support from the Austrian Science Fund (FWF) under the START project BIVISION, No. Y729. The authors would like to thank Dr. Cynthia McCollough, the Mayo Clinic, the American Association of Physicists in Medicine funded by grants EB017095 and EB017185 from the National Institute of Biomedical Imaging and Bioengineering for providing the used data.

References

1. Huang Y, Taubmann O, Huang X, et al. A new weighted anisotropic total variation algorithm for limited angle tomography. Proc IEEE ISBI. 2016; p. 585–8.
2. Huang Y, Taubmann O, Huang X, et al. A new scale space total variation algorithm for limited angle tomography. Proc Int Meeting Image Form X-Ray Comput Tomogr. 2016; p. 149–52.
3. Riess C, Berger M, Wu H, et al. TV or not TV? That is the question. Int Meeting Fully Three-Dimensional Image Reconstr Radiol Nucl Med. 2013; p. 341–4.
4. Würfl T, Ghesu FC, Christlein V, et al. Deep learning computed tomography. Med Image Compute Comput Assist Interv. 2016; p. 432–40.
5. Tomasi C, Manduchi R. Bilateral filtering for gray and color images. Int Conf Comput Vis. 1998; p. 839–46.
6. Dabov K, Foi A, Katkovnik V, et al. Image denoising by sparse 3-D transform-domain collaborative filtering. IEEE Trans Image Process. 2007; p. 2080–95.
7. Rudin LI, Osher S, Fatemi E. Nonlinear total variation based noise removal algorithms. Physica D. 1992;60(1-4):259–68.
8. Bredies K, Kunisch K, Pock T. Total generalized variation. SIAM J Imaging Sci. 2010;3(3):492–526.
9. Chen Y, Yu W, Pock T. On learning optimized reaction diffusion processes for effective image restoration. Proc IEEE CVPR. 2015;07:5261–9.
10. Hammernik K, Knoll F, Sodickson DK, et al. Learning a variational model for compressed sensing MRI reconstruction. Proc Int Magn Reson Med. 2016;24:1088.

Real-Time Virus Size Classification Using Surface Plasmon PAMONO Resonance and Convolutional Neural Networks

Jan Eric Lenssen[1], Victoria Shpacovitch[2], Frank Weichert[1]

[1]Department of Computer Science VII, TU Dortmund University, Germany
[2]ISAS, Leibniz Institut für Analytische Wissenschaften, Dortmund, Germany
janeric.lenssen@tu-dortmund.de

Abstract. Mobile, fast virus detection and classification is of increasing importance in times of epidemic diseases being spread by global traveling and transport. A possible solution is the PAMONO sensor, an optical biological sensor that is able to detect (nanometer-sized) viruses and virus-like particles, utilizing surface plasmon resonance. Captured sensor data is given as image sequences, which can be analyzed by methods from the field of image processing, which is the focus this work. We classify single particles based on their size, using state of the art machine learning techniques, namely convolutional neural networks. This classification allows the measurement of individual particle sizes and the compilation of particle size distributions for a given suspension, which contributes to the goal of classifying different virus types. The classification procedure and estimation of distributions is evaluated using real PAMONO sensor image sequences and particles that simulate viruses. The results show that informative features of the SPR signals can be automatically learned, extracted and used for classification, successfully.

1 Introduction

The emergence and ubiquitary availability of biosensors become important in times of an increasing appearance of pandemic and epidemic diseases. Particularly, efficient and reliable methods for virus detection are needed [1]. This includes diagnosis of a virus infection and the determination of the virus type. In this study, we outline and evaluate a method for particle size classification as part of our image processing pipeline for medical biosensing that fulfills the given requirements. The underlying data is captured by the Plasmon-Assisted Microscopy of Nano-Objects (PAMONO) sensor, which allows the detection of single viruses and virus-like particles, as it was demonstrated by previous studies [2]. The sensor provides plasmon wave signals for each detected particle which can be analyzed further. We use these signals together with interpolated synthetic particle signals to train a convolutional neural network [3])for particle size classification. Based on these classification, we infer particle size distributions for the analyzed suspension.

Outside of our research, image processing methodology for signals measured by intensity-based surface plasmon resonance has only been tackled a few times in literature. One example is time-gradient based detection of plasmon waves as described by Rampazzi et al. [4]. The focus of this approaches lies mainly on the detection part, while we address the classification task. Our task is connected to the general problem of analyzing small structures in images with low signal-to-noise ratio. Surveys about different methods exist for detection [5] and for classification [6]. However, most approaches rely on engineered features while our approach uses trained feature hierarchies by applying convolutional neural networks.

2 Materials and methods

2.1 PAMONO sensor and materials

The PAMONO sensor is an optical biosensor that facilitates the detection of single nano-particles in a given liquid sample [2, 7]. A Kretschmann's scheme for plasmon excitation is utilized to observe the binding of virus-like particles with antibodies applied to a gold surface. A CCD camera observes the surface over time, resulting in captured image sequences. At places of plasmon excitation, intensity steps in consecutive frames can be observed. For our methods, polystyrene nano-particles (Molecular Probes from Life Technologies) of different mean sizes (80 nm, 100 nm, 200 nm, 300 nm and their combinations) were pumped through the sensor cell. Image recording speed was 41-45 images per second, but was kept constant during each experiment. In the following Sections, we outline the image processing methodology of our classification approach. For more information about the PAMONO sensor we refer to the literature [2].

2.2 Processing pipeline summary

An overview about the whole image processing pipeline for PAMONO sensor data analysis is shown in Fig. 1. Applying the signal model developed in [8], the raw images are preprocessed by removing the constant background signal. Thus, only the non-constant parts, particle signals, artifacts and noise, remains in the

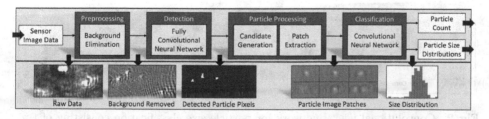

Fig. 1. Overview of the real-time GPU signal processing pipeline. The top row outlines consecutive processing steps. Examples for processed data after these steps are shown below.

images [8]. After preprocessing, we separate particle signals from artifacts, resulting in a binary pixel mask, using a fully convolutional neural network [9]. After the detection step, we extract particle candidates that are visible over several frames [10]. Around these candidates, image patches are extracted and classified by a convolutional neural network, which is shown in Fig. 2 and further detailed in Sec. 2.3. Last, detection and classification results are used to output particle counts and particle size distributions. The whole pipeline is implemented for processing on GPUs and real-time capable, processing approximately 35 sensor images with size of 1100×150 pixels per second.

2.3   Neural network architecture

The estimation of particle size with an image containing a plasmon wave as input is a regression problem. Therefore, we first trained a regression network with the architecture shown in Fig. 2, except for using only one output neuron and sigmoid activation after the last layer. However, our experiments showed that these convolutional regression networks do not reach the accuracy of a convolutional classification network. Thus, we reformulated the regression problem as an ordered classification problem using classes for particle size intervals and a soft ground truth, as described below.

The classification network is shown in Fig. 2. It receives small 32×32 image patches as input and outputs a softmax distribution $\hat{P}(c)$ over 27 classes $c \in \{0, ..., 26\}$ with 10 nm sized bins of particle sizes from 60 to 320 nm as labels. The network consists of two convolutional layers, each followed by a ReLU activation and a MaxPool layer. Then, two fully connected layers perform the classification based on the computed feature maps, followed by a softmax layer. We apply dropout to the first fully connected layer as well as L2-regularization on all weights in order to avoid over-fitting [3]. For training, we synthesize 32×32 image patches for each class $c \in \{2, ..., 24\}$, based on the signal model proposed in [8], using a small set of real seed particle images with four different particle sizes. The synthesis procedure consists of interpolation between particle signals and artificially increases the noise of training images. Instead of training against a binary one-hot ground truth, we soften the ground truth distribution. For a

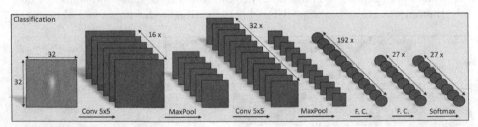

Fig. 2. Convolutional neural network for particle size classification consisting of two convolutional, two MaxPool and two fully connected layers. As a last step, the network output are transformed into a probability distribution by a softmax layer.

labeled image patch with class $c \in \{2, ..., 24\}$ we set

$$P(k) = \begin{cases} 0.44 & \text{if } k = c \\ 0.2 & \text{if } |k - c| = 1 \\ 0.08 & \text{if } |k - c| = 2 \\ 0 & \text{else} \end{cases} \tag{1}$$

for $k \in \{0, ..., 26\}$. The classes $c = 0, 1, 25, 26$ only exist to avoid boundary issues. We motivate the softening by the fact that we have an ordered classification problem and would rather prefer the network to falsely predict a class that is near the correct one, than to predict one which is far away. With this ground truth, false predictions that are far away are punished stronger, resulting in model outputs that are near to normally distributed with the predicted class as mean. We then use the cross entropy between P and $\hat{P}$ as loss function for training. The network is trained using the backpropagation algorithm and stochastic gradient descent [3]. After neural network inference, we evaluated the expected value (EV) as well as the argmax of the distribution to get the particle size of one particle.

3   Results

For evaluation of particle size classification we used three different, disjoint data sets, each containing examples for different particle sizes. The first two data sets are synthetic training and test data sets, generated according to the signal model proposed in [8]. These data sets contain synthetic examples for all 23 classes. For the synthetic test data we used seed images that are disjoint from the training set seeds. The third data set contains real particles as measured by the sensor. These examples are labeled with the mean particle size of the data set, based on a measurement of the employed liquid (Sec. 2.1), resulting in a noisy ground truth. For each class $c \in \{2, ...24\}$, we have 5.000 example image patches in the synthetic training set and 2.500 patches in the synthetic test. The real test set contains 2.500 examples for each class $c \in \{2, 4, 14, 24\}$, which are only labeled approximately, as described above. In addition to exact class accuracy of the network, we calculate a soft accuracy value a^r. Let $c^{\text{pred}}(e)$ be the predicted class and $c^{\text{corr}}(e)$ the correct class of example patch $e \in \mathcal{E}$. Then we define

$$a^r := \frac{|\{e \in \mathcal{E} | |c^{\text{pred}}(e) - c^{\text{corr}}(e)| \leq r\}|}{|\mathcal{E}|} \tag{2}$$

the percentage of predictions that lie in one of the $2 \cdot r + 1$ classes around the correct class. By evaluating the soft accuracy for different r, we can verify if the network predictions only scatter locally (which is good) or if false predictions are far away from the correct value. We also provide accuracy values for both particle size estimation methods. The results are summarized in Tab. 1.

The final goal of particle classification is the calculation of size distribution for a whole image sequence. Thus, for further evaluation, we applied our pipeline

102   Lenssen, Shpacovitch & Weichert

Table 1. Classification accuracy a^0 and soft accuracy a^r for different $r > 0$ from applying the classifying convolutional neural network with 27 classes on different datasets. Two different particle size estimators where tested.

Dataset	Estimator	a^0	a^1	a^2
Synthetic	EV	0.359	0.833	0.969
Training	argmax	0.377	0.828	0.955
Synthetic	EV	0.356	0.816	0.960
Test	argmax	0.365	0.812	0.949
Real	EV	0.289	0.622	0.749
Test	argmax	0.350	0.631	0.731

on whole real PAMONO image sequences, counting particle occurrences for each particle size. Sensor raw data is fed into the pipeline outlined in Fig. 1. The output is a histogram calculated from the numbers of found particles per size, with a bin size of 10. We evaluated four different data sets, three of them having approximately one particle size (80 nm, 200 nm, 300 nm) and one containing a mixture of these three. For comparison of the results shown in Fig. 3, we use particle concentration measurements we performed on the suspensions, before they were analyzed by the PAMONO sensor. These measurements were performed with an LM10 device (Malvern, UK).

4   Discussion

The outcome of our experiments shows the success of the feature training. Despite differences in the distributions, it is evident that information about particle size has been extracted from the image patches and is used for classification. In our distributions, we observe a small overestimation error of 10-20 nm, as a result of our training synthesis procedure. In contrast, our size distributions are

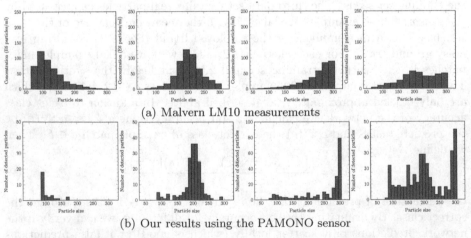

(a) Malvern LM10 measurements

(b) Our results using the PAMONO sensor

Fig. 3. Particle size distributions for the (a) reference data measured by Malvern LM10 and (b) corresponding distributions estimated from the neural networks output. The presented evaluation was performed for four different data sets with target particle sizes of 80 nm, 200 nm, 300 nm and one with all three particles types.

more precise than the reference distributions, indicated by higher concentration of particles in a small amount of bins. The reason is that we classify individual bound particles while the LM10 device observes particle tracks of whole samples. The calculated soft accuracy for classification results increases fast for the first steps of r, showing that prediction values are distributed around the correct label. We do not observe any sudden increases of accuracy while increasing r further, which would indicate a systematic error in the learned model, leading to false predictions that are far away from the correct class. In summary, we confirmed that intensity-based features of surface plasmon resonance waves can be automatically extracted and used for real-time size classification of individual, bound particles. This contributes to the future goal of distinguishing between different types of viruses using the PAMONO sensor.

Acknowledgement. The work on this paper has been supported by Deutsche Forschungsgemeinschaft (DFG) within the Collaborative Research Center SFB 876 "Providing Information by Resource-Constrained Analysis", project B2.

References

1. Baril L. Need for biosensors in infectious disease epidemiology. In: Handbook of Biosensors and Biochips. John Wiley & Sons, Ltd; 2008. p. 1077–84.
2. Shpacovitch V, Temchura V, Matrosovich M, et al. Application of surface plasmon resonance imaging technique for the detection of single spherical biological submicrometer particles. Anal Biochem. 2015;486:62–9.
3. Krizhevsky A, Sutskever I, Hinton GE. ImageNet classification with deep convolutional neural networks. In: Advances in Neural Information Processing Systems 25; 2012. p. 1097–105.
4. Rampazzi S, Danese G, Leporati F, et al. A localized surface plasmon resonance-based portable instrument for quick on-site biomolecular detection. IEEE Trans Instrum Meas. 2016;65:317–27.
5. Smal I, Loog M, Niessen WJ, et al. Quantitative comparison of spot detection methods in fluorescence microscopy. IEEE Trans Med Imaging. 2010;29:282–301.
6. Chatap NJ, Shrivastava AK. A survey on various classification techniques for medical image data. Int J Comput Appl. 2014;97(15):1–5.
7. Zybin A, Kuritsyn YA, Gurevich EL, et al. Real-time detection of single immobilized nanoparticles by surface plasmon resonance imaging. Plasmonics. 2010;5(1):31–5.
8. Siedhoff D, Libuschewski P, Weichert F, et al. Modellierung und Optimierung eines Biosensors zur Detektion viraler Strukturen. Proc BVM. 2014; p. 108–13.
9. Long J, Shelhamer E, Darrell T. Fully convolutional networks for semantic segmentation. IEEE Conf Comput Vis Pattern Recognit. 2015; p. 3431–40.
10. Libuschewski P, Siedhoff D, Timm C, et al. Fuzzy-enhanced, real-time capable detection of biological viruses using a portable biosensor. Biosignals. 2013; p. 169–74.

Fast Pose Verification for High-Speed Radiation Therapy

Andreas Maier[1,2], Susanne Westphal[1], Tobias Geimer[1,2], Peter G. Maxim[3], Gregory King[3], Emil Schueler[3], Rebecca Fahrig[4], Billy Loo[3]

[1]Friedrich-Alexander Universität Erlangen-Nürnberg
[2]Graduate School in Advanced Optical Technologies (SAOT)
[3]Radiation Oncology, Stanford University Medical Center
[4]Radiological Sciences Lab, Stanford University
andreas.maier@fau.de

Abstract. This paper discusses fast pose verification for radiation therapy on a new high-speed radiation therapy device. The PHASER system follows the idea of 4th generation CT imaging and allows fast 360° treatment using a steerable electron beam. Doing so, dose delivery is possible in few seconds. A major problem, however, is fast verification of the patient pose during treatment. In this paper, we suggest to use a projection-based approach that can be evaluated quickly and allows an accuracy below 1 mm as shown by our simulation study based on planning data from six 4D CT data sets.

1   Introduction

Patient motion is a major problem for imaging [1] and radiation therapy [2]. In radiation therapy, dose delivery is typically planned on a 3D CT image [3] and high attention is paid to align the patient's actual position at the treatment site with the planning scan [4]. Due to the long duration of the radiation treatment, there is also motion that cannot be avoided completely. In particular, respiratory motion may cause the target area to move up to 2 cm [5]. Without compensation, this would cause the dose to be delivered to the wrong location, resulting in damaged healthy tissues and more importantly the potential survival of the malignant tumor itself [6]. In order to compensate for this, many approaches have been suggested ranging from implanted gold markers [7] to the use of respiratory surrogate signals [8] and the prediction of dense deformation fields [9]. In summary, these methods are feasible, but come at significant additional efforts.

In this work, we focus on a different treatment device that has been suggested by Maxim and Loo [10]. The Pluridirectional High-Energy Agile Scanning Electron Radiotherapy (PHASER) System is able to deliver the entire treatment dose within only a few seconds and, therefore, provides a treatment duration range that can effectively compensate for respiratory motion by a simple breath hold command. Additionally, in contrast to traditional radiation therapy, electrons instead of photons are used to deliver the radiation dose. This way, energy can be deposited much faster using fewer particles and with higher accuracy [11]. Fig. 1 shows a schematic of the system.

2   Materials and methods

2.1   PHASER system

While delivering such high amounts of dose in such short time has many advantages, it also poses special challenges to the imaging. In order to image the patient quickly, a special CT gantry was designed [12]. The associated detector is curved on a circle segment with a diameter of 1300 mm, an arc length of 1024 mm and a detector height of 192 mm. The detector provides high resolution in the center of the field-of-view (FOV) while offering larger pixels towards the outside of the FOV which typically is of lower interest for the purpose of radiation therapy. Fig. 2 shows the FOV for two typical imaging locations.

2.2   Pose verification

In contrast to typical radiation therapy, the PHASER system allows only very little time to verify the patient pose and deliver the dose. The whole process must be completed within a single breath-hold. As patients often suffer from impaired lung function, we assume this period to be within the range of 12 to 16 seconds [13]. Therefore, computationally expensive approaches that require reconstruction and motion compensation are not applicable [5]. Furthermore, we do not want to create an additional burden to the patients by using e.g. implanted gold markers [14].

The current work-flow on the PHASER system will involve a high-quality CT scan, registration to the planning CT, and an adaptation of the treatment

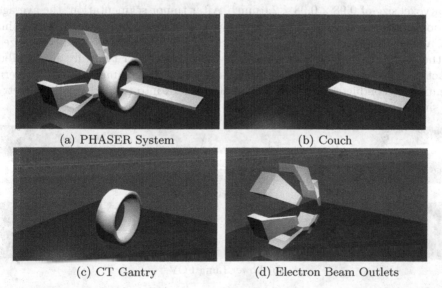

(a) PHASER System   (b) Couch

(c) CT Gantry   (d) Electron Beam Outlets

Fig. 1. A schematic of the PHASER system (a) with its main parts: The couch (b), the CT Gantry (c), and the electron beam outlets (d).

plan [12] to accommodate the current patient position. Hence, we expect the motion during the treatment to emerge only from respiratory motion.

In order to compensate for the current motion state, we propose to use projection-based imaging only, based on projections of the 4D planning CT. In addition, we reuse a lung segmentation that is created during the planing procedure for the pose verification process. In the following, we denote the projection of the mask as $\mathbf{m}_{i,\theta} \in \mathbb{R}^N$ for the ith motion state and projection angle θ where N is the number of pixels. The projection of the planning in state i is denoted as $\mathbf{p}_{i,\theta} \in \mathbb{R}^N$ while the current projection is $\mathbf{p}_\theta \in \mathbb{R}^N$. This allows us to identify the two motion states i_1^* and i_2^* that are closest to $\mathbf{p}_\theta$ using

$$i^* = \operatorname{argmin}_i = f(\mathbf{p}, i) = \sum_\theta ||\mathbf{m}_{i.\theta} \cdot (\mathbf{p}_{i,\theta} - \mathbf{p}_\theta)||_1 \qquad (1)$$

where $\cdot$ denotes the element-wise vector product. For the experimental evaluation, we chose to sample θ at 18 eqiangular positions over $360°$ of gantry rotation. The estimated tumor position $\hat{\mathbf{t}} \in \mathbb{R}^3$ can now be estimated as the weighted mean position between $\mathbf{t}_{i_1^*}$ and $\mathbf{t}_{i_2^*}$.

2.3   Patient data

Patient data from six patients that underwent regular lung tumor radiation therapy using a traditional CT scanner were used to investigate the accuracy of the proposed approach. For each patient, there were two 4D CT scans with 10 motion states in each available, one scan from the beginning of the treatment and one four weeks later, after the therapy was finished. The volumes were sampled at a voxel size of $0.98 \times 0.98 \times 2.0 \, \text{mm}^3$. After tumor segmentation, the average tumor centroid motion in these patients was determined at $2.50 \pm 2.10 \, \text{mm}$. This low amount of motion is related to the fact that the tumors were mainly localized in the top of the lung and that patients with lung cancer typically also exhibit functional losses associated with low changes in lung volume (Fig. 3). Experiments were conducted projecting the patient data into the PHASER geometry by simulation.

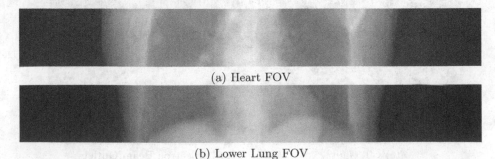

(a) Heart FOV

(b) Lower Lung FOV

Fig. 2. The CT detector that was developed for the PHASER system offers a larger field-of-view than a traditional CT detector which makes projection-based motion state verification possible.

Table 1. Localization accuracy using leave-one-motion-state-out-evaluation.

Patient ID	Acquisition Date	RMSE [mm]	$\mathbf{t}_{max}$ [mm]
Patient 1	2015-10	0.64 ± 0.31	2.0
Patient 1	2015-11	0.62 ± 0.30	2.0
Patient 2	2015-11	1.01 ± 0.71	7.0
Patient 2	2015-12	0.82 ± 0.48	7.0
Patient 3	2013-11	0.98 ± 0.62	1.5
Patient 3	2013-12	0.72 ± 0.56	1.5
Patient 4	2014-12	1.18 ± 0.75	2.0
Patient 4	2015-01	1.12 ± 0.78	2.0
Patient 5	2014-06	0.36 ± 0.22	0.5
Patient 5	2014-07	0.40 ± 0.18	0.5
Patient 6	2014-04	0.83 ± 0.59	2.0
Patient 6	2014-05	0.80 ± 0.58	2.0
Average		0.80 ± 0.25	2.50 ± 2.10

3   Results

Fig. 3 shows the behavior of the measure proposed in (1) compared to the relative change in lung volume for Patient 1. It can be observed that states with a similar lung volume also show similar values in $f(\mathbf{p}, i)$. We observed a similar relation in the other five patients.

In a second experiment, we excluded one of the breathing phases from the data and performed a leave-one-out evaluation to estimate the accuracy of unknown breathing motion. Tab. 1 presents these localization accuracies. We observe that the average error is much below the maximal tumor motion. This results in an average error of 0.80 ± 0.25 mm compared to 2.50 ± 2.10 mm maximal tumor motion. In the case with the largest tumor motion of 7 mm the error is reduced down to 0.83 mm.

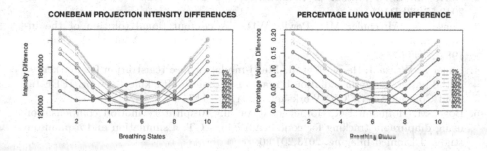

Fig. 3. The proposed measure (left) exhibits a high correlation with the relative volumetric change between two breathing states (right).

4   Discussion

From the experimental results, we observed that the localization accuracy is on average below 1 mm. Compared to current clinical safety margins of about 7 mm even for motion compensated treatment, this is a great reduction. However, one has to be careful with the interpretation of the results, as the average motion in our patients was only 2.50 ± 2.10 mm. Thus, our error is well below the maximal motion, but also higher than one would expect given that the motion was sampled ten times. This is related to the resolution of our 4D CT scan that had a voxel size of $0.98 \times 0.98 \times 2.0$ mm^3. In case of our patients, the main magnitude of motion occurs along the z axis, i.e. our results lie below the accuracy of one voxel. In future studies, we will have to verify whether this low amount of motion occurs in more patients with lung cancer. As a result, we would have to increase the resolution of the planning CT in the affected directions to alleviate the problem. Nonetheless even with the current setup, patients with large tumor motion benefit greatly from the method.

The current approach for interpolation of the motion state is very simple and will produce suboptimal results in the full inhale and full exhale position. However, with the small amount of motion in the study, this is not a major problem at present.

Another challenge that we plan to investigate in future work is continuous treatment using precomputed 4D treatment plans for patients such as young children who cannot follow breathing commands. With the current system setup, we would be able to select the correct treatment plan for the current motion state in real-time.

References

1. Nehmeh SA, Erdi YE.   Respiratory motion in positron emission tomography/computed tomography: a review.   Semin Nucl Med Dev Instrum. 2008;38(3):167–76.
2. Korreman SS.   Motion in radiotherapy: photon therapy.   Phys Med Biol. 2012;57(23):R161.
3. Censor Y, Altschuler MD, Powlis WD.   A computational solution of the inverse problem in radiation-therapy treatment planning.   Appl Math Comput. 1988;25(1):57–87.
4. Bauer S, Wasza J, Haase S, et al. Multi-modal surface registration for markerless initial patient setup in radiation therapy using microsoft's kinect sensor. IEEE Int Conf Comput Vis (ICCV) Workshops. 2011; p. 1175–81.
5. Bögel M, Hofmann HG, Hornegger J, et al.   Respiratory motion compensation using diaphragm tracking for cone-beam c-arm CT: a simulation and a phantom study. J Biomed Imaging. 2013;2013:6.
6. Shepard DM, Ferris MC, Olivera GH, et al. Optimizing the delivery of radiation therapy to cancer patients. SIAM Rev. 1999;41(4):721–44.
7. Huang CY, Tehrani JN, Ng JA, et al. Six degrees-of-freedom prostate and lung tumor motion measurements using kilovoltage intrafraction monitoring. Int J Radiat Oncol Biol Phys. 2015;91(2):368–75.

8. Wasza J, Fischer P, Leutheuser H, et al. Real-Time respiratory motion analysis using 4-D shape priors. IEEE Trans Biomed Eng. 2016;63(3):485–95.

9. Taubmann O, Wasza J, Forman C, et al. Prediction of respiration-induced internal 3-D deformation fields from dense external 3-D surface motion. Comput Assist Radiol Surg (CARS) 28th Int Congr Exhib. 2014; p. 33–4.

10. Maxim PG, Loo BW. Pluridirectional High-Energy Agile Scanning Electron Radiotherapy (PHASER): Extremely Rapid Treatment for Early Lung Cancer. DTIC Document; 2015.

11. Bazalova-Carter M, Qu B, Palma B, et al. Treatment planning for radiotherapy with very high-energy electron beams and comparison of VHEE and VMAT plans. Med Phys. 2015;42(5):2615–25.

12. Kemmerling EMC, Wu M, Yang H, et al. Optimization of an on-board imaging system for extremely rapid radiation therapy. Med Phys. 2015;42(11):6757–67.

13. Rosenzweig KE, Hanley J, Mah D, et al. The deep inspiration breath-hold technique in the treatment of inoperable non–small-cell lung cancer. Int J Radiat Oncol Biol Phys. 2000;48(1):81–7.

14. Chen S, Lu Y, Hopfgartner C, et al. 3-D printing based production of head and neck masks for radiation therapy using ct volume data: a fully automatic framework. Proc IEEE Int Symp Biomed Imaging. 2016; p. 403–6.

Fourier Consistency-Based Motion Estimation in Rotational Angiography

Mathias Unberath[1,2], Martin Berger[1], André Aichert[1], Andreas Maier[1,2]

[1]Pattern Recognition Lab, Friedrich-Alexander-University Erlangen-Nuremberg
[2]Graduate School in Advanced Optical Technologies, Erlangen
mathias.unberath@fau.de

Abstract. Rotational coronary angiography allows for volumetric imaging but requires cardiac and respiratory motion management to achieve meaningful reconstructions. Novel respiratory motion compensation algorithms based on data consistency conditions are applied directly in projection domain and, therefore, overcome the need for uncompensated reconstructions. Earlier, we combined single-frame background subtraction and epipolar consistency conditions to compensate for respiratory motion. In this paper, we show that background subtraction also enables motion estimation via optimization of novel Fourier consistency conditions. The proposed method is evaluated in a numerical phantom study. Compared to the uncompensated case, we found a reduction in residual root-mean-square error of 89 % when Fourier consistency conditions were used. The results are promising and encourage experiments on clinical data.

1 Introduction

Providing physicians with models of the 3D anatomy of arterial trees is considered beneficial for diagnostic assessment and interventional guidance [1]. In the context of minimally invasive treatment of coronary artery disease, rotational angiography is an increasingly popular acquisition protocol that allows for 3D reconstruction of the vasculature [1, 2].

Due to the low temporal resolution of clinical C-arm cone-beam CT (CBCT) scanners straight-forward 3D reconstruction is not always possible. Rotational angiography sequences are acquired over multiple seconds and, thereby, are corrupted by cardiac and respiratory motion. As a consequence, both motion patterns must be incorporated into reconstruction algorithms. Cardiac motion is high frequency and, as multiple recurrences are observed throughout the acquisition, is effectively handled by phase gating [1, 2].

In contrast, respiratory motion is very low frequency and, consequently, quasi non-recurrent which imposes a need for intra-scan respiratory motion compensation. Most state-of-the-art methods rely on 3D-2D registration and assume that, albeit motion-induced inconsistencies prevail, meaningful initial reconstructions are possible [1]. This assumption, however, is a serious limitation to the applicability of aforementioned methods in presence of substantial motion.

To overcome this limitation, we recently proposed a motion compensation algorithm that operates directly in projection domain. The method is based on virtual single-frame material decomposition that enables motion estimation using data consistency conditions (CC) [3]. Recently, epipolar CC [4] were used to assess the craniocaudal component of intra-scan respiratory motion [3]. In this work, we show that single-frame material decomposition also allows for the application of novel Fourier CC [5, 6]. We compare the results obtained with both data consistency measures to a manually extracted ground-truth in a numerical phantom study based on XCAT [7].

2 Material and methods

We describe an algorithm for consistency-based motion assessment in rotational coronary angiography. First, non-truncated images of the contrasted lumen are obtained using virtual single-frame background subtraction. Second, novel Fourier consistency conditions are used to estimate detector domain shifts parallel to the rotation axis.

2.1 Virtual single-frame material decomposition

As the thorax extends beyond the 3D field of view of conventional C-arm CT scanners, rotational angiography acquisitions are truncated. Consequently, data consistency measures cannot be applied directly because scans exhibiting truncation are inherently inconsistent. While the thorax as a whole may be truncated, the contrast-filled coronary arteries only occupy the central volume and are, therefore, not truncated. We briefly restate the method proposed in [3] that allows for the single-frame separation of contrast agent and background in the sense of digital subtraction angiography.

Contrasted vessels manifest as small tubular structures that are bright with respect to the background. Filters enhancing these properties have been found effective for vessel segmentation. Here, we use a combination of morphological and Hessian-based filters to obtain a binary segmentation mask $\mathcal{W}_i$ of projection image $\mathcal{I}_i$, where $\mathcal{W}_i(\boldsymbol{u}) = 1$ if $\boldsymbol{u} \in \mathbb{R}^2$ belongs to the background and 0 otherwise.

We seek to estimate a background image $\mathcal{B}_i$ that constitutes a non-contrast version of $\mathcal{I}_i$ to be used for digital subtraction. To this end, all evidence of contrast agent is removed from $\mathcal{I}_i$ yielding corrupted images $\mathcal{G}_i(\boldsymbol{u}) = \mathcal{I}_i(\boldsymbol{u}) \cdot \mathcal{W}_i(\boldsymbol{u}) \overset{!}{=} \mathcal{B}_i(\boldsymbol{u}) \cdot \mathcal{W}_i(\boldsymbol{u})$. Estimating $\mathcal{B}_i$ in spatial domain may lead to a patchy and unnatural appearance. Therefore, background estimation is performed in frequency domain by iterative deconvolution. Finally, the background estimate is subtracted from the contrasted projection, yielding a virtual digital subtraction angiogram $\mathcal{D}_i(\mathbf{u})$ that, ideally, only shows the contrasted vessels and is not truncated. Intermediate results of the pipeline are visualized in Fig. 1.

2.2   Fourier consistency

The background subtracted images $\mathcal{D}_i$, $i = 1, \ldots, M$ are not truncated and can be processed using data consistency conditions. Up to now, consistency measures based on the epipolar geometry [4] were used to estimate detector domain shifts that optimize consistency.

However, consistency among projections cannot only be formulated in terms of epipolar geometry, but also in the Fourier domain of the sinogram. Edholm *et al.* [8] showed that there exist triangular regions in the Fourier transform (FT) of parallel-beam sinograms that have an absolute value close to zero, a property that enables the definition of Fourier Consistency Conditions (FCC). Recently, Berger *et al.* [6] proposed a heuristic extension of FCC for cone-beam geometries based on Brokish *et al.* [9]. In presence of motion, however, the triangular regions are not vacant. This property can, therefore, be exploited to correct for motion.

The exact shape of the vacant regions depends on the acquisition geometry as well as the object's maximum extent r_p. For the fan-beam case it is given by

$$\left| \frac{\omega}{\omega - \xi \cdot D_{\mathrm{SD}}} \right| > \frac{r_p}{D_{\mathrm{SI}}} \tag{1}$$

where D_{SD}, D_{SI} are the source-to-detector and source-to-isocenter distances, and ω, ξ are frequency variables associated with the projection angles and the detector rows, respectively. Let ψ be the frequency variable corresponding to the vertical detector direction. As changes in shape of the triangular regions at different ψ are negligible [9], Berger *et al.* proposed to extend the fan-beam condition stated in Eq. 1 in the direction of ψ creating vacant regions for the 3D FT [6]. Similar to [3], we consider a motion model that consists of detector domain shifts in vertical direction that is parametrized by a sequence of shifts $\boldsymbol{\gamma} = (\gamma_1, \ldots, \gamma_M)^{\top}$. The consistency metric that has to be optimized is given by

$$\mathrm{FC}(\boldsymbol{\gamma}) = \| \mathbf{W} \left(\mathbf{F} \cdot \mathbf{d}(\gamma) \right) \|_2^2 \tag{2}$$

where $\mathbf{d}(\gamma) \in \mathbb{R}^K$ are the projection images $\mathcal{D}_i$ in vector format shifted according to γ, $\mathbf{F} \in \mathbb{C}^{K \times K}$ is a symmetric matrix that performs the 3D FT, and

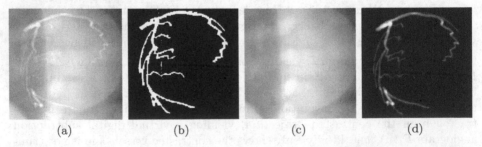

(a)   (b)   (c)   (d)

Fig. 1. Intermediate results and final digital subtraction angiogram of the numerical phantom data set. Fig. 1(a) to 1(d) show the original projection, the segmentation mask, the background estimate, and the digital subtraction angiography image, respectively.

$W \in \mathbb{R}^{K \times K}$ is a diagonal matrix that represents the 3D mask for the vacant regions. Moreover, $K = M \cdot U_1 \cdot U_2$, and $U_{1/2}$ is the size of the images $\mathcal{D}_i$ in $u_{1/2}$-direction, respectively. If the motion consists of projection domain shifts only as is the case here, the consistency metric defined in Eq. 2 can be implemented very efficiently as the shifts can be applied in the 2D Fourier domain according to the shift theorem [5, 6], yielding

$$FC(\gamma) = \| W (F_i (T(\gamma) \cdot F_u \cdot d)) \|_2^2 \qquad (3)$$

F_i and F_u are in $\mathbb{C}^{K \times K}$ and correspond to a 1D FT over the angles, and a 2D FT over the projections, respectively. The detector domain shifts along the u_2 direction are encoded as phase factors in $T(\gamma) \in \mathbb{C}^{K \times K}$, such that

$$
\begin{aligned}
T(\gamma) = \mathrm{diag}\Big(& \exp(-i2\pi\psi_1\gamma_1), \dots, \exp(-i2\pi\psi_{U_2}\gamma_1), \\
& \exp(-i2\pi\psi_1\gamma_2), \dots, \dots, \exp(-i2\pi\psi_{U_2}\gamma_M) \Big)
\end{aligned}
\qquad (4)
$$

where $\mathrm{diag}(\cdot)$ converts a vector to a matrix having the vector elements on the diagonal, and d is in row-major order. The derivative of Eq. 4 with respect to γ_i can be computed analytically, allowing for an efficient gradient-based optimization of Fourier CC [6].

2.3 Experiments

We evaluate the proposed algorithm on a numerical thorax phantom based on XCAT, i.e. Cavarev [7]. The data set contains 128 projection images with 960×960 pixels with an isotropic pixel size of 0.308 mm. The acquisition is corrupted by substantial respiratory and cardiac motion, the respective surrogate signals are shown in Fig. 2. Motion patterns are modeled such that no motion state is observed multiple times.

Projection images are processed according to Sec. 2.1 yielding non-truncated images of the contrasted lumen. Subsequently, detector domain shifts along the u_2-direction γ^{FCC} are estimated by optimization of Fourier consistency following Sec. 2.2. Moreover, we extract shifts that optimize epipolar CC γ^{ECC} following the method described in [3].

To enable quantitative evaluation, we manually tracked the position of two vessel bifurcation points over the acquisition, yielding a sequence of displacements. This step became necessary because, unfortunately, Cavarev does not include ground-truth motion patterns. For evaluation, we use the average displacement $\bar{\gamma}^{Man}$ and compute the root-mean-square error (RMSE) between $\bar{\gamma}^{Man}$ and the shifts extracted using Fourier and Epipolar CC, respectively.

3 Results

Shifts obtained by optimization of both data consistency measures are plotted in Fig. 2 together with the respective motion phase that is stated using

114   Unberath et al.

Table 1. Root-mean-square error (RMSE) between the manually extracted shifts and the displacements obtained by optimization of Epipolar and Fourier CC, respectively. The results are stated in mm.

	Uncompensated	Epipolar CC	Fourier CC
RMSE	10.3 ± 5.9	1.01 ± 0.83	1.11 ± 1.15

normalized time. It becomes apparent that all three motion patterns, namely $\bar{\gamma}^{Man}$, γ^{ECC}, and γ^{FCC} are very similar and exhibit global and local extrema at approximately the same positions. When considering the surrogate signals, one observes that the low frequency, high amplitude motion pattern correlates well with the respiratory phase. Moreover, local maxima occur around systole and suggest compensation of the craniocaudal displacement of the heart during contraction [3, 10]. However, shifts estimated using Fourier CC exhibit less pronounced local extrema. This observation is also reflected in a higher RMSE that is stated in Tab. 1. While optimization of both consistency metrics resulted in RMSEs that are substantially lower than for the uncompensated case, the results obtained using epipolar CC are closer to the ground-truth.

4 Discussion

We showed that background subtracted rotational angiography images can be input to novel data consistency conditions based on Fourier properties of the sinogram. We evaluated the proposed approach in a numerical phantom study on a XCAT-like phantom and obtained promising results. The shifts obtained by optimizing Fourier CC are in very good agreement with both, the ground-truth and the displacements obtained on the same data set with a method that optimizes epipolar consistency. Currently, consistency-based motion assessment in rotational angiography requires a sophisticated preprocessing pipeline to obtain

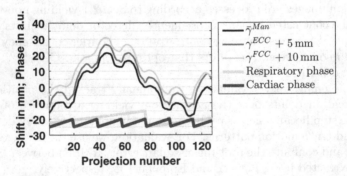

Fig. 2. We show shifts obtained by optimization of Fourier and Epipolar consistency, and the manually extracted ground-truth shifts. The motion patterns are slightly repositioned to avoid overlap and improve visualization: $\bar{\gamma}^{Man}$, γ^{ECC}, and γ^{ECC} are offset by 0, 5, and 10 mm, respectively. Normalized times indicating the respiratory and cardiac phase are shown at the bottom of the plot.

an estimate of non-truncated images of the contrasted lumen. This requirement is a serious limitation for the applicability of consistency-based methods. Consequently, future work will investigate possibilities for less complex preprocessing. Finally, we plan to evaluate consistency-based motion assessment algorithms on real clinical data.

Acknowledgement. The authors gratefully acknowledge funding of DFG MA 4898/3-1 "Consistency Conditions for Artifact Reduction in Cone-beam CT", the Research Training Group 1773 "Heterogeneous Image Systems", and the Erlangen Graduate School in Advanced Optical Technologies (SAOT) by the German Research Foundation (DFG) in the framework of the German excellence initiative.

References

1. Çimen S, Gooya A, Grass M, et al. Reconstruction of coronary arteries from x-ray angiography: a review. Med Image Anal. 2016;32:46–68.
2. Unberath M, Achenbach S, Fahrig R, et al. Exhaustive graph cut-based vasculature reconstruction. Proc ISBI. 2016; p. 1143–6.
3. Unberath M, Aichert A, Achenbach S, et al. Single-frame subtraction imaging. Proc CT Meet. 2016; p. 89–92.
4. Aichert A, Berger M, Wang J, et al. Epipolar consistency in transmission imaging. IEEE Trans Med Imaging. 2015;34(10):2205–19.
5. Berger M, Maier A, Xia Y, et al. Motion Compensated Fan-Beam CT by Enforcing Fourier Properties of the Sinogram. In: Proc. CT Meeting; 2014. p. 329–32.
6. Berger M. Motion-Corrected Reconstruction in Cone-Beam CT of Knees Under Weight-Bearing Conditions. Friedrich-Alexander-University Erlangen-Nuremberg; 2016.
7. Rohkohl C, Lauritsch G, Keil A, et al. CAVAREV : an open platform for evaluating 3D and 4D cardiac vasculature reconstruction. Phys Med Biol. 2010;55(10):2905–15.
8. Edholm PR, Lewitt RM, Lindholm B. Novel properties of the fourier decomposition of the sinogram. Proc SPIE 0671. 1986; p. 8–18.
9. Brokish J, Bresler Y. Sampling requirements for circular cone beam tomography. In: Proc. NSS. vol. 5. IEEE; 2006. p. 2882–4.
10. Shechter G, Resar JR, McVeigh ER. Displacement and velocity of the coronary arteries: cardiac and respiratory motion. IEEE Trans Med Imaging. 2006;25(3):369–75.

Towards Understanding Preservation of Periodic Object Motion in Computed Tomography

Franziska Schirrmacher[1,*], Oliver Taubmann[1,2,*], Mathias Unberath[1,2], Andreas Maier[1,2]

[1]Pattern Recognition Lab, Department of Computer Science,
Friedrich-Alexander-University Erlangen-Nuremberg, Germany
[2]Graduate School in Advanced Optical Technologies (SAOT), Erlangen, Germany
*These authors contributed equally to this work.
franziska.schirrmacher@fau.de

Abstract. In this paper, we study periodic object motion in computed tomography. Specifically, we investigate the phenomenon that motion may–in a sense–be preserved even in a standard analytical reconstruction that assumes a static object. In fact, these preserved motion patterns reappear in a forward-projection of the allegedly static reconstruction. In numerical simulations abstracting the cardiac anatomy, we show that not only the type of motion, but also the sharpness of the boundary of the moving object affects how much of the motion is preserved.

1 Introduction

Computed tomography (CT) imaging of the heart typically entails a challenging image reconstruction problem. While the radiation source rotates around a patient, their heart beats. This leads to inconsistencies in the acquired data and results in artifacts when performing a straight-forward reconstruction [1, 2, 3]. Different types of motion may be observed in a cardiac scan; the ventricles contract periodically, whereas the coronary arteries or catheters inserted into the heart mostly exhibit translational motion caused by the contraction [4]. Naturally, the sizes and shapes of the moving objects vary considerably as well. Arteries and catheters are narrow, elongated structures with a relatively sharp response characteristic, i. e. the image gradient at the object edges is high, and they are often displaced by a distance at least as large as their own diameter, while their shape remains mostly unaffected. In contrast, the ventricles usually do not have boundaries that are as well-defined and they describe a pulsating motion pattern, causing the object to change its size and shape.

In a standard reconstruction that assumes a static object, these differences lead to the ventricles appearing blurred, while arteries or catheters tend to cause streaking artifacts [3]. Curiously, in a forward projection of such an image using the same trajectory, the ventricles appear largely stationary while the catheter follows its original motion to a certain extent. An illustrative example is shown in Fig. 1. In this paper, we aim to identify properties relevant to this phenomenon and quantify their influence using numerical simulations.

116

Fig. 1. Frames of a rotational angiogram (a, b) and corresponding digitally reconstructed radiographs (DRR) obtained via projection of a *static* reconstruction (c, d).
Note that the catheter still follows its original motion (red) in the DRR, whereas the
left ventricle no longer pulsates (yellow). The full scan covers ca. 27 heart beats.

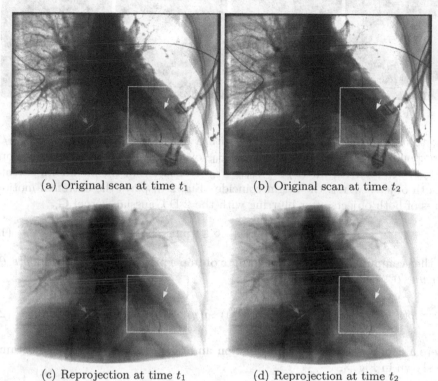

(a) Original scan at time t_1 (b) Original scan at time t_2

(c) Reprojection at time t_1 (d) Reprojection at time t_2

2   Materials and methods

2.1   A simple dynamic phantom

The phantom used in our simulations consists in a temporally varying circle.
Blurring the edges of the circle by convolution with a Gaussian filter kernel
yields different versions with varying sharpness. Modifiable parameters for each
circle are its center $\mu = (\mu_x, \mu_y)^\top$, its radius r, the number of motion periods f
during the acquisition, and the standard deviation of the Gaussian σ.

These parameters allow for a dynamic simulation adapted to the properties
of cardiac motion.

We define motion by two extremal states between which a parameter oscil-
lates following a sinusoidal curve. As a consequence, $r(t)$, $\mu(t) \propto \cos(2\pi \cdot f \cdot t)$
are time dependent, with $t \in [0, 1]$ being the time relative to the complete acquisition.

Two different dynamic objects, $\mathbf{O}_\text{puls}$ and $\mathbf{O}_\text{shift}$, are considered, which roughly
mimic the behavior of ventricles and arteries/catheters, respectively. $\mathbf{O}_\text{puls}$ is
centered at the origin, $\mu = (0, 0)^\top$, and pulsates with its radius ranging from

Fig. 2. Extremal states of the motion patterns of both considered objects $\widehat{\mathbf{O}}_{\mathrm{puls}}$ (a, b) and $\widehat{\mathbf{O}}_{\mathrm{shift}}$ (c, d), with $\sigma = 5$.

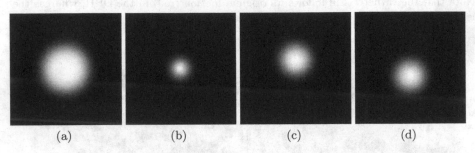

(a)   (b)   (c)   (d)

$r_{\min}$ to $r_{\max}$. $\mathbf{O}_{\mathrm{shift}}$ retains its shape with a fixed radius $r_{\mathrm{c}} = (r_{\max} + r_{\min})/2$ corresponding to the mean radius of $\mathbf{O}_{\mathrm{puls}}$ over time. Its position ranges from $(0, -\mu_{\mathrm{s}})^{\top}$ to $(0, \mu_{\mathrm{s}})^{\top}$, where $\mu_{\mathrm{s}} = r_{\max} - r_{\mathrm{c}}$ to ensure that the maximum extents of both objects w. r. t. the origin coincide. Fig. 2 displays the extremal motion states of both objects after blurring with the 2-D Gaussian kernel $\mathbf{G}_{\sigma}$

$$\widehat{\mathbf{O}}_{\diamond} = \mathbf{O}_{\diamond} * \mathbf{G}_{\sigma}, \quad \diamond \in \{\mathrm{puls}, \mathrm{shift}\} \tag{1}$$

We then compute the Radon transform to obtain a parallel-beam sinogram $p(s, \theta)$ over $\theta \in [0°, 180°]$

$$p(s, \theta \mid \widehat{\mathbf{O}}_{\diamond}) = \iint \widehat{\mathbf{O}}_{\diamond}(\boldsymbol{\mu}(t_\theta), r(t_\theta)) \cdot \delta(y \cos(\theta) + x \sin(\theta) - s) \, \mathrm{d}x \, \mathrm{d}y \tag{2}$$

where δ denotes the Dirac delta function and $t_\theta = \theta/180°$. Example sinograms are shown in Fig. 3.

2.2   Reconstruction and reprojection

Filtered back-projection using the standard Ram-Lak convolver [5] is employed to obtain a (motion-corrupted) reconstruction $\mathbf{R}_{\diamond}$ from each sinogram. Subsequently, we project the reconstructed image forward again with the same acquisition geometry. Although generated from a static image, it can be observed that this reprojected sinogram may retain a fraction of the original motion. It is,

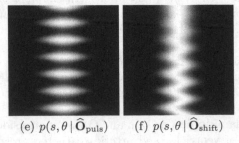

(e) $p(s, \theta \mid \widehat{\mathbf{O}}_{\mathrm{puls}})$ (f) $p(s, \theta \mid \widehat{\mathbf{O}}_{\mathrm{shift}})$

Fig. 3. Sinograms for $f = 23$ and $\sigma = 5$. The angular range $\theta \in [0°, 50°]$ is shown.

Fig. 4. Plots of the fraction of preserved motion q over the frequency f for different values of σ, which controls the edge sharpness.

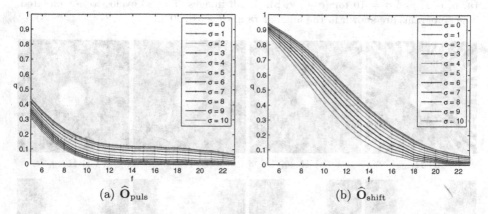

(a) $\hat{\mathbf{O}}_{\text{puls}}$ (b) $\hat{\mathbf{O}}_{\text{shift}}$

therefore, compared to the original sinogram in terms of the amount of periodic motion it still contains.

To obtain a quantitative measure for this property, we consider the point $(0, r_c)^{\top}$, located on the boundary of both objects in their mean state of motion, and collect all line integrals through this point observed in both the original and reprojected sinograms as two sequences s_{orig}, s_{reproj}, respectively. On both sequences, the 1-D Fourier transform $\mathcal{F}$ is performed to obtain the energy associated with the frequency f of the simulated motion. To increase the robustness of the measure, nearby frequencies are considered as well. More precisely, the Fourier-transformed sequences are multiplied element-wise with a 1-D Gaussian function with mean f and standard deviation of unity and, finally, summed up as $\xi_f(\mathcal{F}\{s_{\text{orig}}\})$ and $\xi_f(\mathcal{F}\{s_{\text{reproj}}\})$. To quantify the remaining motion in the reprojected sinogram, we compute their ratio

$$q = \frac{\xi_f(\mathcal{F}\{s_{\text{reproj}}\})}{\xi_f(\mathcal{F}\{s_{\text{orig}}\})} \tag{3}$$

2.3 Parameter values

We set $r_{\min} = 5$ and $r_{\max} = 20$, resulting in $r_c = 12.5$ and $\mu_s = 7.5$. For σ and f all integers in the ranges $[0, 10]$ and $[5, 23]$ are considered, respectively. Frequencies $f \leqslant 4$, for which a period would cover at least $45°$ of the trajectory, were not evaluated to keep the focus on cases where the motion is markedly faster than rotational effects. For all possible combinations of both of these parameters, q is calculated to comprehensively assess their influence on the amount of motion preserved. The phantom images are 300×300 pixels large. The acquisition was simulated with an angular spacing of $0.5°$ and 500 detector elements.

Fig. 5. Reconstructed images (top row) and reprojected sinograms (bottom row) displayed with a bright, high-contrast windowing to emphasize artifacts, where $\sigma = 5$ for (a, b, e, f) and $\sigma = 10$ for (c, d, g, h). In all images, $f = 23$ cycles were simulated. The sinograms are shown in the angular range $\theta \in [0°, 50°]$.

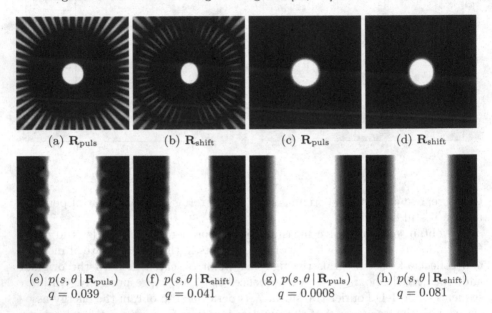

(a) $\mathbf{R}_{\mathrm{puls}}$ (b) $\mathbf{R}_{\mathrm{shift}}$ (c) $\mathbf{R}_{\mathrm{puls}}$ (d) $\mathbf{R}_{\mathrm{shift}}$

(e) $p(s, \theta \,|\, \mathbf{R}_{\mathrm{puls}})$ (f) $p(s, \theta \,|\, \mathbf{R}_{\mathrm{shift}})$ (g) $p(s, \theta \,|\, \mathbf{R}_{\mathrm{puls}})$ (h) $p(s, \theta \,|\, \mathbf{R}_{\mathrm{shift}})$
 $q = 0.039$ $q = 0.041$ $q = 0.0008$ $q = 0.081$

3 Results

The quantitative results of the simulation are summarized in Fig. 4. For both motion types, higher fractions q of the original motion are retained for lower frequencies f. The predominant trend is that this effect is much stronger for the translational than for the pulsating movement, which is intuitively in line with what can be observed from catheters and ventricles in real data (Fig. 1).

However, it is important to note that at higher frequencies, the influence of edge sharpness gradually increases and finally surpasses that of the motion type. E. g., for $f = 23$, a sharper $\widehat{\mathbf{O}}_{\mathrm{puls}}$ at $\sigma = 5$ exhibits substantially more motion after reconstruction and reprojection than a smoother $\widehat{\mathbf{O}}_{\mathrm{shift}}$ at $\sigma = 10$, both in terms of the quantitative measurement and visual impression (Fig. 5). In fact, the difference in edge sharpness is more likely to explain what is observed in Fig. 1 as the real scan covers 27 cycles, falling into a similar frequency regime.

In addition, looking at the reconstructed images Fig. 5(a) and Fig. 5(b), it seems reasonable to assume that the preservation of motion in the static image is closely linked to the streaking artifacts typically observed in motion-corrupted scans. In other words, the streaks "encode" the original motion, which could be a valuable insight when designing methods to deal with this effect. A practical consequence of this issue, seen in Fig. 5(e), is the angle-dependence of the preserved motion due to the rotational asymmetry of Fig. 5(a). It also implies that the grid size contributes to the occurrence of this effect.

4   Discussion

In summary, this work is concerned with the phenomenon that periodic motion of a dynamic object may be preserved even within a static reconstruction. We were able to reproduce observations made in complex real-world data sets within a simple simulation framework, where we quantified the contribution of two properties of the dynamic object on this effect: The type of motion (translational vs. pulsating) and the sharpness of its boundaries. While both were influential, we found that the relative strength of their influence is highly dependent on the motion frequency.

Our findings can help foster a better understanding of the applicability and limitations of techniques which directly rely on a static reconstruction of dynamic objects as an intermediate step. Prominent examples are the artifact reduction method by McKinnon and Bates [6], prior image constrained compressed sensing [7], or joint bilateral filtering using a static guidance image [8]. Considering the importance of edge sharpness discovered in our simulations, investigating specialized reconstruction filters may be worthwhile, the design of which could be informed by artifact models in the spirit of, e.g., prior work on perfusion imaging [9].

References

1. Hansis E, Schäfer D, Dössel O, et al. Projection-based motion compensation for gated coronary artery reconstruction from rotational x-ray angiograms. Phys Med Biol. 2008;53(14):3807–20.
2. Schwemmer C, Rohkohl C, Lauritsch G, et al. Residual motion compensation in ECG-gated interventional cardiac vasculature reconstruction. Phys Med Biol. 2013;58(11):3717–37.
3. Müller K, Maier A, Schwemmer C, et al. Image artefact propagation in motion estimation and reconstruction in interventional cardiac C-arm CT. Phys Med Biol. 2014;59(12):3121–38.
4. Unberath M, Aichert A, Achenbach S, et al. Virtual single-frame subtraction imaging. Proc Intl Conf Image Form Xray CT. 2016; p. 89–92.
5. Zeng GL. Medical Image Reconstruction : A Conceptual Tutorial. Springer; 2010.
6. Mc Kinnon GC, Bates RHT. Towards imaging the beating heart usefully with a conventional CT Scanner. IEEE Trans Biomed Eng. 1981;BME-28(2):123–7.
7. Chen GH, Tang J, Leng S. Prior image constrained compressed sensing (PICCS): a method to accurately reconstruct dynamic CT images from highly undersampled projection data sets. Med Phys. 2008;35(2):660–3.
8. Taubmann O, Maier A, Hornegger J, et al. Coping with real world data: artifact reduction and denoising for motion-compensated cardiac C-arm CT. Med Phys. 2016;43(2):883–93.
9. Fieselmann A, Dennerlein F, Deuerling-Zheng Y, et al. A model for filtered backprojection reconstruction artifacts due to time-varying attenuation values in perfusion C-arm CT. Phys Med Biol. 2011;56(12):3701–17.

The Impact of Semi-Automated Segmentation and 3D Analysis on Testing New Osteosynthesis Material

Rebecca Wöhl[1], Michaela Huber[1], Markus Loibl[1], Birgit Riebschläger[2], Michael Nerlich[1], Christoph Palm[3,4]

[1]Department of Trauma Surgery, University Medical Center Regensburg
[2]Department of Neurology, University Medical Center Regensburg
[3]Regensburg Medical Image Computing (ReMIC),
Ostbayerische Technische Hochschule Regensburg (OTH Regensburg)
[4]Regensburg Center of Biomedical Engineering (RCBE),
OTH Regensburg and Regensburg University
rebecca.woehl@klinik.uni-regensburg.de

Abstract. A new protocol for testing osteosynthesis material postoperatively combining semi-automated segmentation and 3D analysis of surface meshes is proposed. By various steps of transformation and measuring, objective data can be collected. In this study the specifications of a locking plate used for mediocarpal arthrodesis of the wrist were examined. The results show, that union of the lunate, triquetrum, hamate and capitate was achieved and that the plate is comparable to coexisting arthrodesis systems. Additionally, it was shown, that the complications detected correlate to the clinical outcome. In synopsis, this protocol is considered beneficial and should be taken into account in further studies.

1 Introduction

Semi-automated segmentation is considered an important tool in various fields of surgery. Whether it is used for simulating the complex 3D anatomies in the field of teaching [1] or for pre- and intraoperative planning in fracture treatment [2]. In contrast there are only few studies taking these tools for postoperative evaluation and in vivo studies into account [3, 4]. The aim of this study was testing a new locking plate in vivo used in hand surgery. Patients who suffer from scaphoid non-union or a lesion of the scapholunate ligament after wrist trauma develop radiocarpal arthrosis over time. One option of treatment is the scaphoidectomy and midcarpal fusion of the lunate, triquetrum, hamate and capitate. The four corner fusion can be performed using K-wires, compression screws or (locking) plates. The arthrodesis is considered successful if a bony union is detected six weeks after surgery and if no complications occur [5]. In this study a new protocol of examination was established. First a semi-automated segmentation of CT scans of the wrist was performed. The plate, screws and the four carpals fused were included in the volumes of interest (VOI). Afterwards the

122

semi-automatically generated surface meshes were analysed in a 3D environment and selected features from the manufacture's brochure were inquired. All these findings were correlated to the clinical outcome.

2 Materials and methods

All eleven patients, who received a midcarpal arthrodesis between August 2011 and July 2014, were included in the study. The indication for surgery was a progressing radiocarpal arthrosis after rupture of the scapholunate ligament in eight cases and after scaphoid non-union in three cases. Ten patients received the standard size of the 2.0/2.3 Four Corner Fusion Aptus Plate (Medartis, Basel, Switzerland), one patient the small size plate. All surgeries were conducted at our institute by the same hand surgeon. The six month follow up consisted of clinical examination and X-ray imaging. In addition, six weeks after surgery a CT scan of the operated wrist was performed. For semi-automated segmentation the software ITK Snap (Open Source, Version 3.4.0, www.itksnap.org) [6] was used, which is based on Geodesic Active Contours [7] and Region Competition [8] embedded in a level-set framework.

The axial CT layers were used to create a multiplanar visualisation. After defining the region of interest (ROI) the first step comprised of defining thresholding limits. For the ROI of the four carpals the lower threshold was set at 220 Hounsfield Units (HU), the upper one at 2000 HUs. Respectively the ROI of the osteosynthesis material was determined just by a lower threshold of 2000 HUs. To initialize the active contour segmentation circles of various sizes were placed within the ROI so each structure is addressed. The software transferred those into 3D bubbles automatically and the user could correct them after controlling the location in the multiplanar visualisation. After that the segmentation evolved automatically. Since additional pathologies were found in two cases they were included as segmentation results. After segmentation all surface meshes were saved as STL files.

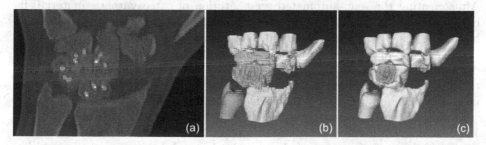

Fig. 1. After semi-automated segmentation and manual correction (a) the ROIs (red) were transformed into surface meshes (b). Subsequently they were processed with cleaning and remeshing filters in order to prepare for 3D analysis. For demonstration purpose smoothing filters were applied and the structures were coloured depending on the type of material (c).

Especially for the segmentation of the carpals and metacarpals the bubbles have to be set anatomically correct. If they exceed the anatomic contour of the bone in just one layer of the multi planar visualisation, highly inaccurate outcomes occur because thereby the small cartilaginous border is overstepped and two different structures will be treated as one. This problem also happens if the iteration count of the automated segmentation is set to high. If it is shut down after too few iterations holes occur, so the user has to strike a compromise. Unfortunately, there are no standards for bubble placement or iteration count, so it depends on individual anatomic knowledge and segmentation experience how fast a reasonable image can be created. Nonetheless, all transverse, sagittal and coronal planes of the four carpals fused were scrolled through and each slice was edited manually as well to ensure anatomic accuracy which is indispensable for the following tests.

The 3D analysis and transformation of the meshes were conducted with Meshlab (Open Source, Version 1.3.3, meshlab.org) [9]. This process consisted of cleaning, remeshing and creating a watertight mesh. The union of the carpals fused and the detection of the screw position could be proven just by visualisation in a 3D environment. To verify the multidirectional angle of 15 degrees a cone with the same specifications was built as a surface mesh. To show the mono- or bicortical ply of the screws the surface mesh of the four carpals fused depicting the outer shell of the corticalis was remeshed using a uniform mesh resampling filter to create the inner shell of the corticalis. With the software netfabb Basic (netfabb Basic, netfabb GmbH, Lupburg, Germany) measurements and volumes were detected automatically. Solely for visualisation purposes the surfaces were post processed. A depth and laplacian smoothing filter was applied and afterwards the meshes were coloured by the per mesh colour option using the RGB colour code for bone and metal (Fig. 1).

3   Results

After creating the semi-automated segmentation of osteosynthesis material, it became apparent that this step is not challenging because of its clear defined hounsfield scale. On the other hand, segmenting small bones with a complex shape e.g. carpals can be quite time consuming because there are only small distances of less than one millimetre of cartilage separating them. Depending on the anatomical knowledge and the skill to imagine the 3D geometry it can take up to several hours generating the surfaces meshes.

Union of the lunate, triquetrum, hamate and capitate could be proven in 100% of all cases in the CT scans. This result could also be verified by visualization of the surface meshes of the carpals. In in all but one cases it could be shown that at least two screws per carpal can be applied: 87 of 88 possible screws were drilled into lunate, triquetrum, capitate and hamate of eleven patients. If the standard size plate is used, even three screws per carpal can be placed except for two cases. On average seven screws had a bicortical ply (Fig. 2). One overlong screw in the triquetrum led to an irritation of the pisotriquetral joint

(Fig. 3a). The multidirectional angle of 15 degrees, which is important to ensure the locking of the screw, could be substantiated for all 125 screws employed.

The dimensions of the plate with 1.45 cm in length and width and 1.25 cm for the standard and the small size plate, respectively, are suitable compared to the mean 3.67 cm length and 3.41 cm width of the four carpals. To avoid impingement between radius and plate, a mean margin of 6.1 mm between lunate and plate and 8.2 mm between triquetrum and plate should be observed. Due to proximal positioning of the plate the radiocarpal joint was impaired in one case (Fig. 3b). The placement of the plate and screws led to reduction of bony substance of maximum 7.5%, which had no effect on union. The complications found in medical imaging correlated 100% to the clinical findings. Those two

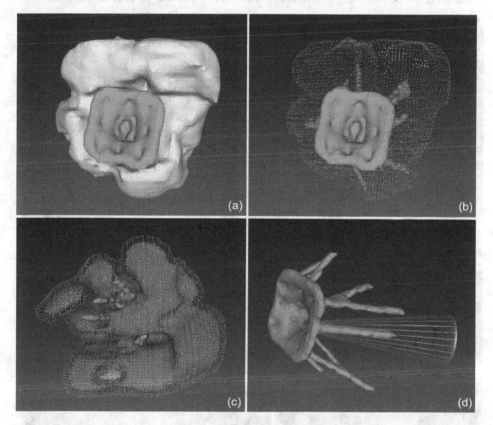

Fig. 2. The anatomical knowledge combined with the models (a) of the four carpals fused (white) and the osteosynthesis material (grey) allowed to identify the carpal the screw was position in by studying the models in a 3D testing environment (b). After using a uniform mesh resampling filter, the inner shell of the corticalis (red) could be visualised (c). So even in borderline cases, we were able to distinguish between a mono- or bicortical ply of the screws. The multidirectional angle of 15 degrees could be proven, if the screw lay within a cone (green) of the same defaults and in the direction of the normal vector of the plate (d).

patients complained about severe pain and restrictions in movement even six months after surgery. Both pathologies were not detected in the X-ray images (Fig. 3c,d) postoperatively.

4   Discussion

Due to this new protocol of testing objective proof was determined: the plate can keep up to the manufacturer's promises and it can compare to traditional fixation methods. The 3D visualisation allowed to proof bony union of the four carpals fused six weeks after surgery. The relations of anatomical structures were visualized and even complications arising were detected, so it is a valuable tool

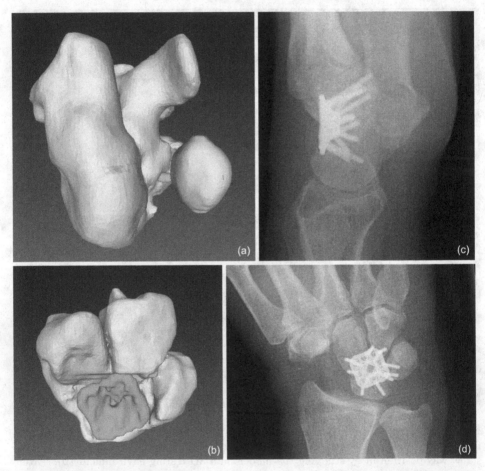

Fig. 3. Due to semi-automated segmentation and 3D analysis complications could be depicted. In one case an overlong screw (red) impaired the pisotriquetral joint (a). In another case the proximal positioning of the plate led to irritations of the radiocarpal joint (b). These pathologies (arrow) could not have been substantiated in the 2D display of the postoperative x-ray pictures (c, d).

for evaluating surgeons and their outcome as well as for testing osteosynthesis material. In conclusion a CT scan followed by semi-automated segmentation and visualisation should be contemplated to search for correlates if the patient complains about severe pain postoperatively. With the supplemental information gathered it was even possible to distinct intraoperative pitfalls. The placement of the plate is very important, so despite reaming the plate free hand, as the manufacturer suggests, the surgeon should utilize a reaming guide to avoid proximal positioning. Yet this protocol comprises many steps of manual labour. Generating a protocol fast and easy to use both applicable to surgeons and professionals in medical image processing is desirable. Especially an improvement of the automated segmentation of the carpals and metacarpals would be time saving. Addtionally, automated segmentation would result in observer independend meshes. However, existing semi-automated segmentation and 3D analysis tools are on the market and should be acknowledged more often. The impact of these tools in clinical practise to find reasons for postoperative complications as well as in testing new osteosynthesis material was shown here.

Acknowledgement. This work was funded as a part of the BMBF project HaptiVisT: Entwicklung und Evaluierung eines haptisch-visuellen Lernsystems für chirurgische Eingriffe.

References

1. Gehrmann S, Höhne K, Linhart W, et al. A novel interactive anatomic atlas of the hand. Clin Anat. 2006;19(3):258–66.
2. Olsson P, Nysjö F, Hirsch JM, et al. A haptics-assisted cranio-maxillofacial surgery planning system for restoring skeletal anatomy in complex trauma cases. Int J Comput Assist Radiol Surg. 2013;8(6):887–94.
3. Baan F, Liebregts J, Xi T, et al. A new 3D tool for assessing the accuracy of bimaxillary surgery: the orthognathicanalyser. PloS one. 2016;11(2):e0149625.
4. Anderst WJ, Baillargeon E, Donaldson III WF, et al. Validation of a non-invasive technique to precisely measure in vivo three-dimensional cervical spine movement. Spine. 2011;36(6):E393.
5. Ashmead D, Watson HK, Damon C, et al. Scapholunate advanced collapse wrist salvage. J Hand Surg Am. 1994;19(5):741–50.
6. Yushkevich PA, Piven J, Cody Hazlett H, et al. User-guided 3D active contour segmentation of anatomical structures: significantly improved efficiency and reliability. Neuroimage. 2006;31(3):1116–28.
7. Caselles V, Kimmel R, Sapiro G. Geodesic active contours. Int J Comput Vis. 1997;22:61–79.
8. Zhu S, Yuille A. Region competition: unifying snakes, region growing, and Bayes/MDL for multiband image segmentation. IEEE Trans Pattern Anal Mach Intell. 1996;18(9):884–900.
9. Cignoni P, Callieri M, Corsini M, et al. Meshlab: an open-source mesh processing tool. Eurograph Ital Chap Conf. 2008; p. 129–36.

Pathology-Related Automated Hippocampus Segmentation Accuracy

M. Liedlgruber[2], K. Butz[1,4], Y. Höller[1], G. Kuchukhidze[1], A. Taylor[1],
A. Thomschewski[1,4], O. Tomasi[3], E. Trinka[1,4], A. Uhl[2]

[1]Department of Neurology, Christian Doppler Medical Centre and Centre for
Cognitive Neuroscience, Paracelsus Medical University, Salzburg, Austria
[2]Department of Computer Sciences, University of Salzburg, Austria
[3]Department of Neurosurgery, Paracelsus Medical University, Salzburg, Austria
[4]Spinal Cord Injury and Tissue Regeneration Center Salzburg, Austria
uhl@cosy.sbg.ac.at

Abstract. Hippocampal segmentation accuracy of out-of-the-box software tools (FreeSurfer, AHEAD, BrainParser) is analysed wrt. potential variability in populations with different pathologies. Findings confirm variabilities wrt. different pathologies but also human rater ground truth and single pathologies exhibit significant variability as well.

1 Introduction

Mild cognitive impairment (MCI) is a condition of cognitive deterioration that is difficult to classify as normal aging or as a prodromal stage to dementia [1]. Despite considerable progress of research, current endeavours are still focused on accurate and early diagnosis of MCI [2]. Similarly, the diagnosis of temporal lobe epilepsy (TLE) was [3] and still is based on clinical assessment and electroencephalographic (EEG) examination, sometimes being inconclusive. Both diseases need to be treated and handled adequately, in order to prevent massive memory decline or hazards by seizures. From a structural point of view, the hippocampus is an area of the brain that links the two conditions [4]. It is therefore worth evaluating techniques for the diagnosis of these conditions that are based on distinctive features of this structure of the brain. Segmentation of the hippocampi is of course a prerequisite for such approaches.

Since manual definition of the borders of the hippocampus is tedious and time-consuming work, many techniques for automated hippocampus segmentation have been published over the last years [5, 6, 7] including state-of-the-art algorithms based on multi-atlas segmentation (MAS)[8].

In this paper, we look into the accuracy of out-of-the-box segmentation software (which is highly attractive for research groups interested in segmentation results but not segmentation algorithm development) applied to hippocampi when differentiating patients diagnosed with MCI and TLE and comparing the results to a healthy control group. Previous work [9] revealed significant variability wrt. various aspects of hippocampal segmentation however being restricted to an overall analysis without differentiating different subject groups. As a hypothesis, one might conjecture that automated segmentation tools tend to commit more errors in subjects suffering from MCI or TLE as the atlases they base their segmentation on usually consist of healthy subjects. In Section 2, we describe the employed data set (including the rare availability of a three human rater ground truth significantly surpassing [9]) and automated segmentation tools used in this study. Section 3 outlines experimental setup and present results, while a conclusion is given in Section 4.

2   Materials and methods

2.1   Dataset and manual ground truth

In this work we use a data set that has been acquired at the Department of Neurology, Paracelsus Medical University Salzburg and consists of 58 T1-weighted MRI volumes, including patients with mild cognitive impairment (MCI, 20 subjects), with temporal lobe epilepsy (TLE, 17 subjects), and a healthy control group (CG, 21 subjects). The dataset contains 28 males (18-76 years, mean age 53 ± 19 years) and 30 females (23-71 years, mean age 54 ± 14 years). We defined patients with amnestic MCI according to level three of the global deterioration scale for aging and dementia. Diagnosis was based on multimodal neurological assessment, including imaging (high resolution 3T magnetic resonance tomography, and single photon emission computed tomography with Hexamethylpropylenaminooxim), and neuropsychological testing.

Manual segmentations have been performed by 3 experienced raters (one senior neurosurgeon and two junior neuroscientists supervised by a senior neuroradiologist) on a Wacom Cintiq 22HD graphic tablet device (resolution 1920x1200) using a DTK-2200 pen and employing the 32-bit 3DSlicer software for Windows (v. 4.2.2-1 r21513) to delineate hippocampus voxels for each slice separately. The raters independently used consensus on anatomical landmarks/boarders of the hippocampus based on Henry Duvemoy's hippocampal anatomy [10]. The procedure used was to depict the hippocampal outline in the view of all planes in the following order: sagittal – coronal – axial with subsequent cross line control through all planes.

2.2   Hippocampus segmentation software packages

In contrast to most of the algorithms presented in literature, e.g. [7], all employed software packages are already pre-compiled and available for free [9]:

- *FreeSurfer* (FS)[1] is a set of tools which allow an automated labelling of subcortical structures in the brain. Such a subcortical labelling is obtained by using the volume-based stream which consists of five stages [5]. The result is a label volume, containing labels for various different subcortical

---

[1] v. 51.0, available at http://surfer.nmr.mgh.harvard.edu

structures (e.g. hippocampus, amygdala, and cerebellum). FreeSurfer is a highly popular tool to assess clinical hypotheses [11] or to compare to newly proposed segmentation techniques (e.g. [7]).

- *Automatic Hippocampal Estimator using Atlas-based Delineation* (AHEAD)[2] is specifically targeted at an automated segmentation of hippocampi [6]. Based on multiple atlases and a statistical learning method, the final segmentation is obtained.
- Although *BrainParser* (BP)[3] is usually able to label various different subcortical structures, we use a version which is specifically tailored to hippocampus segmentation. The tool uses a deformable registration between the input and the reference volume and subsequent corresponding input volume labeling.

In case of BrainParser and AHEAD the MNI152 atlas has been used as provided with the software. For FreeSurfer we used the MNI305 atlas.

2.3   Metrics used to assess segmentation quality

In the following the automated segmentation is denoted by S, the ground truth segmentation is called G, and $v(\cdot)$ is a volume operator which computes the volume of a voxel volume with respect to the actual dimensions of a voxel.

- *Symmetric Hausdorff distance* (SHD): This metric is based on the actual structure of a voxel volume. It is defined as

$$SHD(G, S) = \max(HD(G, S), HD(S, G)) \tag{1}$$

where

$$HD(X, Y) = \max_{x \in X}(\min_{y \in Y} d(x, y)) \tag{2}$$

is the non-symmetric Hausdorff distance, x and y are vectors in $\mathbb{R}^3$ and $d(\cdot, \cdot)$ denotes the Euclidean distance between two vectors.

- *Relative overlap* (RO): The relative overlap (also known as the Jaccard similarity coefficient) represents the fraction of voxels in the union of G and S which are also contained in the intersection of G and S

$$RO(G, S) = \frac{v(G \cap S)}{v(G \cup S)} \tag{3}$$

While low values in $[0, 1]$ correspond to little similarity or quality for RO, the SHD produces large values (differences) between dissimilar segmentations.

---

[2] version 1.0, available at http://www.nitrc.org/projects/ahead
[3] available at http://www.nitrc.org/projects/brainparser

Table 1. Summary of normalised hippocampus volumina (in percent of the entire brain volume) as obtained from the three human raters and the three software packages, averaged over all subjects of each pathology class also showing standard deviation.

	V_{CG}	V_{MCI}	V_{TLE}
Rater 1	0.482±0.092	0.383±0.065	0.442±0.060
Rater 2	0.450±0.125	0.360±0.079	0.393±0.078
Rater 3	0.556±0.086	0.457±0.058	0.514±0.073
FreeSurfer	0.542±0.135	0.499±0.086	0.579±0.120
AHEAD	0.333±0.031	0.304±0.049	0.348±0.075
BrainParser	0.366±0.116	0.363±0.057	0.376±0.067

3 Results

The following results are always based on both hippocampi simultaneously (both hippocampi from each scan are treated as one segmentation object).

First, we provide quantitative results in terms of normalised hippocampus volumina in Tab. 1 (i.e. the percentage of the entire brain volume of each subject is given). As the hippocampus in known to be atrophic in MCI and dementia [12] and is sclerotic in specific subtypes of epilepsy [13] we expect reduced volumina for MCI and TLE (V_{MCI}, V_{TLE}) respectively, as compared to the volume of healthy subjects (V_{CG}).

We clearly have $V_{CG} > V_{TLE} > V_{MCI}$ as the main result seen for all three raters consistently, thus, results are corresponding well with the expectations at first sight. However, this is only true when looking at the raters' results individually. However, cross-rater differences are significant and volumes among raters vary by up to 20%. Additionally, partially high standard deviations among subjects obliterate the clear trend as seen from the averaged values.

For the automated segmentation tools we observe a different, still clear ordering as displayed in the table: $V_{TLE} > V_{CG} > V_{MCI}$. This of course does not correspond to the expectations. While the known over-segmentation of FS [11] is also reflected in our results (making the comparison with AHEAD and BP volumina impossible), we also find clear cross-tool variation between AHEAD and BP as well as significant standard deviations (see e.g. FS and BP for CG and FS for TLE). Thus, in terms of volumina, human rater results are closer to the expected values, however, for both human raters as well as automated segmentation tools we notice significant inter-rater and inter-tool variability as well as high subject variability as indicated by high standard deviations.

The following Tab. 2 provides a more qualitative view when comparing the segmentation results. We compare the results of the automated tools with the human rater ground truth (which is a voxel-based majority vote among the three raters) in terms of the two metrics, SHD and RO, respectively. Apart from differences in volume also shape differences are reflected by these metrics, where SHD indicates shape differences in the most pronounced manner.

Table 2. Summary of segmentation assessment metrics (SHD and RO) computed between the automated segmentations and the ground truth (majority voted among three raters), averaged over all subjects of each pathology class.

SHD Results	Overall	CG	MCI	TLE
FreeSurfer	7.73±2.27	6.95±1.36	7.74±1.98	8.93±3.00
AHEAD	7.78±14.03	11.31±24.13	5.30±0.98	6.89±2.61
BrainParser	9.64±16.29	14.43±26.87	7.38±9.11	8.10±3.41
RO Results				
FreeSurfer	0.63±0.06	0.66±0.03	0.62±0.05	0.59±0.09
AHEAD	0.62±0.08	0.59±0.12	0.64±0.03	0.61±0.05
BrainParser	0.59±0.17	0.54±0.23	0.61±0.15	0.59±0.09

The upper half of Tab. 2 shows results wrt. SHD. FS results meet the expectations in that lowest distance to human raters is seen for CG subjects. The largest distance (i.e. error) to the ground truth is seen for TLE patients. The other two segmentation tools exhibit a different behaviour: While the relation between TLE and MCI patients is identical to FS segmentations, CG subjects exhibit the largest distance to the ground truth. While this result is highly unexpected, we need to consider the extremely high standard deviation in the CG results of AHEAD and BP. It seems that the data set contains CG subjects for which those two segmentation tools are highly erroneous, while for others the results are quite good.

The lower half of Tab. 2, showing the results of the RO metric, basically confirms the findings of the SHD metric. Again, FS results corresponds to the expectations (higher similarity for CG subjects as compared to MCI and TLE patients), while AHEAD and BP results show the CG subjects as those with lowest similarity to the ground truth. By perfect analogy to the SHD metric also RO results rate segmentations of MCI patients more similar to ground truth as compared to TLE patients **and** we observe very high standard deviations in the metric values for AHEAD and BP considering CG subjects.

4   Discussion

For FS segmentations, we find more errors in subjects suffering from MCI and TLE, compared to errors in the CG population. However, AHEAD and BP segmentations exhibit lowest correspondence to human ground truth for CG subjects on average, although for this population a very high standard deviation is present in the results. All three tools commit more errors in subjects suffering from TLE as compared to the MCI patient population.

All these results have to be taken with great caution, as the variability in the results of the three human raters is found to be very high, i.e. the inter-rater variability in terms of hippocampal volume of the same pathology class (CG, MCI, or TLE) is in the same order of magnitude as the inter-pathology volume difference of a single rater.

Acknowledgement. This work has been funded by the Austrian Science Fund (FWF) under Project No. KLI 00012.

References

1. Hänninen T, Soininen H. Age-associated memory impairment. Normal aging or warning of dementia? Drugs Aging. 1997;11:480–9.
2. Lei B, Chen S, Ni D, et al. Discriminative learning for alzheimer's disease diagnosis via canonical correlation analysis and multimodal fusion. Front Aging Neurosci. 2016;8(77).
3. Tharp B. Recent progress in epilepsy. Diagnostic procedures and treatment. Calif Med. 1973;119:19–48.
4. Höller Y, Trinka E. What do temporal lobe epilepsy and progressive mild cognitive impairment have in common? Front Syst Neurosci. 2014;8(58).
5. Fischl B, van der Kouwe A, Destrieux C, et al. Automatically parcellating the human cerebral cortex. Cereb Cortex. 2004;14(1):11–22.
6. Suh JW, Wang H, Das S, et al. Automatic segmentation of the hippocampus in T1-weighted MRI with multi-atlas label fusion using open source software: evaluation in 1.5 and 3.0T ADNI MRI. Proc Int Soc Magn Reson Med Conf. 2011; p. 3844.
7. Zarpalas D, Gkontra P, Daras P, et al. Accurate and fully automatic hippocampus segmentation using subject-specific 3D optimal local maps into a hybrid active contour model. IEEE J Transl Eng Health Med. 2014;2:1–16.
8. Leung KK, Barnes J, et al. Automated cross-sectional and longitudinal hippocampal volume measurement in mild cognitive impairment and Alzheimer's disease. Neuroimage. 2013;51(4):1345–59.
9. Liedlgruber M, Butz K, Höller Y, et al. Variability issues in automated hippocampal segmentation. A study on out-of-the-box software and multi-rater ground truth. Proc IEEE CBMS. 2016; p. 191–6.
10. Kuzniecky R, Jackson GD. Magnetic Resonance in Epilepsy. New York: Raven Press; 1995.
11. Cherbuin N, Anstey1 KJ, Réglade-Meslin C, et al. In vivo hippocampal measurement and memory. A comparison of manual tracing and automated segmentation in a large community-based sample. PLoS ONE. 2009;4:1–10.
12. Fotuhi M, Do D, Jack C. Modifiable factors that alter the size of the hippocampus with ageing. Nat Rev Neurol. 2012;8:189–202.
13. Malmgren K, Thom M. Hippocampal sclerosis. Origins and imaging. Epilepsia. 2012;53:19–33.

Interaktive Planung von Gesichtsimplantaten

Jan Egger[1,2], Markus Gall[1], Jürgen Wallner[3], Knut Reinbacher[3]
Katja Schwenzer-Zimmerer[3], Dieter Schmalstieg[1]

[1]Institut für Maschinelles Sehen und Darstellen, TU Graz
[2]BioTechMed, Graz
[3]Klinische Abteilung für Mund-, Kiefer- und Gesichtschirurgie, Meduni Graz
egger@icg.tugraz.at

Kurzfassung. In diesem Beitrag wird eine neue Methode zur computerunterstützten Behandlungsplanung von knöchernen Gesichtsschädelbrüchen unter der Verwendung von Miniplatten vorgestellt. Diese Art von Implantaten wird verwendet, um Knochenbrüche im Gesicht zu behandeln. Nach dem derzeitigen Stand der Technik verwendete Methoden wie die Plattenadaption an stereolithischen Modellen oder auf Basis einer computerunterstützten Planung weisen allerdings eine geringere Flexibilität, Mehrkosten oder hygienische Risiken auf. Mit der hier vorgestellten Software ist es den Chirurgen möglich, das Resultat vorab in nur wenigen Minuten an einem computervisualisierten Modell zu planen und anschließend als STL-Datenformat zu exportieren, um es so in der zukunftsträchtigen 3D-Drucktechnologie verwenden zu können. Dadurch werden Chirurgen in die Lage gesetzt, das generierte Implantat oder eine entsprechende Biegevorlage flexibel für jeden visualisierten Defekt im Behandlungszentrum präzise innerhalb weniger Stunden zu erstellen.

1 Einleitung

Die Rekonstruktion von Deformationen im Gesichtsbereich auf Grund knöcherner Frakturen ist Teil der täglichen Routine eines Chirurgen im Bereich der Mund-, Kiefer- und Gesichtschirurgie. Die Frakturen können als Folge von Unfällen im Sport, Straßenverkehr, auf Grund von Rohheitsdelikten oder im Rahmen von pathologischen Prozessen wie Tumoren oder Knochenzysten auftreten [1]. Bei vielen Rekonstruktionen von Knochendefekten kommen so genannte Miniplatten zur Anwendung. Mit dem Ziel, das betroffene (defekte) Gebiet zu stabilisieren, werden die Miniplatten über der Fraktur an der Knochenoberfläche beider Fragmente platziert und mit Schrauben befestigt. Da allerdings die Implantate in ihrer Ausgangsform gerade sind, müssen sie an die Knochenstruktur entsprechend angepasst werden. Dies geschieht intraoperativ durch passive Adaption unmittelbar vor der Plattenfixierung. In der klinischen Routine kann dieser Vorgang ein erhebliches Maß an Operationszeit in Anspruch nehmen und auch zusätzlich ein hygienisches Problem darstellen. Im Allgemeinen verlangt die Plattenadaption eine mehrmalige Anpassung und Korrektur, um ein zufriedenstellendes Ergebnis zu erzielen. Dabei wird das Implantat immer wieder an die knöcherne Struktur angelegt und muss bei ungenügender Passung wieder erneut adaptiert und nachgebogen werden. Eine andere Methode, die vor allem bei der Planung komplexer Frakturen eingesetzt wird, verwendet stereolithographische Modelle. Diese 3D-Modelle werden anhand von computertomographischen (CT) Bildern generiert, um daran die verwendeten Implantate präoperativ zu adaptieren [2]. Im Gegensatz zur intraoperativen Plattenadaption verschiebt sich damit der Zeitaufwand in die präoperative Planungsphase. Neben den katalogisierten Implantaten gibt es computerunterstützte Planungssoftware, die es ermöglicht, patientenspezifische Implantate zu generieren [3]. Die meisten dieser Produkte legen ihren Fokus allerdings auf die Repositionierung von Knochenfragmenten – im Gegensatz zur Generierung von konventionell erhältlichen Implantaten [4]. Obwohl diese Softwaretools professionelle und umfassende Pakete zur präoperativen Planung von Gesichtsdefekten bereitstellen, bieten sie in der klinischen Routine lediglich limitierte Optionen für die praktische Anwendung. Zusätzlich sind kommerzielle Softwareprogramme (z.B. von Materialise) mit komplexen Arbeitsabläufen verbunden, die keine Möglichkeit zur individuellen Anpassung der Software oder Erweiterungen im Rahmen von Forschungsvorhaben bieten. Außerdem sind die käuflich zu erwerbenden Programme lizenzgeschützt, ihre Beschaffung und Wartung sind mit hohem finanziellen Aufwand verbunden. Im Gegensatz dazu präsentiert unser Beitrag eine neue, einfache und adaptierbare Methode zur computerunterstützten Planung für die Behandlung von Gesichtsdefekten unter MeVisLab [5].

2   Material und Methoden

Für diese Studie wurden Standard (512x512)-Computertomographiedaten mit einer maximalen Schichtdicke von einem Millimeter verwendet. Diese wurden im Rahmen der klinischen Routine zur Diagnosesicherung und Behandlungsplanung bei Gesichtsschädelbrüchen in der Abteilung für Mund-, Kiefer- und Gesichtschirurgie der Medizinischen Universität Graz erstellt. Als Implementierungsgrundlage wurde die Prototyping Plattform MeVisLab eingesetzt, die ein Interface für den Aufbau einfacher und fortgeschrittener Anwendungen und Algorithmen mit Hilfe eines modularen Systems bietet. Um einem Benutzer unserer Anwendung eine einfache und klar verständliche Oberfläche zur Verfügung zu stellen, wurde mit Hilfe der Mevis Description Language und dem fachlichem Input unserer klinischen Partner aus mehreren Meetings ein übersichtliches Userinterface implementiert und realisiert. Abb. 1 zeigt in einem Ablaufdiagramm die implementierten Algorithmen, wie sie bei der Planung der Gesichtsrekonstruktion angewendet werden. Zuerst muss der Datensatz des Patienten in das Programm geladen werden, um dann einen initialen Marker mittels linkem Mausklick zu setzen. Dieser Marker definiert das Zentrum des Implantats und wird außerdem zur Berechnung der sogenannten Basislinie verwendet. Die Basislinie dient als simplifiziertes, aber dennoch genaues und klar erkennbares Modell des gewünschten Implantats. Außerdem werden durch die Basislinie die langen Rechenzeiten, die durch die Konstruktion des vollständigen geometri-

136   Egger et al.

schen Implantats entstehen, eingespart. Diese Vorgehensweise ermöglicht eine
interaktive Echtzeitpositionierung eines abstrakten Implantats (Basislinie) auf
der Patientenoberfläche. Abhängig vom initialen Marker, der durch das Maus-
rad vorgegebenen Richtung und dem gewählten Implantatmodell wird die Basislinie automatisch berechnet, positioniert und visualisiert. Dabei basiert die
Erstellung der Linie auf der Berechnung des Strahl/Dreieck-Schnittpunktes, vorgestellt durch Möller und Trambone [6, 7]. Zusammengefasst wird eine Kaskade
von Strahlen, abhängig vom Oberflächennormalvektor des Dreieckes des initialen Punktes, ausgesendet und auf Schnitte mit Oberflächendreiecken geprüft.
Die Oberflächenschnittpunkte werden anschließend linear miteinander verbunden und ergeben die Basislinie. Hat sich die Basislinie an gewünschter Position

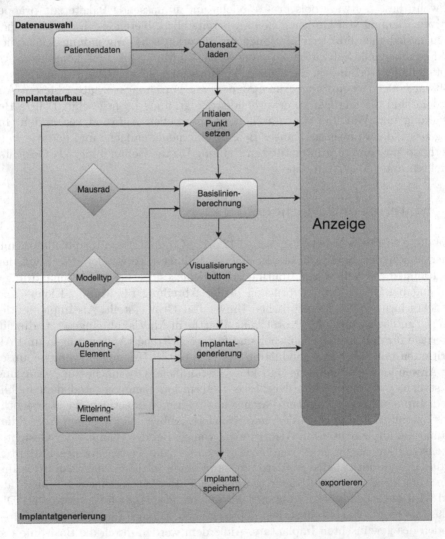

Abb. 1. Ablaufdiagramm der Planungssoftware.

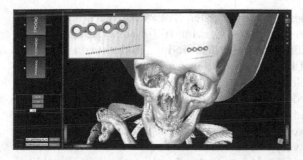

Abb. 2. Die Benutzeroberfläche besteht aus einem Kontrollfenster und einem Visualisierungsfenster. Visualisiert ist ein Datensatz (weiß) mit einer Basislinie (grüne Punkte) und einem schon geplanten Implantat an einer anderen Position (Gold).

an die Oberfläche des Datensatzes angelegt, wird das fertige Modell durch Betätigen des Visualisierungsbuttons generiert. Zuerst werden vorgefertigte Ringteile auf die gewünschte Position registriert, um in einem weiteren Schritt die Stege zwischen den Ringen durch Verwendung der Delaunay-Triangulation zu erstellen. Das erstellte Implantat kann für die aktuelle Sitzung gespeichert werden, um weitere Miniplatten, z.B. bei multiplen Frakturen, zu planen. Abschließend können alle generierten Implantate durch Betätigen des Export-Buttons lokal auf dem Rechner gespeichert werden. Dieses Format erlaubt u.a. das Generieren eines physischen Modells mittels 3D-Drucktechnologie. Die Software wurde mit Hilfe von Endanwendern verschiedener Expertisen getestet und evaluiert. Darunter befanden sich Versuchspersonen aus dem Bereich der Softwareentwicklung und Chirurgen einer Abteilung für Mund-, Kiefer- und Gesichtschirurgie, die regelmäßig Patienten mit Brüchen des Gesichtsschädels behandeln. Um die Tests durchzuführen, wurde ein Testfall zusammengestellt, bei dem es galt, eine mediane mandibulare Fraktur mittels zweier verschiedener Modelle an Miniplatten zu versorgen. Einen Fragebogen, welcher aus der ISO NORM 9241/10 zur Software-Ergonomie auf einer Siebener-Likert-Skala abgeleitet wurde, galt es anschließend zu beantworten und auszuwerten (Abb. 4).

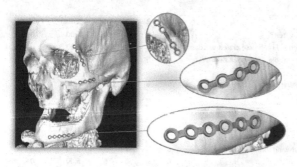

Abb. 3. Planungsergebnisse von drei unterschiedlichen Miniplattenmodellen (Gold) an häufig auftretenden Frakturstellen.

3   Ergebnisse

Die entwickelte Software und das Benutzerinterface werden in Abb. 2 präsentiert. Dabei besteht die Benutzeroberfläche aus einem Kontroll- (links) und einem Visualisierungsfenster (rechts). In Abb. 2 wurde ein Datensatz aus der klinischen Routine geladen, bei dem eine Basislinie (grüne Punkte) und ein Implantat

(Gold) unabhängig voneinander platziert wurden. Außerdem wird eine Detail-
ansicht der Basislinie und des Implantats gezeigt (rote Box). Auf der linken
Seite können verschiedene Miniplatten aus der Modus 2.0-Serie von MedArtis
(www.medartis.com) für eine Planung ausgewählt werden. Abb. 3 zeigt drei verschiedene Implantatmodelle (Gold), die an im klinischen Alltag häufig auftretenden Frakturstellen geplant wurden. Die Software wurde von zwei Kieferchirurgen,
einem Biomedizintechniker und einem Informatiker evaluiert. Dazu wurde allen
vier Benutzern die Software vorgeführt (Trainingsphase). Danach nahmen die
Benutzer eine eigene Planung vor, beginnend mit dem Laden eines Datensatzes
bis hin zum Speichern/Exportieren des geplanten Implantats (Zeit T in Minuten). Anschließend wurden die Benutzer gebeten, einen Evaluationsfragebogen
auszufüllen: von trifft nicht zu"(0) bis trifft zu"(6) (Abb. 4).

4 Diskussion

In diesem Beitrag haben wir den Prozessablauf von Gesichtsfrakturbehandlungen
unter der Verwendung von konventionellen Miniplatten vorgestellt. Dabei können mit unserem Ansatz verschiedene Implantate interaktiv und in kürzester Zeit
über unterschiedlichen Frakturen an beliebigen Positionen im Gesicht/Schädel
platziert werden.Die Evaluierung des in dieser Untersuchung durchgeführten
Prozessablaufes mit Hilfe eines Fragebogens zeigte, dass alle Nutzer die Software
auf Grund kurzer Trainingszeiten, kurzer Anwendungszeit, Genauigkeit, Präzisi-
on der Plattenadaption und ihrer Benutzerfreundlichkeit als effektives computer-
unterstütztes interaktives Planungsprogramm zur Generierung von Implantaten
am Gesichtsschädel beurteilten. Zukünftige Arbeiten beinhalten die Möglichkeit
der Generierung von patientenindividuellen Implantaten, die nach ihrer virtuellen bild- und computergestützten Konstruktion mit Hilfe eines 3D-Druckers oder

Nr.	Fragen	1	2	3	4	Median	Fehler
Q1	Benötigt die Software wenig Einarbeitungszeit?	6	6	6	6	6,00	0
Q2	Können mit der Software zufriedenstellende Ergebnisse erzielt werden?	6	6	6	6	6,00	0
Q3	Stellt die Software genügend Funktionen für die Aufgabe bereit?	6	5	6	6	5,75	0,22
Q4	Ist die Software leicht zu bedienen?	4	6	6	6	5,50	0,43
Q5	Wie zufrieden sind Sie mit der Benutzeroberfläche (Gestaltung, Style, Übersichtlichkeit)?	6	6	6	6	6,00	0
Q6	Wie präzise konnte das Implantat platziert werden?	6	6	6	6	6,00	0
Q7	Wie zufrieden sind Sie mit dem erzielten Resultat?	6	6	6	6	6,00	0
Q8	Wie einfach war es, das Implantat anzupassen (Position, Orientierung, Modell, ...)?	5	6	6	5	5,50	0,25
Q9	Wie zufrieden waren Sie mit dem Zeitaufwand (ohne Training)?	6	6	6	6	6,00	0
Q10	Wie ist Ihr Gesamteindruck?	6	6	6	6	6,00	0
Q11	Angenommen, das 3D-gedruckte Implantat würde mir wenigen Korrek- turen passen, würden Sie dann die Software in der täglichen Routine benutzen?	6	6	6	6	6,00	0
T	Wieviel Zeit (in Minuten) haben Sie benötigt, um ein zufriedenstellen- des Ergebnis zu erzielen?	4,0	5,5	3,5	4,2	4,30	0,37

Abb. 4. Evaluationsfragebogen inklusive Benutzerergebnissen: Biomedizintechniker
(1), Kieferchirurg (2), Kieferchirurg (3), Informatiker (4).

einer Fräse hergestellt werden können. Außerdem soll die vorgestellte Arbeit auf Frakturen in anderen Körperteilen – etwa der Wirbelsäule – adaptiert [8] und in ein AR-System zur visuellen Unterstützung eingebunden werden [9].

Danksagung. Diese Arbeit erhielt Förderung von BioTechMed-Graz und der 6. Ausschreibung der kompetitiven Anschubfinanzierung der TU Graz (İnteraktive Planung und Rekonstruktion von Gesichtsdefekten", PI: Dr. Dr. Jan Egger). Dank gilt auch Frau Edith Egger-Mertin für das Korrekturlesen des Beitrags. Ein Video der interaktiven Planung von Gesichtsimplantaten finden Sie unter folgendem YouTube-Kanal: http://www.youtube.com/c/JanEgger/videos

Literaturverzeichnis

1. Ritacco L, Milano F. Computer-assisted Musculoskeletal Surgery. Thinking and Executing in 3D. 2016;1:1–326.
2. Bell R. A Comparison of Fixation Techniques in Oro-Mandibular Reconstruction utilizing Fibular free Flaps. J Oral Maxillofac Surg. 2007;65(9):39.
3. Peng L, Wei T, Chuhang L, et al. Clinical Evaluation of Computer-assisted Surgical Technique in the Treatment of Comminuted Mandibular Fractures. J Oral Maxillofac Surg Medicine and Pathology. 2015;27(3):332–6.
4. Chapuis J, Schramm A, Pappas I, et al. A new System for Computer aided preoperative Planning and intraoperative Navigation during Corrective Jaw Surgery. IEEE J Biomed Health Inf. 2007;11(3):274–87.
5. Egger J, Tokuda J, Chauvin L, et al. Integration of the OpenIGTLink network protocol for image-guided therapy with the medical platform MeVisLab. Int J Med Robot. 2012;8(3):282–90.
6. Möller T, Trumbore B. Fast, Minimum Storage Ray-Triangle Intersection. Journal of Graphics Tools. 1997;2(1):21–8.
7. Egger J, et al. Fast self-collision detection and simulation of bifurcated stents to treat abdominal aortic aneurysms (AAA). IEEE EMBC. 2007; p. 6231–4.
8. Chen X, Xu L, Yang Y, et al. A semi-automatic computer-aided method for surgical template design. Sci Rep. 2016;20280:1–18.
9. Chen X, Xu L, Wang Y, et al. Development of a Surgical Navigation System based on Augmented Reality using an Optical see-through Head-mounted Display. J Biomed Inform. 2015;55:124–31.

Abstract: Automatic Image Registration for 3D Cochlea Medical Images

Ibraheem Al-Dhamari, Sabine Bauer, Dietrich Paulus, Friedrich Lissek,
Roland Jacob

MTI, University of Koblenz and Landau, Koblenz, Germany
idhamari@uni-koblenz.de

A Prior knowledge of the cochlea's characteristics helps for selecting the suitable cohlear implants for different patients. Cochlea medical images provide such prior knowledge. Doctors use a manual procedure for image registration and segmentation which is time consuming. The cochlea's small size and complex structure reveals a big challenge for the automated registration of multi-modal cochlea images [1]. An automatic Cochlea image registration (ACIR) method for multi-modal human cochlea images is proposed in this paper. This method uses the adaptive stochastic gradient descent (ASGD) optimizer [2] and Mattes's mutual information (MMI) metric [3]. The state of the art medical image registration optimizers published over the last two years are studied and compared. ACIR requires only a few seconds to align cochlea images automatically. The source code is based on the tool elastix [4]. Another contribution of this work is a proposed public cochlea standard dataset called HCD. ACIR and HCD can be downloaded for free from a public server. Fig. 1. shows a sample of our results.

References

1. Hajnal H Hill. Medical Image Registration. CRC Press; 2001.
2. Klein, Pluim, Staring, et al. Adaptive stochastic gradient descent optimisation for image registration. Int J Computer Vis. 2009;81(3):227–39.
3. Mattes, Haynor, Vesselle, et al. Non-rigid multimodality image registration. Proc SPIE Med Imaging. 2001; p. 1609–20.
4. Klein, Staring, Murphy, et al. Elastix: a toolbox for intensity-based medical image registration. IEEE Trans Med Imaging. 2010;29(1):196–205.

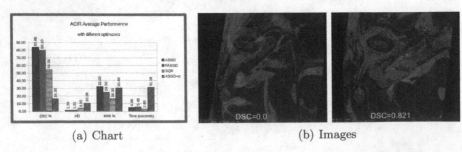

(a) Chart   (b) Images

Fig. 1. Sample results. The CBCT image is registered to the MR image.

Barrett's Esophagus Analysis Using SURF Features

Luis Souza[1,2], Christian Hook[2], João P. Papa[1], Christoph Palm[2,3]

[1]Department of Computing,
Faculty of Sciences, São Paulo State University
[2]Regensburg Medical Image Computing (ReMIC),
Ostbayerische Technische Hochschule Regensburg (OTH Regensburg)
[3]Regensburg Center of Biomedical Engineering (RCBE),
OTH Regensburg and Regensburg University
luis.souza@fc.unesp.br

Abstract. The development of adenocarcinoma in Barrett's esophagus is difficult to, detect by endoscopic surveillance of patients with signs of dysplasia. Computer assisted diagnosis of endoscopic images (CAD) could therefore be most helpful in the demarcation and classification of neoplastic lesions. In this study we tested the feasibility of a CAD method based on Speeded up Robust Feature Detection (SURF). A given database containing 100 images from 39 patients served as benchmark for feature based classification models. Half of the images had previously been diagnosed by five clinical experts as being "cancerous", the other half as "non-cancerous". Cancerous image regions had been visibly delineated (masked) by the clinicians. SURF features acquired from full images as well as from masked areas were utilized for the supervised training and testing of an SVM classifier. The predictive accuracy of the developed CAD system is illustrated by sensitivity and specificity values. The results based on full image matching where 0.78 (sensitivity) and 0.82 (specificity) were achieved, while the masked region approach generated results of 0.90 and 0.95, respectively.

1 Introduction

In the last decades, the incidence of adenocarcinoma in patients with Barrett's esophagus has increased significantly in Western populations. The dismal prognosis of the disease can be largely improved through early identification and surgical treatment of high-grade dysplasia and non-metastatic stages of cancer [1, 2, 3]. Therefore, strong emphasis is being placed on the computer assisted diagnosis (CAD) of endoscopy images. Some studies have already been carried out to classify lesions of the esophagus, based on conspicuous color and textural anomalies [4]. Benefitting from substantial improvements in the field of image analysis and artificial intelligence, methods like Speed-Up Robust Features (SURF) [5] and Deep Learning [6] are increasingly applied. The aim of the current study was to investigate the feasibility of a support vector machine

(SVM) to classify dysplastic and cancerous lesions in Barrett's esophagus based on SURF descriptors.

2   Materials and methods

This section demonstrates the steps to develop a computerized system for the detection, delineation and characterization of endoscopic images obtained from individuals with clinically manifest tissue abnormalities in the esophagus. Based on a given set of endoscopic photographs (benchmark database). SURF descriptors are utilized for the training and validation of an SVM classifier.

2.1   Image database

The set of images used as benchmark database was provided at the MICCAI 2015 EndoVis Challenge (https://endovissub-barrett.grand-challenge.org). It is composed of 100 endoscopic pictures of the lower esophagus, captured from 39 individuals, 17 of them being diagnosed with early stage Barrett's, and 22 displaying signs of esophageal adenocarcinoma. From each proband several endoscopic images were available, ranging from one to a maximum of eight. The database contained a total of 50 images displaying cancerous tissue areas (C2 labeled images), plus 50 images showing dysplasia without signs of cancer (C0 labeled images). Suspicious lesions observed in the C2 images had been delineated individually by five endoscopy experts. Some of the expert's demarcations in identical images exhibited substantial regional deviations. Therefore all delineated (masked) areas were combined to employ a gold standard for definitive states of adenocarcinoma.

2.2   SURF

The SURF algorithm operates on integral images to detect dominant structures and their spatial orientation. To ensure scale and spatial invariance the SURF seeks for maxima of the determinant of Hessian, demarcating specific key-points in the image, which are further explored in their local neighborhood. These sub-regions are evenly split into square patches while their wavelet responses in horizontal and vertical directions generate the elements of a high-dimensional feature vector of size 64 [5].

2.3   Interest points

Interest point (IP) acquisition was performed with the SURF algorithm provided in MATLAB using the OpenCV interface support package. The assessment of suitable IPs was based on two approaches. The first approach simulated "real life situations" lacking detailed information about tissue abnormalities. This analysis worked on the original full images. Two attributes were defined for the SVM training process: Class 0 images (C0, non-cancerous but with possible signs of early dysplasia), and class 2 images (C2, exhibiting cancerous tissue regions). The second approach was based on designated spatial annotations provided by five endoscopy experts, denoted as regions S_1 to S_5. In order to define a secure gold standard despite considerably dissenting delineations (Fig. 1), the area of intersection from all demarcated regions in the same image was denoted as class 2 area (C2, "cancerous"). Tissue linings which had been inconsistently marked as cancerous or as non-cancerous were labelled as class 1 (C1, "fuzzy regions"). Epithelium diagnosed by all experts in unison as negative was labelled as class 0 (C0, "non-cancerous"), cf. Equations 1-3

$$\text{Cancer}: C2 = \bigcap_{i=1,\dots,5} S_i \tag{1}$$

$$\text{Fuzzy}: C1 = \bigcup_{i=1,\dots,5} S_i \backslash C_2 \tag{2}$$

$$\text{Non-cancer}: C0 = 1 - (C_2 \bigcup C_1) \tag{3}$$

Full image approach. Each image j, $(j = 1, \dots, 100)$ is mapped to an average vector $\boldsymbol{r}(j) \in \mathbb{R}^{64}$ composed of n_{IP} (n_{IP} = number of IP in image j) individual SURF feature vectors $\boldsymbol{f}(j,k) \in \mathbb{R}^{64}; k = 1,\dots, n_{IP}$ (Fig.2, top)

$$\boldsymbol{r}(j) = \frac{1}{n_{IP}} \cdot \sum_{k=1}^{n_{IP}} \boldsymbol{f}(j,k) \tag{4}$$

Masked image approach. The process applied to full images is similarly applied to the segmented areas labelled with class codes C0, C1, C2, respectively. Each region is compressed to a mean feature vector, normalized by the number of selected SURF interest points $n_{IP}(i)$ of the corresponding region. Consequently, each image j $(j = 1, \dots, 50)$ belonging to the cancer subset is mapped to three feature vectors $\boldsymbol{r}(i,j), (i = 0, 1, 2)$ (Fig.2, bottom)

$$\boldsymbol{r}(j,i) = \frac{1}{n_{IP}(i)} \cdot \sum_{k=1}^{n_{IP}(i)} \boldsymbol{f}(j,k,i), i = 0, \dots, 2 \tag{5}$$

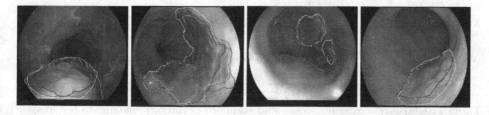

Fig. 1. Five different experts annotation from four different cancer images.

2.4 Classification

An SVM classifier was selected to discriminate between C0 and C2 type epithelium. The classification steps were performed in two different ways. In the first approach, SVM training as well as testing was performed using averaged features obtained from the full images. In the second approach, SVM training and test runs worked on average feature vectors of masked image regions. In both cases the conventional leave-one-patient-out cross validation (LOPO-CV) was applied using SVM parameters $\gamma = 0.02$, cost $c = 5$ with an RBF kernel.

3 Results

According to the number of patients in the database, 39 computations were performed for each approach. It should be clear that leaving out a certain patient

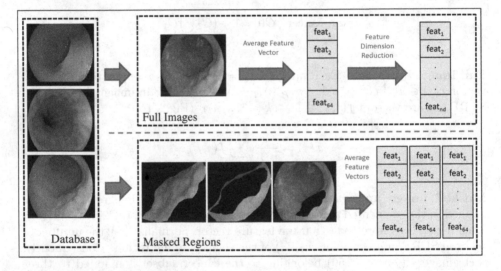

Fig. 2. Mapping full images and masked areas to feature vectors.

TrainingSets	TestSets	Sensitivity	Specificity
Full Images	Full Images	0.78 ($\sigma = 0.37$)	0.82 ($\sigma = 0.33$)
Masked Regions C0, C1, C2	Masked Regions C0, C1, C2	0.90 ($\sigma = 0.17$)	0.95 ($\sigma = 0.18$)
Masked Regions C0, C1, C2	Masked Regions C2	0.91 ($\sigma = 0.24$)	0
Masked Regions C0, C1, C2	Masked Regions C0	0	0.95 ($\sigma = 0.18$)

Table 1. Classification results (mean and standard deviation) referring to full images and masked regions.

Fig. 3. SVM hyperplanes separating C0 and C2 in a fictitious three-dimensional feature space. Points in (a), (b) and (c) indicate average feature vectors extracted from masked C0 and C2 regions, (d) and (e) refer to mean SURF features assessed from full images.

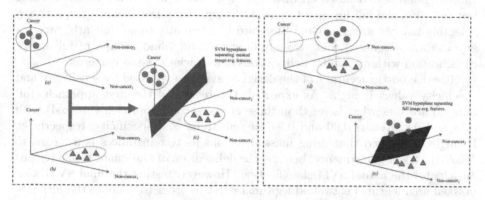

from the training set implies that all available images from this patient are removed from the training set. In order to comprehend the results summarized in Tab. 3, we consider a feature space spanned by only three variables. Let two features reflect specific properties of the masked non-cancerous regions (C0), and a single feature being indicative for masked cancerous regions (C2). Presuming adequate separability of C0 and C2 points (Figs. 3a, b) the SVM hyperplane might be positioned as shown in Fig. 3c. A high predictive accuracy of the classifier is expected if the test data are also supplied from masked image regions. SURF feature vectors calculated from full images will of course be located in other regions of the feature space (Figs. 3d, e), resulting in an essentially different SVM hyperplane. Moreover, test vectors scatter considerably due to non-distinctive features contained in the full images. Note that hyperplanes generated from masked regions will definitely not cope with test features obtained from full images, and vice versa. The sensitivity and specificity mean values above 78% and 90% for full image and masked image classification, respectively, confirm these considerations (Tab. 3).

4   Discussion and conclusions

The presented CAD system is a promising approach to evaluate various types and stages of epithelial lesions in patients suffering from Barrett's esophagus. The method uses SURF to exploit hidden structural patterns embedded in endoscopy images. This technique was applied to full images as well as to masked image regions which provide a gold standard for the identification of malignant lesions. Both approaches require a reference database comprising endoscopy images from patients with non-cancerous (C0) and cancerous (C2) linings in the esophagus. In order to develop a classifier with high predictive accuracy, an SVM was trained with a sufficiently large subset of the original endoscopy images. The CAD performance can be improved if the SURF and SVM algorithms operate on delineated (masked) tissue regions. The geometric boundaries

146   Souza Jr et al.

separating malignant parts of the mucosa from early dysplastic stages must be
provided by clinical experts. Note that the SVM classifier should be trained,
validated and tested based on instances from the same set, i.e. either utilizing
features from the full image set or from the set of masked regions, respectively.
Selecting masked areas as Gold Standard is inherently somewhat arbitrary (as
any medical diagnosis), but strongly improves the 'blind' results of full image
classification without similar delineations of suspicious tissue patterns.

The diagnostic accuracy of the designed system expressed by sensitivity and
specificity values is high. As expected, the results of the first approach (full
images) are somewhat lower than those of the second approach (masked) with
0.78 and 0.82 versus 0.90 and 0.95 for sensitivity and specificity, respectively.
It might be argued that using masked regions as test instances is a means to
"fake" the SVM performance, because the delineation of malignant tissue regions
anticipates the actual SVM classification. However, testing the final SVM with
masked area features is twofold legitimate: 1st in order to validate the ultimate
classifier on a higher level (as compared with simple LOPO-CV), and 2nd to rate
attempts of a yet unexperienced clinician (or even an experienced one) to circum-
scribe a cancerous tissue area. While our recent MICCAI Endovis approach was
based on textural (i.e. Haralick) features [7] characterizing local tissue anomalies,
the present study is focussed on the evaluation and classification of structural
(i.e. SURF) features. Motivated by the good results, we will fuse both feature
sets in a further study, expecting a considerable accuracy improvement.

References

1. Dent J. Barrett's esophagus: a historical perspective, an update on core practicali-
   ties and predictions on future evolutions of management. J Gastroenterol Hepatol.
   2011;26:11–30.
2. Sharma P, Bergman JJGHM, Goda K, et al. Development and validation of a classification system to identify high-grade dysplasia and esophageal adenocarcinoma
   in Barretts' esophagus using narrow-band imaging. Gastroenterol. 2016;150:591–8.
3. Phoa KN, Pouw RE, Bisschops R, et al. Multimodality endoscopic eradication for
   neoplastic Barrett's esophagus: results of an european multicentre study (EURO-II).
   Gut. 2015.
4. Sommen FVD, Zinger S, Curvers WL, et al. Computer-aided detection of early
   neoplastic lesions in Barrett's esophagus. Endoscopy. 2016;48(7):617–24.
5. Bay H, Ess A, Tuytelaars T, et al. Speeded-up robust features (SURF). Comput
   Vis Image Underst. 2008;110(3):346–59.
6. Shin HC, Roth HR, Gao M, et al. Deep convolutional neural networks for computer-
   aided detection: CNN architectures, dataset characteristics and transfer learning.
   IEEE Trans Med Imaging. 2016;35(5):1285–98.
7. Palm C. Color texture classification by integrative co-occurrence matrices. Pattern
   Recognit. 2004;37(5):965–76.

Unterstützte Handerkennung in Thermographiebildern zur Validierung der hygienischen Händedesinfektion

Manfred Smieschek[1], André Stollenwerk[1], Stefan Kowalewski[1],
Thorsten Orlikowsky[2], Mark Schoberer[2]

[1]Informatik 11 – Embedded Software, RWTH Aachen University
[2]Scktion Neonatologie, Klinik für Kinder- und Jugendmedizin, Uniklinik RWTH
Aachen
smieschek@embedded.rwth-aachen.de

Kurzfassung. Bei der Verbreitung und Übertragung von Infektionen im Krankenhaus sind die Hände ein zentraler Infektionsweg. Die korrekt ausgeführte hygienische Händedesinfektion ist deshalb entscheidend, um nosokomiale Infektionen zu verhindern. Unser Prototyp, aus voran gegangenen Arbeiten, bewertet die Händedesinfektion mit Hilfe von Infrarotthermographie. Ziel ist dem medizinischen Personal im Krankenhausalltag unmittelbare Rückmeldung über die Qualität ihrer Händedesinfektion zu geben. Dazu ist es essentiell die Hände im Wärmebild zu detektieren, was bei ähnlicher Umgebungs- und Handoberflächentemperatur nicht möglich ist. Hier stellen wir eine Erweiterung unseres Systems vor, welche die benötigte Handdetektion in einem Farbbild robust ermöglicht und transformieren die Ergebnisse anschließend ins Wärmebild.

1 Einleitung

Nosokomiale Infektionen sind Infektionen, die auf einen Krankenhausaufenthalt oder eine Behandlung in einer Pflegeeinrichtung zurückzuführen sind. Sie treten in Europa jährlich bei rund 4 Millionen Patienten auf und sind für rund 37.000 Todesfälle pro Jahr verantwortlich [1]. Schätzungen zufolge könnte ein Drittel aller Krankenhausinfektionen durch bessere Handhygiene verhindert werden. Hierbei stellt die hygienische Händedesinfektion mit Desinfektionsmitteln auf Alkoholbasis die effektivste und kostengünstige Möglichkeit dar [2]. Eine Reinigung der Hände mit Wasser und Seife wird explizit nur bei sichtbarer Verschmutzung der Hände empfohlen [3]. Typische Fehlverhalten bei der Händedesinfektion sind das vollständige Auslassen der Desinfektion, sowie das unzureichende Verteilen des Desinfektionsmittels, wodurch in den Benetzungslücken potentiell pathogene Erreger auf den Händen verbleiben. Wir adressieren an dieser Stelle ausdrücklich nur den Fall der unzulänglichen hygienischen Händedesinfektion. Dazu stellen wir eine Erweiterung unseres Systems vor, welches mittels Infrarotthermographieaufnahmen der Hände vor und nach der Desinfektion Benetzungslücken detektieren kann. Die vorgestellte Erweiterung fokussiert sich auf das Ermöglichen einer Segmentierung der Hände im Wärmebild.

2 Material und Methoden

Bei der Händedesinfektion werden in der Regel Desinfektionsmittel auf Alkoholbasis verwendet. Diese sind sehr flüchtig und verdunsten während des Desinfektionsvorgangs. Dieser Vorgang entzieht der Umgebung Energie und lässt sie abkühlen, auch bekannt als Verdunstungskälte. Vorarbeiten haben gezeigt, dass sich die Thermographie eignet diesen Temperaturunterschied aufzuzeichnen [4]. Der hierfür von uns entwickelte Prototyp besteht aus einer Infrarotkamera (PIR uc 180, InfraTec), die zentral im Aufbau montiert ist. Der Aufbau ist bis auf einen kleinen Schlitz zum Einführen der Hände verschlossen. Dadurch sollen ungewollte Störgrößen wie Lichteinfall und Reflektionen verringert werden. Das Verfahren sieht vor, dass der Benutzer seine Hände vor und nach der Händedesinfektion in diesen Aufbau einführt, um jeweils ein Wärmebild aufzuzeichnen. Anschließend wird die Temperaturdifferenz bestimmt, um so Benetzungslücken zu erkennen. Hierbei ist ein pixelweises Differenzieren der gemessenen Temperaturen zur Bestimmung der Temperaturveränderung nicht möglich, da man davon ausgehen muss, dass sich die Handpositionen zwischen den Aufnahmen verändert haben. Aus diesem Grund müssen die Hände in den Aufnahmen detektiert und segmentiert werden. Insgesamt wird jede Hand in 20 Segmente aufgeteilt, die in Anlehnung an die Fingerknochen des Menschen definiert wurden. Der Handteller wurde in sechs Segmente unterteilt. Alle extrahierten Segmente werden gegen ein Handmodel registriert. Im folgenden Schritt berechnen wir die durchschnittliche Temperatur für die einzelnen Segmente und bilden die Differenz zwischen der Vorher- und Nachher-Aufnahme [4].

Für die Extraktion der Hände haben wir bisher die Wärmebilder binarisiert. Dieses Vorgehen ist jedoch problematisch, wenn die Handoberflächentemperatur und die Temperatur des Hintergrunds zu ähnlich sind. Abb. 1 zeigt links ein grauwertkodiertes Wärmebild und rechts daneben das dazugehörige binarisierte Bild. Es ist deutlich zu sehen, dass durch den geringen Temperaturunterschied zwischen Handoberfläche und Hintergrund bei der Binarisierung zwischen den beiden nicht unterschieden werden kann und das resultierende Binärbild für eine anschließende Segmentierung unbrauchbar ist. Dies ist ein fundamentales Problem der Thermographie, dass im Wärmebild selbst nicht gelöst werden kann.

Zur Evaluation unseres Verfahrens haben wir initial eine Webcam (Logitech C910, Logitech) zusammen mit der Infrarotkamera installiert, um unsere Ergeb-

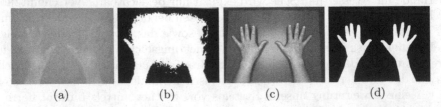

(a)   (b)   (c)   (d)

Abb. 1. (a) Grauwertkodiertes Wärmebild, (b) zum Wärmebild gehöriges Binärbild, (c) parallel aufgenommenes Farbbild, (d) Binärbild des Rotkanals des Farbbildes.

nisse mit der zur klinischen Hygieneschulung etablierten Fluoreszenzmethode vergleichen zu können [4, 5]. Diese Webcam nutzen wir, um parallel zu den Wärmebildern auch Farbbilder der Hände vor und nach der Händedesinfektion aufzunehmen. Den Untergrund unseres Aufbaus haben wir grün gefärbt, so dass sich im Farbbild die Hände mittels Chroma Keying zuverlässig erkennen lassen, da der Hintergrund einen geringen Rotanteil hat und die Hautfarbe der Hände einen hohen Rotanteil hat. Abb. 1 zeigt mittig rechts das Farbbild, welches parallel zum links abgebildeten grauwertkodierten Wärmebild aufgenommen wurde, und ganz rechts das entsprechende Binärbild gewonnen aus dem Rotkanal des Farbbildes. Die auf diese Weise erkannten Hände können, wie vorher beschrieben, segmentiert und gegen ein Handmodel registriert werden.

Da die Bildebenen der Thermographiekamera und Webcam versetzt sind, können die im Farbbild extrahierten Hände nicht direkt in das Wärmebild übertragen werden, sondern müssen durch eine entsprechende Transformation projiziert werden. Eine einfache Form der Projektion bietet eine Homographie-Matrix, zu deren Berechnung korrespondierende Punkte in beiden Bildern benötigt werden. Zu diesem Zweck haben wir ein Kalibrierungsobjekt erarbeitet, das sowohl im Farb- als auch im Wärmebild ausreichend gut sichtbar ist. Das Kalibrierungsmuster wurde analog zu Lagüela et al. [6] erstellt. Es enthält 36 Schrauben, die im asymmetrischen 4 × 9 Muster an einem Holzbrett angebracht wurden. Die Schrauben sind auf der Unterseite über einen Draht miteinander verbunden und können durch Zufuhr von elektrischen Strom erhitzt werden. In Abb. 2 zeigt das linke Bild das Kalibrierungsobjekt im Farbbild. Die dunklen Schraubenköpfe heben sich deutlich vom hellen Holz ab. Das rechte Bild zeigt die aufgewärmten Schraubenköpfe im graukodierten Wärmebild. Auch hier sind die Schraubenköpfe gut erkennbar. Durch ihre runde Form sind sie auch automatisch als Punkte mittels Schwerpunktfindung aus den Bildern extrahierbar.

Da das Brett des Kalibrierungsmusters auf einem Lasercutter (Epilog Zing 6030, cameo Laser Franz Hagemann GmbH), mit ausreichender Genauigkeit (1000 dpi), nach einer bekannten Vorlage gefertigt wurde, lassen sich mit den extrahierten Punktkorrespondenzen zum einen die intrinsischen Kameraparameter

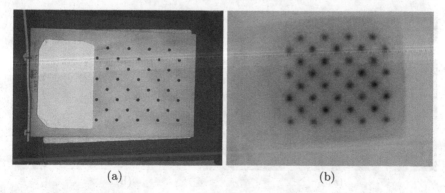

(a)   (b)

Abb. 2. (a) Farbbild des erarbeiteten Kalibrierungsobjekts, (b) grauwertkodiertes Wärmebild des aufgeheizten Kalibrierungsobjekts.

der beiden Kameras (K_a und K_b), i. e. Brennweite, Bildmittelpunkt und Pixels-
kalierung, und zum anderen die erwähnte Homographie-Matrix (H_{ba}) berechnen.
Mit diesen drei Matrizen ist es möglich einen Punkt p_a, der von Kamera a aufgenommen wurde, in den korrespondierenden Punkt p_b im Bild von Kamera b
zu transformieren, falls sich dieser Punkt in derselben Ebene in den Weltkoordi-
naten befindet, für die die Kalibration durchgeführt wurde. Die Transformation
erfolgt nach der Formel

$$p_a = K_a \cdot H_{ba} \cdot K_b^{-1} \cdot p_b \tag{1}$$

Das veränderte Vorgehen sieht vor die Hände im Farbbild zu erkennen, in
die 20 Segmente aufzuteilen, und anschließend in das Wärmebild zu projizieren.
Abb. 3 zeigt links beispielhaft ein Farbbild, das vor der Händedesinfektion aufgenommen wurde. Im Farbbild wurden die Hände wie beschrieben durch Binarisierung erkannt, segmentiert und registriert. Die segmentierten Hände wurden
anschließend mit der Gleichung (1) in das parallel aufgenommene Wärmebild
projiziert. Abb. 3 zeigt rechts das graukodierte Wärmebild überlagert mit den
projizierten 20 Handsegmenten. Die signifikant höhere Auflösung der Webcam
(640×480 Pixel) gegenüber der Thermographiekamera (160×120 Pixel) ermöglicht die Handposition in der Thermographiebildebene subpixelgenau zu bestimmen. Für diesen Vorgang muss nur einmalig vorher die Kalibrierung durchgeführt werden, um die Homographie und die intrinsischen Kameraparameter zu
berechnen.

3   Ergebnisse

Im Zuge der Entwicklung unseres Prototypen zur Handdesinfektionsvalidierung
wurden 198 Händedesinfektionen durch medizinisches Personal in Kooperation
mit Mitarbeitern der Kinderklinik des UK Aachen aufgenommen. Dazu wurde
ein Händedesinfektionsmittel auf Propanol-Basis (Sterillium classic pure, Bode Chemie GmbH, Hamburg) unter Zusatz von, des zur Evaluation benötigten,

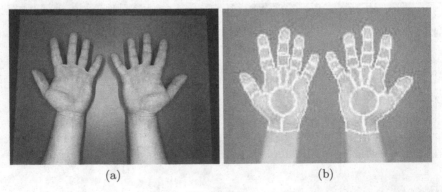

(a)   (b)

Abb. 3. (a) Beispiel für ein Farbbild vor der Händedesinfektion, (b) das entsprechende
graukodierte Wärmebild mit überlagerter Segmentierung der Hände.

unter UV-Licht fluoreszierendem, Farbstoff (Visirub Concentrat, Bode Chemie GmbH, Hamburg), verwendet. Von den 198 Aufnahmen konnten 8 nicht ausgewertet werden, da die Finger nicht genügend gespreizt waren und es Überlagerungen bei den Fingern gab, so dass die Registrierung gegen das Handmodel nicht durchgeführt werden konnte. Bei der Auswertung mussten wir feststellen, dass der Großteil der übrigen 190 Aufnahmen ebenfalls nicht auswertbar ist.

Bei 110 Aufnahmen war die gemessene Hauttemperatur nach der Desinfektion höher als vorher. Dies führen wir auf Reibungswärme zurück. Medizinisches Personal wird in der Ausbildung angewiesen das Desinfektionsmittel solange auf den Händen zu verteilen, bis die Hände trocken sind. Die entstehende Reibungswärme negiert den Effekt der Verdunstungskälte vollständig. Aber auch bei den Aufnahmen, in denen eine Abkühlung festgestellt wurde, müssen wir davon ausgehen, dass Reibungswärme mit eingeflossen ist.

Bei 130 Aufnahmen führte die vorgestellte Projektion zu Fehlern. Abb. 4 zeigt links das Farbbild und rechts das grauwertkodierte Wärmebild mit überlagerter Projektion der Handsegmente. Im rechten Bild ist deutlich zu sehen, dass die Fingerspitzen der erkannten Hand über die reale Hand hinausragen. Als Grund konnten wir die angewinkelte Handstellung ausmachen. Die von uns angewandte Transformationsvorschrift gilt nur für die Ebene in der die beiden Kameras zueinander kalibriert wurden. Die Fingerspitzen verlassen in diesen Fällen die Kalibrierungsebene, was in Abbildungsfehlern resultiert. Als Konsequenz wird in die berechnete Durchschnittstemperatur der betrachteten Segmente zum Teil der Hintergrund mit einbezogen, was die gemittelte Temperatur verfälscht.

4 Diskussion

Wir haben ein Verfahren untersucht um die Position der Hände robust in Wärmebildern zu bestimmen. Dafür haben wir eine Thermographiekamera und eine Webcam gegeneinander kalibriert. Die daraus gewonnene Transformationsvorschrift konnten wir in eigenen Versuchen erfolgreich dazu nutzen Hände im

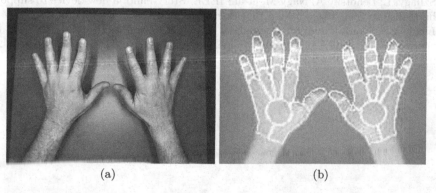

(a)   (b)

Abb. 4. (a) Beispiel für ein Farbbild mit angewinkelten Händen, (b) das entsprechende graukodierte Wärmebild mit Projektionsfehlern der überlagerten Segmentierung.

Wärmebild zu detektieren, die sonst wegen zu geringem Temperaturunterschied zum Hintergrund nicht hätten erkannt werden können.

Eine erste Benutzerstudie zeigte jedoch, dass es häufig zu signifikanten Projektionsfehlern kommt, weil die berechnete Homographie nur für die Kalibrierungsebene gilt. Zur Lösung des Problems streben wir eine 3D Kalibrierung an, damit frei wählbare Handpositionen korrekt in die Thermographiebildebene projiziert werden können. Hierzu ist eine Erweiterung des Aufbaus um eine zweite Webcam nötig.

Die Untersuchungen haben gezeigt, dass neben physiologischen und Umgebungsfaktoren die Durchführung der Händedesinfektion selbst erheblichen Einfluss auf den Wärmeunterschied vor und nach der Desinfektion hat. Die Wärmeerzeugung durch Reibung zwischen den gegeneinander geriebenen Handteilen wirkt dem kühlenden Effekt der Verdunstung entgegen und übersteigt diesen. Insofern hat sich gezeigt, dass untersucht werden muss zu welchem Zeitpunkt des aktuell geschulten Desinfektionsablaufs das hier vorgestellte Verfahren anzuwenden ist, um zu bestmöglichen Ergebnissen zu führen.

Literaturverzeichnis

1. Gastmeier P, Geffers C, Herrmann M, et al. Nosokomiale Infektionen und Infektionen mit multiresistenten Erregern. Häufigkeit und Sterblichkeit. Dtsch Med Wochenschr. 2016;141(06):421–6.
2. Pittet D, Hugonnet S, Harbarth S, et al. Effectiveness of a hospital-wide programme to improve compliance with hand hygiene. J Lancet. 2000;356(9238):1307–12.
3. Centers for Disease Control and Prevention. Guideline for hand hygiene in healthcare settings: recommendations of the healthcare infection control practices advisory committee and the HICPAC/SHEA/APIC/IDSA hand hygiene task force. MMWR CDC Surveill Summ. 2002;51(8):1–59.
4. Smieschek M, Stollenwerk A, Jüptner P, et al. Evaluating hand disinfection with alcohol-based hand sanitizers using thermal imaging. Proc CEUR. 2016;1559(2):174–81.
5. Szilágyi L, Lehotsky Á, Nagy M, et al.; IEEE. Stery-hand: a new device to support hand disinfection. Procs J Med Biol Eng. 2010; p. 4756–9.
6. Lagüela S, González-Jorge H, Armesto J, et al. Calibration and verification of thermographic cameras for geometric measurements. Infrared Phys. 2011;54(2):92–9.

Abstract: Quantitative Photoakustische Tomografie durch lokale Kontextkodierung

Janek Gröhl, Thomas Kirchner, Lena Maier-Hein

Abteilung für Computer-assistierte Medizinische Interventionen, DKFZ Heidelberg
j.groehl@dkfz.de

Photoakustische Tomografie (PAT) ist eine neue strukturelle und funktionale Bildgebung, welche die Darstellung von optischen Absorbern im Gewebe ermöglicht. Im Gegensatz zu anderen weit verbreiteten Modalitäten ermöglicht PAT die Aufnahme von Bildern in Echtzeit und ohne Strahlungsbelastung. Dabei bietet PAT eine hohe räumliche und zeitliche Auflösung. Anders als etablierte optische Bildgebungsverfahren ist PAT in der Lage, optische Parameter mehrere Zentimeter tief im Gewebe zu messen. Jüngste Studien zeigen vielversprechende klinische Anwendungen, unter anderem die Darstellung von Wächterlymphknoten [1] oder die Beobachtung der Aktivität von entzündlichen Prozessen bei Morbus Crohn [2].

Eine der Hauptherausforderungen für die klinische Anwendbarkeit von PAT ist, dass optische Eigenschaften des Gewebes nicht zuverlässig quantifiziert werden können. Dies ist jedoch eine wichtige Voraussetzung für viele multispektrale Anwendungen wie beispielsweise die Schätzung der lokalen Blutsauerstoffsättigung. Das gemessene Signal ist nicht nur proportional zum optischen Absorptionskoeffizienten des Gewebes, sondern zusätzlich abhängig von der optischen Fluenz, welche wiederum von den optischen Eigenschaften des Gewebes und der Art der Beleuchtung abhängig ist. Bisherige Ansätze in der Literatur für die Korrektur für diesen Term scheitern an geringer Robustheit und langen Rechenzeiten.

In diesem Beitrag präsentieren wir einen neuartigen Ansatz zur Quantifizierung von PAT. Mittels einer Methode zur Schätzung der Fluenz in jedem Voxel aus lokaler Kontextinformation kann das PAT Signal korrigiert werden. Erste in silico Experimente zeigen eine hohe Genauigkeit und Robustheit des neuen Konzepts bei um Größenordnungen geringeren Rechenzeiten im Vergleich zu verwandten Verfahren. Sollte eine ähnliche Performanz in vivo erreicht werden, ist das Potential des neuen Ansatzes für die klinische Anwendung enorm.

Literaturverzeichnis

1. Erpelding TN, Garcia-Uribe A, Krumholz A, et al.; International Society for Optics; Photonics. A dual-modality photoacoustic and ultrasound imaging system for noninvasive sentinel lymph node detection: preliminary clinical results. SPIE BiOS. 2014; p. 894359.
2. Waldner MJ, Knieling F, Egger C, et al. Multispectral optoacoustic tomography in Crohn's disease: non-invasive imaging of disease activity. Gastroenterol. 2016.

3D Histograms of Oriented Gradients zur Registrierung von regulären CT mit interventionellen CBCT Daten

Barbara Trimborn[1,4], Ivo Wolf[1], Denis Abu-Sammour[2], Thomas Henzler[3], Lothar R. Schad[4], Frank G. Zöllner[4]

[1]Institut für Medizinische Informatik, Hochschule Mannheim
[2]Institut für Instrumentelle Analytik und Bioanalytik, Hochschule Mannheim
[3]Institut für Klinische Radiologie und Nuklearmedizin,
Medizinische Fakultät Mannheim, Universität Heidelberg
[4]Lehrstuhl für Computerunterstütze Klinische Medizin,
Medizinische Fakultät Mannheim, Universität Heidelberg
b.trimborn@hs-mannheim.de

Zur Unterstützung onkologischer Interventionen können durch die Registrierung präoperativer Bildaten zu intraoperativen Cone-Beam-Computertomographieaufnahmen (CBCT) zusätzliche Informationen über die Anatomie und Morphologie des Patienten erhalten werden. In der vorliegenden Arbeit wird eine neuartige Metrik für die gradientenbasierte Bildregistrierung vorgestellt. Grundlage dieser Metrik ist die lokale Bestimmung von Histograms of Oriented Gradients (HOG) [1], welche die Basis für einen Merkmalsvektor bilden. Die Metrik wurde zur Registrierung präinterventioneller CT-Daten zu intrainterventionellen CBCT-Daten einer transateriellen Chemoembolisation verwendet und die Ergebnisse mit den Resultaten bei Verwendung einer normierten Kreuzkorrelationsmetrik verglichen. Als Vergleichsgrundlage diente hierbei die Bestimmung des Capture Range der Metrik basierend auf dem mittleren Registrierungsfehler [2]. Die Ergebnisse zeigen, dass die auf HOG beruhende Metrik mit etablierten Methoden bzgl. der Registrierungsgenauigkeit konkurrieren kann.

Literaturverzeichnis

1. Dalal N, Triggs B. Histograms of oriented gradients for human detection. Proc IEEE Comput Soc Conf Comput Vis Pattern Recognit. 2005;1:886–93.
2. van de Kraats EB, Penney GP, Tomazevi D, et al. Standardized evaluation methodology for 2-D-3-D registration. IEEE Trans Med Imaging. 2005;24(9):1177–89.

A Kernel Ridge Regression Model for Respiratory Motion Estimation in Radiotherapy

Tobias Geimer[1,2], Adriana Birlutiu[3], Mathias Unberath[1,2],
Oliver Taubmann[1,2], Christoph Bert[2,4], Andreas Maier[1,2]

[1]Pattern Recognition Lab, Friedrich-Alexander-Universität Erlangen-Nürnberg
[2]Graduate School in Advanced Optical Technologies (SAOT), Erlangen
[3]Computer Science Department, "1 December 1918" University of Alba Iulia,
Romania
[4]Department of Radiation Oncology, Universitätsklinikum Erlangen,
Friedrich-Alexander-Universität Erlangen-Nürnberg
tobias.geimer@fau.de

Abstract. This paper discusses a kernel ridge regression (KRR) model
for motion estimation in radiotherapy. Using KRR, dense internal motion
fields are estimated from high-dimensional surrogates without the need
for prior dimensionality reduction. We compare the proposed model to a
related approach with dimensionality reduction in the form of principal
component analysis and principle component regression. Evaluation was
performed in a simulation study based on nine 4D CT patient data sets
achieving a mean estimation error of 0.84 ± 0.21 mm for our approach.

1 Introduction

Respiratory motion is of concern for several medical procedures in the thoracic
and abdominal areas. In external beam radiation therapy, intra-fractional motion may lead to underdosing the clinical target volume (CTV), if not addressed
properly [1]. The patient is irradiated according to a treatment plan based on
CT imaging, defining an optimized dose distribution. However, respiratory motion typically leads to displacement of the CTV, resulting in insufficient dose in
the target and thus the potential survival of malignant cells. One option is to introduce additional margins covering the extent of the CTV's motion at the cost
of higher dose to healthy tissue. More preferably, real-time motion estimation
can be used to either restrict exposure time to certain parts of the respiratory
cycle (gating) or adjust the beam according to the target volume (tracking).

For real-time motion estimation, a patient-specific motion model can be
trained pre-procedurally connecting a highly correlated external surrogate signal to the corresponding internal deformation [2]. The ground-truth deformation field is usually obtained from 4D imaging by registration to a reference
phase. In recent literature, various methods for ground-truth-to-surrogate correspondence estimation such as (multi-)linear regression [3] are employed. Then,
intra-procedural acquisition of just the surrogate signal allows for inference of
the internal motion field [2].

Wilms et al. [3] investigated multi-variate regression approaches based on range imaging among other surrogates. While these approaches operate directly on the acquired data, others also based on multi-linear regression incorporate an additional generalization step in the form of Principal Component Analysis (PCA) to describe both the internal and external variation of a patient's breathing cycle [4, 5]. As an additional benefit, the reduced dimensionality in feature space also reduces the complexity of the regression problem. Another way of dealing with high-dimensional domains is to incorporate kernels into the regression. Li and Xing [6] investigated kernel-based respiratory motion estimation but only used a 1-D surrogate. The major benefit of such a kernel approach is its ability to represent non-linear mappings between internal and external motion.

In this work, we present a correlation model based on Kernel Ridge Regression (KRR) to estimate dense internal motion fields from two marker-less high-dimensional surrogates: range imaging [7] and X-ray fluoroscopy. We evaluate our approach in a simulation study on 4D CT data of nine cancer patients and compare it to Principal Component Regression (PCR).

2   Materials and methods

First, we will introduce our notation. Then, the two correlation approaches will be covered: a) related work in the form of PCR and b) KRR without prior dimensionality reduction. An overview of our data and evaluation methods will conclude the section.

2.1   Data matrices

The respiratory motion model can be trained pre-procedurally from 4D imaging such as the planning CT for radiotherapy. Performing demons-based non-rigid registration [8], n internal deformation fields $\{t_1, \ldots, t_n\}, t_i \in \mathbb{R}^{d_t}$ are obtained, that are stored column-wise in the data matrix $T \in \mathbb{R}^{d_t \times n}$. Similarly, $S \in \mathbb{R}^{d_s \times n}$ denotes the n corresponding surrogate observations $s_i \in \mathbb{R}^{d_s}$. These can either be the patient's thorax surface motion fields or fluoroscopic images at the same breathing phase. For training purposes, they are extracted from the 4D CT as well (Sec. 2.4).

2.2   Principal component regression

Principal component analysis. PCA is a popular linear dimensionality reduction technique [9]. It can be used to decompose a given data set into mutually orthogonal modes of variation, called principal components. With the first few components often being sufficient to represent more than 90% of the variance present in the data set, the number of basis vectors is less than that of the original domain. Using PCA, the data sets $S \in \mathbb{R}^{d_s \times n}$ and $T \in \mathbb{R}^{d_t \times n}$ can, therefore, be represented by a set of features $F_S \in \mathbb{R}^{p_s \times n}$ and $F_T \in \mathbb{R}^{p_t \times n}$ of reduced dimensionality.

Multi-linear regression. Let $F_S \in \mathbb{R}^{p_s \times n}$ and $F_T \in \mathbb{R}^{p_t \times n}$, where n is the number of observations and p_s, d_t denote feature dimensionality chosen for the PCA. Correlation between the target and the surrogate domain can be formulated as a multi-linear regression problem [4]. Combined with Tikhonov regularization, this is also known as (standard) Ridge Regression with the corresponding objective function

$$\underset{W}{\operatorname{argmin}} \left(\frac{1}{2}\|WF_S - F_T\|_{\mathcal{F}}^2 + \alpha\frac{1}{2}\|W\|_{\mathcal{F}}^2 \right) \tag{1}$$

where $\|\cdot\|_{\mathcal{F}}$ is the Frobenius norm. The closed-form solution involves the Moore-Penrose pseudo-inverse

$$W = \underbrace{F_T F_S^\top}_{p_t \times p_s} (\underbrace{F_S F_S^\top}_{p_s \times p_s} + \alpha \mathbb{I}_{p_s})^{-1} \in \mathbb{R}^{p_t \times p_s} \tag{2}$$

which is computed using singular value decomposition (SVD). For low-dimensional feature spaces $(p_s, p_t \leq n)$ W can be calculated explicitly.

2.3   Kernel ridge regression

The KRR method [9] is a regularized least squares method for classification and regression. For high-dimensional data T and S an explicit computation of W as presented in (2) without prior dimensionality reduction is computationally expensive (as $d_s, d_t \gg p_s, p_t$). Fortunately, (2) can be rewritten to

$$W = \underbrace{TS^\top}_{d_t \times d_s} (\underbrace{SS^\top}_{d_s \times d_s} + \alpha \mathbb{I}_{d_s})^{-1}$$

$$= \underbrace{T}_{d_t \times n} (\underbrace{S^\top S}_{n \times n} + \alpha \mathbb{I}_n)^{-1} \underbrace{S^\top}_{n \times d_s} \tag{3}$$

Making use of the kernel trick, the observations s_i are implicitly mapped to an even higher-dimensional Reproducing Kernel Hilbert space [10]

$$\Phi = \left[\phi(s_1), \ldots, \phi(s_n) \right] \tag{4}$$

When predicting a target t_{pred} from a new observation s_{new}, explicit access to Φ is never actually needed

$$t_{\text{pred}} = T \left(\Phi^\top \Phi + \alpha \, \mathbb{I}_n \right)^{-1} \Phi^\top \phi(s_{\text{new}})$$

$$= T \left(K + \alpha \, \mathbb{I}_n \right)^{-1} \kappa \left(s_{\text{new}} \right) \tag{5}$$

With $K_{ij} = \phi(s_i)^\top \phi(s_j)$ and $\kappa(s_{\text{new}})_i = \phi(s_i)^\top \phi(s_{\text{new}})$, the prediction can be described entirely in terms of inner products in the higher-dimensional space. Not only does this approach work on the original data sets as well as the principal component representations, it also opens up ways to introduce non-linear mappings into the regression.

2.4 Data and evaluation

Evaluation was conducted on nine 4D CT data sets of lung tumor patients treated at UK Erlangen. Each data set provided nine respiratory deformation fields of spacing $0.97 \times 0.97 \times 2.5\,\text{mm}^3$, which were manually cropped to an internal region of interest (ROI) to represent the ground truth. For simulating the range imaging surrogate data, the fields were interpolated at a surface mesh directly extracted from the CT acquisition at the reference phase. This provided between 2252 and 4667 surface points for each patient. For fluoroscopy, Digitally Reconstructed Radiographs (DRR) with 1024×768 pixels and $0.39\,\text{mm}$ pixel spacing were generated by forward-projecting the 4D CT volumes.

Leave-one-out evaluation was performed for each of the patients individually. Each phase was subsequently tested and, for this purpose, removed from the training sample together with its two neighbors. Estimation accuracy was assessed by the L2-norm of the residual vectors between estimated field and ground truth. Parameters for regularization and the Gaussian kernel were determined using grid search in the same leave-one-out manner. Similarly, internal model accuracy was determined, given perfect estimation of the weights from the surrogate. For PCR, the generalization ability of the internal model is the limiting factor. For KRR, each deformation field t_i was compared to the optimal guess $t_{i,\text{optim}} = T a_i$, where $a_i = \operatorname{argmin}_{\tilde{a}_i} \left(\|T \tilde{a}_i - t_i\|_2^2 \right)$. This deformation field arises from interpolation weights that are optimal in a least-squares sense. As a result, we have a lower bound on the estimation error (dashed lines in Fig. 3).

3 Results

Fig. 1 shows the grid search result for PCR. Estimation error decreases for higher internal model dimensionality as more components also explain a higher amount of variance present in the data. The need for regularization was low for both surrogate types. The overall estimation error averaged over all patients and

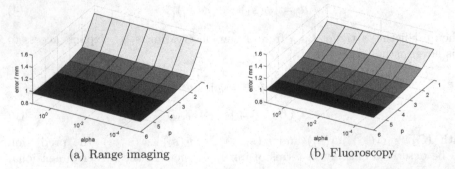

(a) Range imaging   (b) Fluoroscopy

Fig. 1. Estimation error using surrogates from range imaging (a) and fluoroscopy (b) for $p = 1, \ldots, 6$ components and different regularization strengths.

phases is plotted in Fig. 2. For a more detailed look, Fig. 3 shows the estimation error of a single patient for each breathing phase for the surface surrogate only, including the breathing magnitude and the inherent model error for each phase.

In general, all proposed methods are suitable for motion estimation with a mean estimation error of around 1.0 ± 0.22 mm compared to a reference mean magnitude of 2.48 ± 0.81 mm without compensation. Data-based KRR for the surface surrogate achieved the best average estimation error of 0.84 ± 0.21 mm.

4   Discussion

Contrary to expectation, no significant benefits could be observed from applying non-linear KRR instead of PCR. This may be due to the low number of 6 phases available to train the models. Special attention should be given to the way the internal motion is reconstructed for PCR and KRR, respectively. In the case of KRR, the new phase is a linear interpolation between all observed phases. For PCR, the regression result yields the weights for the principal components from which the internal motion field is reconstructed as a linear combination of eigenvectors. Thus, PCA introduces an additional generalization step not present in data-based KRR. However, from the dashed lines in Fig. 3 it can be seen that the principal components lack the variation to describe an entire cycle. Because of our 6 : 3 split for training and evaluation, the internal model only observed two thirds of a breathing cycle. This is particularly obvious for phases near end-exhale where the magnitude of breathing is low. Here, both PCR and Gaussian kernel produce errors higher than the reference magnitude. Only surface-based linear KRR was able to cope with low-magnitude phases near end-exhale. For the fluoroscopy surrogate, however, this trend could not be observed.

In summary, all mean estimation errors were close to their respective lower bound. Thus, the major bottleneck seems to be the reconstruction of the new phase from the internal model rather than the correlation problem itself.

For future work, an extended evaluation of both PCR and KRR is necessary. Using a patient's planning CT to train on an entire breathing cycle with evaluation on a potential follow-up CT will bring evaluation closer to the actual

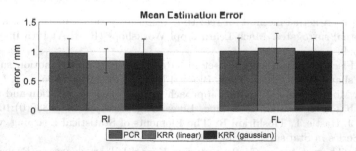

Fig. 2. Mean estimation error using PCR and KRR with a linear and a Gaussian kernel for the surface (RI) and the fluoroscopy (FL) surrogate.

Fig. 3. Surface-based estimation error for each phase of patient 9. The black bars show the mean magnitude of the ground truth deformation field, while the dashed black lines indicate the lower bound for the mean error achievable with the respective model.

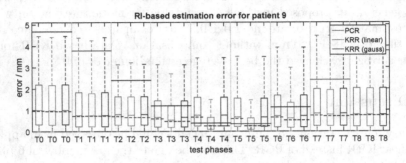

application case, where the treatment is performed days or even weeks after the planning images were acquired. This will also give a good indication whether the additional generalization step of PCA will proof beneficial in comparison to the phase interpolation of KRR.

References

1. Keall PJ, Mageras GS, Balter JM, et al. The management of respiratory motion in radiation oncology report of AAPM Task Group 76. Med Phys. 2006;33(10):3874–900.
2. McClelland JR, Hawkes DJ, Schaeffter T, et al. Respiratory motion models: a review. Med Image Anal. 2013;17(1):19–42.
3. Wilms M, Werner R, Ehrhardt J, et al. Multivariate regression approaches for surrogate-based diffeomorphic estimation of respiratory motion in radiation therapy. Phys Med Biol. 2014;59(5):1147.
4. Taubmann O, Wasza J, Forman C, et al. Prediction of respiration-induced internal 3-D deformation fields from dense external 3-D surface motion. Proc CARS. 2014; p. 33–4.
5. Geimer T, Unberath M, Taubmann O, et al. Combination of markerless surrogates for motion estimation in radiation therapy. 30th Trans Comput Assist Radiol Surg (CARS). 2016; p. 59–60.
6. Li R, Xing L. A kernel method for real-time respiratory tumor motion estimation using external surrogates. Mach Learn Appl Workshops (ICMLA) 10th Int Conf. 2011;2:206–9.
7. Wasza J, Fischer P, Leutheuser H, et al. Real-time respiratory motion snalysis using 4-D shape priors. IEEE Trans Biomed Eng. 2016;63(3):485–95.
8. Fischer B, Modersitzki J. A unified approach to fast image registration and a new curvature based registration technique. Linear Algebra Appl. 2004;380(0):107–24.
9. Friedman J, Hastie T, Tibshirani R. The Elements of Statistical Learning. vol. 1. Springer Series in Statistics, Berlin; 2001.
10. Berlinet A, Thomas-Agnan C. Reproducing Kernel Hilbert Spaces in Probability and Statistics. Springer Science & Business Media; 2011.

Low Rank-&-Sparse Matrix Decomposition as Stroke Segmentation Prior: Useful or Not?
A Random Forest-Based Evaluation Study

René Werner[1], Daniel Schetelig[1], Thilo Sothmann[1], Eike Mücke[1],
Matthias Wilms[2], Bastian Cheng[3], Nils D. Forkert[4]

[1]Department of Computational Neuroscience,
University Medical Center Hamburg-Eppendorf
[2]Institute of Medical Informatics, University of Lübeck
[3]Department of Neurology, University Medical Center Hamburg-Eppendorf
[4]Department of Radiology & Hotchkiss Brain Institute, University of Calgary
r.werner@uke.de

Abstract. Manual ischemic stroke lesion segmentation in MR image
data is a time-consuming task subject to inter-rater variability. Reliable
automated lesion segmentation is of high interest for clinical trials and research in ischemic stroke. However, recent segmentation challenges (e.g.
ISLES 2015) illustrate that current state-of-the-art approaches still lack
accuracy and ischemic stroke segmentation remains a complicated problem. Within this context, low rank-&-sparse matrix decomposition (also
known as robust PCA, RPCA) and RPCA-based non-linear subject-to-
atlas registration could provide valuable segmentation prior information.
The aim of this study is to evaluate the suitability of RPCA and RPCA-
based registration for ischemic stroke segmentation in follow-up FLAIR
MR data sets. Building on a top-ranked segmentation approach of ISLES
2015, the performance of RPCA sparse component image information as
random forest (RF) feature is evaluated. A comprehensive feature-by-
feature comparison of the segmentation performance with and without
RPCA sparse component information as RF feature illustrate the potential of low rank-&-sparse decomposition to improve stroke segmentation.

1 Introduction

Ischemic stroke has been reported to be the most common cerebrovascular disease, a leading cause of death and disability worldwide [1], and is, consequently,
the subject of many clinical trials and research projects. Stroke-related studies
often require segmenting the stroke lesions in mono- or multi-modal MR images
(e.g. for computation of the lesion volume as trial end-point or co-variate [2]).
The segmentation is usually performed manually by a clinical expert. As this is
a time-consuming process and associated to high inter-rater differences, reliable
and reproducible automatic stroke lesion segmentation is of high interest.

An overview of state-of-the-art approaches for automatic stroke lesion segmentation methods is, for example, described in the MICCAI ischemic stroke

lesion segmentation (ISLES) challenge [3]. ISLES revealed that especially automatic segmentation of sub-acute lesions (SISS part of the challenge) lacks accuracy, which motivates developing novel and extending existing methods.

In this context, low rank-&-sparse matrix decomposition (also known as robust PCA, RPCA) could prove valuable. Already commonly applied, e.g., for foreground-background separation in computer vision, RPCA has recently gained increasing interest in medical image computing. For instance, Liu et al. proposed incorporating RPCA into a registration framework to enable unbiased atlas generation in the presence of pathologies [4]. The main idea was to decompose a matrix of patient images into a low-rank matrix that contains population-consistent intensity information and a sparse matrix that ideally captures only the pathologies of the different patients. The low rank matrix information was then used for registration purposes. However, Liu *et al.* also suggested that the sparse matrix information could be used as spatial prior for tumor segmentation. This hypothesis, which has not been tested in detail so far, can also be transferred to the task of stroke lesion segmentation. Consequently, building on one of the best performing approaches of the SISS subchallenge of ISLES 2015, we investigate whether the RPCA sparse component(s) of stroke lesion MR images provide valuable information for random forest-based stroke lesion segmentation.

2   Materials and methods

2.1   Low rank-&-sparse matrix decomposition

Interpreting a series of mono-modal MR data sets $I_i : \Omega \subset \mathbb{R}^3 \to \mathbb{R}$ of the patients $i = 1, \ldots, p$ in discrete and vector shape form $\tilde{I}_i \in \mathbb{R}^m$ (m: number of voxels) as a 'corrupted' (here: pathology-affected) measurement matrix $I = \left(\tilde{I}_1 \ldots \tilde{I}_p \right) \in \mathbb{R}^{m \times p}$, low rank-&-sparse matrix decomposition reads

$$\{L_0, S_0\} = \underset{L,S}{\arg\min} \ (\mathrm{rk}\,(L) + \lambda \|S\|_0) \ \text{s.t.} \ L + S = I$$

$$\approx \underset{L,S}{\arg\min} \ (\|L\|_* + \lambda \|S\|_1) \ \text{s.t.} \ L + S = I \tag{1}$$

As written before, equation (1) aims at separating inter-patient consistent image information and patient-specific anomalous appearance into $L_0 \in \mathbb{R}^{m \times p}$ and $S_0 \in \mathbb{R}^{m \times p}$, respectively. The nuclear norm $\|L\|_* := \sum_i \sigma_i (L)$, i.e. the sum of the singular values σ_i of L, and the l_1-norm of S approximate the desired 'low rank' $\mathrm{rk}(L)$ and the l_0-norm sparsity to allow for convex optimization. Here, the augmented Lagrangian multiplier approach of [5] was used to solve (1).

Application of (1) requires aligning the images I_i to avoid that inter-patient positioning and anatomical differences lead to S_0 contributions. Since image alignment and matrix decomposition influence each other, Liu et al. proposed integrating the decomposition into an *iterative* non-linear registration framework [4]. A similar approach was used in the current work, resulting in two main parameters to be chosen: a factor $\lambda \in \mathbb{R}_+$, controlling the amount of information separated into S_0, and the number of decomposition-registration-steps n_{Its}.

2.2 Random forest-based lesion segmentation

Even after registration-based compensation of positioning differences and parts of the anatomical variability, some variability and also undesired non-stroke pathologies remain in S_0, which prevents direct stroke lesion segmentation. Therefore, combining the information in S_0 with additional image information for stroke lesion segmentation appears valuable. Here, we build on the work of Halme et al. and their random forest (RF)-based lesion segmentation approach. Halme et al. proposed using four image features per image modality [6]:

1. Z-score normalized image intensity,
2. voxel-wise Z-score deviation from global average,
3. image intensity after Gaussian smoothing of original images,
4. voxel-wise hemispheric asymmetry of Gaussian-smoothed image intensities.

Binary lesion segmentations were finally obtained by post-processing the RF likelihood maps using the contextual clustering approach described in [7].

In the current study, the suitability of RPCA and the respective S_0 component information to improve stroke segmentation accuracy is investigated by evaluating RF-based segmentation performance when considering the S_0 image intensities (patient-specifically rescaled to an intensity range [0;255]) as an RF feature – either as single feature or in combination with features 1-4.

2.3 Image data and study design

29 fluid-attenuated inversion recovery (FLAIR) MR images (Siemens 1.5T scanners) of patients with an ischemic stroke acquired approximately three days after stroke symptom onset and respective expert-drawn stroke lesion segmentations were available for this work. All FLAIR images were resampled to isotropic image resolution of 2 mm and affinely registered to the MNI152 atlas [8]. The same atlas served as reference image of the non-linear registration steps (using ANTs [9]) of the RPCA-based iterative registration framework [4].

For RF-based lesion segmentation, the ranger C++ package was used [10] (Gini impurity as split criterion; randomness injected by random training set sampling; 100 trees, unlimited tree growth). All combinations of the five features (aforementioned features 1-4, evaluated for affinely aligned FLAIR images, plus S_0; i.e. $2^5 - 1 = 31$ combinations) were analyzed. Segmentation performance was evaluated in a leave-one patient-out (LOO) manner, i.e. the RF training was performed on 28 datasets and the resulting RF used for lesion segmentation in the left-out FLAIR image. Like [6], 300 lesion voxels and 600 non-lesioned brain voxels were randomly selected for each of the 28 training data sets to define the feature values used for RF training. To further account for uncertainties due to the injected randomness, RF training and evaluation was repeated 5-times for each feature combination. To focus on the feature contributions to RF-based lesion segmentation accuracy (rather than the influence of the post-processing), the applied contextual clustering was limited to one iteration, using a threshold of 0.85 for conversion of the likelihood into binary maps (see [6, 7] for details).

Following the ISLES study, segmentation accuracy was quantified by the average symmetric surface distance (ASSD), the Dice coefficient (DICE), and the Hausdorff distance (HD) comparing the RF and the expert segmentation [3].

3   Results

3.1   Influence of low rank-&-sparse decomposition parameters

The influence of the low rank-&-sparse decomposition parameters on the appearance of the sparse component images is illustrated in Fig. 1. The sparse component images in the upper row represent the results of a decomposition directly after affine registration ($n_{\mathrm{Its}} = 0$). The amount of anatomical variability compensated by the iterative decomposition-non-linear registration becomes obvious by comparing the upper and the lower row sparse component images. In terms of RF lesion segmentation accuracy based on only the S_0 information, the four iteration steps result in an increase of the Dice coefficient from $(49.1\pm0.2)\%$ to $(50.4\pm0.2)\%$ (for $\lambda = 0.0015$; average of mean values of the five repeat runs), $(50.9\pm0.6)\%$ to $(54.2\pm0.0)\%$ ($\lambda = 0.0020$) and $(52.0\pm0.6)\%$ to $(56.0\pm0.3)\%$ (for

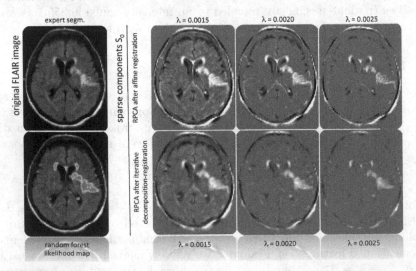

Fig. 1. Illustration of low rank-&-sparse matrix decomposition parameter influence. Left: original FLAIR data set and ground truth segmentation (top) and RF likelihood map (bottom; red = high lesion probability; LOO-training with S_0 image information as single RF feature [$\lambda = 0.0025$, $n_{\mathrm{Its}} = 4$]). Columns 2-4: corresponding sparse components S_0 after decomposition with different λ and n_{Its} values.

Low Rank-&-Sparse Decomposition   165

Table 1. Segmentation accuracy measures, evaluated for each feature combination. The values are given as mean ± std of the mean values of the five repeat runs. Bold entries indicate measure-specific superior segmentation accuracy, evaluated per row; in addition, '*' indicates Bonferroni-corrected $p \leq 0.05$ for t-test comparison of the mean values of the five repeat runs obtained by (1) the original feature sets and (2) the original features sets plus S_0 information. If ASSD or HD entries read 'n/a', RF segmentation failed for at least one dataset. For feature description see section 2.2.

Features	Only original features			Original features + S_0		
	ASSD [mm]	Dice [%]	HD [mm]	ASSD [mm]	Dice [%]	HD [mm]
None[1]	—	—	—	11.4 ± 0.1	50.4 ± 0.2	81.2 ± 1.0
None[2]	—	—	—	10.5 ± 0.1	54.2 ± 0.0	81.6 ± 0.9
None[3]	—	—	—	10.5 ± 0.2	56.0 ± 0.3	81.4 ± 1.0
1	12.6 ± 0.2	52.4 ± 0.3	77.3 ± 0.3	**9.5 ± 0.3***	**61.0 ± 0.3***	**72.4 ± 1.0***
2	12.6 ± 0.3	52.5 ± 0.3	78.0 ± 0.6	**9.2 ± 0.1***	**61.4 ± 0.1***	**74.5 ± 1.6***
3	n/a	13.3 ± 0.6	n/a	**9.0 ± 0.1***	**56.9 ± 0.3***	**72.3 ± 0.5***
4	10.3 ± 0.1	50.7 ± 0.3	82.4 ± 2.7	**6.0 ± 0.1***	**65.6 ± 0.2***	**75.0 ± 0.8***
1+2	12.4 ± 0.1	52.6 ± 0.2	76.9 ± 0.7	**9.4 ± 0.1***	**61.0 ± 0.2***	**72.4 ± 0.7***
1+3	11.0 ± 0.4	55.4 ± 0.6	76.1 ± 1.5	**9.3 ± 0.1***	**61.0 ± 0.4***	**71.9 ± 1.9***
1+4	6.8 ± 0.2	67.2 ± 0.3	69.6 ± 2.1	**6.1 ± 0.2***	**68.5 ± 0.2***	**68.6 ± 2.2**
2+3	11.1 ± 0.2	55.3 ± 0.4	75.5 ± 1.3	**9.1 ± 0.1***	**61.4 ± 0.0***	**71.4 ± 1.5***
2+4	6.6 ± 0.3	67.3 ± 0.3	69.4 ± 1.2	**5.7 ± 0.2***	**68.6 ± 0.2***	**67.7 ± 0.8**
3+4	8.4 ± 0.1	52.9 ± 0.6	73.6 ± 1.9	**4.9 ± 0.1***	**66.6 ± 0.2***	**70.5 ± 1.7**
1+2+3	11.0 ± 0.1	56.1 ± 0.2	75.1 ± 0.9	**9.5 ± 0.4***	**60.8 ± 0.4***	**72.3 ± 1.1***
1+2+4	6.7 ± 0.1	67.3 ± 0.1	69.7 ± 0.8	**6.1 ± 0.2***	**68.5 ± 0.5***	**69.0 ± 1.7**
1+3+4	6.4 ± 0.4	67.6 ± 0.2	68.4 ± 1.5	**5.4 ± 0.2***	**68.1 ± 0.6**	**67.5 ± 0.6**
2+3+4	5.9 ± 0.3	67.6 ± 0.4	**65.9 ± 1.4**	**5.3 ± 0.2***	**68.4 ± 0.3***	66.5 ± 2.8
1+2+3+4	6.6 ± 0.6	67.4 ± 0.2	**68.4 ± 1.6**	**5.4 ± 0.2***	**68.5 ± 0.3***	68.8 ± 1.9

[1]: S_0 obtained by $\lambda = 0.0015 \wedge n_{\text{Its}} = 4$; [2]: $\lambda = 0.0020 \wedge n_{\text{Its}} = 4$; [3]: $\lambda = 0.0025 \wedge n_{\text{Its}} = 4$

$\lambda = 0.0025$). As already reflected by these numbers, increasing λ from 0.0015 to 0.0025, which enforces increased sparsity of S_0, also results in higher Dice values and segmentation accuracy (Tab. 1 for additional numbers).

3.2 Combination of S_0 information and features of Halme et al.

Continuing with $\lambda = 0.0025$ and $n_{\text{Its}} = 4$ as low rank-&-sparse decomposition parameters, a detailed overview of the segmentation accuracy numbers for the $2^5 - 1 = 31$ feature combinations is given in Tab. 1. Bold entries in the table indicate – line-by-line, i.e. separately for each combination of the features proposed by Halme et al. – whether the information contained in S_0 improves the RF segmentation accuracy or not. Almost all bold entries can be found in the columns 5-7. Thus, the sparse component images appear to add valuable information, which especially holds true when combining S_0 information and hemispheric asymmetry (feature 4). The differences decrease, however, with increasing the number of features used for RF prediction; for larger sets, some of the differences in, e.g., HD are no longer statistically significant.

4   Discussion

The present work describes the first comprehensive evaluation study of the suitability of low rank-&-sparse matrix decomposition and the resulting sparse component information for stroke lesion segmentation in MR images. Direct comparison of single feature RF segmentation performance illustrate the sparse component information potential: A Dice coefficient of 56% for the S_0 image information (third row of Tab. 1) is, for instance, significantly higher than corresponding numbers for features 1-4. From that perspective, the opening question ("Is the sparse component information useful in the given context?") can be answered with "yes". However, the overall gain in RF segmentation performance is rather limited when adding S_0 information as "yet another feature" to a series of established features. Thus, the opening question is difficult to answer conclusively and motivates further studies. As the current work focussed on stroke lesion segmentation using only FLAIR images, it would, for example, be interesting to transfer the presented approach to multi-modal image databases and to verify our results using accepted publicly available images such as the ISLES data set.

References

1. WHO methods and data sources for global causes of death 2000-2012. WHO; 2014.
2. Maier O, Schröder C, Forkert ND, et al. Classifiers for ischemic stroke lesion segmentation: a comparison study. PLoS One. 2015;10(12):e0145118.
3. Maier O, Menze BH, von der Gablentz J, et al. ISLES 2015: a public evaluation benchmark for ischemic stroke lesion segmentation from multispectral MRI. Med Image Anal. 2016;35:250–69.
4. Liu X, Niethammer M, Kwitt R, et al. Low-rank atlas image analyses in the presence of pathologies. IEEE Trans Med Imaging. 2015;34(12):2583–91.
5. Lin Z, Liu R, Si Z. Linearized alternating direction method with adaptive penalty for low rank representation. Proc NIPS 2011. 2012; p. 612–20.
6. Halme HL, Korvenoja A, Salli E. ISLES (SISS) challenge 2015: segmentation of stroke lesions using spatial normalization, random forest classification and contextual clustering. Lect Notes Computer Sci. 2016;9556:211–21.
7. Salli E, Aronen HJ, Savolainen S, et al. Contextual clustering for analysis of functional MRI data. IEEE Trans Med Imaging. 2001;20(5):403–14.
8. Mazziotta JC, Toga AW, Evans A, et al. A probabilistic atlas of the human brain: theory and rationale for its development. The international consortium for brain mapping (ICBM). Neuroimage. 1995;2(2):89–101.
9. Avants BB, Epstein CL, Grossman M, et al. Symmetric diffeomorphic image registration with cross-correlation: evaluating automated labeling of elderly and neurodegenerative brain. Med Image Anal. 2008;12(1):26–41.
10. Wright MN, Ziegler A. Ranger: a fast implementation of random forests for high dimensional data in C++ and R. J Stat Softw. 2016;in press.

Automatic Layer Generation for Scar Transmurality Visualization

S. Reiml[1,4], T. Kurzendorfer[1,4], D. Toth[2,5], P. Mountney[6], M. Panayiotou[2], J. M. Behar[2,3], C. A. Rinaldi[2,3], K. Rhode[2], A. Maier[1], A. Brost[4]

[1]Pattern Recognition Lab, University Erlangen-Nuremberg, Germany
[2]Department of Biomedical Engineering, King's College London, United Kingdom
[3]Department of Cardiology, Guy's and St. Thomas' NHS Foundation Trust
[4]Siemens Healthcare GmbH, Forchheim, Germany
[5]Siemens Healthcare Ltd, London, United Kingdom
[6]Medical Imaging Technologies, Siemens Healthcare, Princeton, NJ, USA
sabrina.reiml@fau.de

Abstract. In 2014, about 26 million people were suffering from heart failure. Symptomatic heart failure is treated by cardiac resynchronization therapy. However, 30 % to 50 % do not clinically respond after the implantation of a biventricular pacemaker. To improve the success rate, the quantification of a patient's scar burden is very important. Late-gadolinium-enhanced magnetic resonance imaging is used to visualize regions of scarring in the left ventricle. Scar is very hard to visualize and interpret in 3D. To solve this, an automated scar layer generation method is proposed. The scar is divided into layers and an interactive scrolling is provided. This method allows for precise treatment planning. With the scar layer visualization, eight clinical experts were asked to decide if the scar is epicardial or endocardial. The correct location was identified in 93.75 % of the cases using the scar layer visualization.

1 Introduction

Heart failure affected in 2014 about 26 million people worldwide [1]. Symptomatic heart failure is often treated by cardiac resynchronization therapy (CRT). Patients eligible for CRT undergo a minimally invasive procedure for implantation of a biventricular pacemaker, often called CRT device [2].

The localisation and quantification of scar tissue in the myocardium of the left ventricle (LV) is crucial to increase the success rate of CRT [3, 4]. However, the myocardial scar distribution can be challenging to interpret, in particular the transmurality. Transmurality is present when the scar extends from the endocardium to the epicardium. The problem in CRT is that about 30 % to 50 % of the patients do not respond clinically [5]. One of the main reasons of non response is considered to be suboptimal placement of the left ventricular pacing lead. Pacing in areas of myocardial infarction has less effect, because scar tissue is not electrical conductive. To improve the success rate, precise scar information is required for choosing the optimal pacing location.

The state-of-the-art for assessing the viability of the myocardium is late-gadolinium-enhanced magnetic resonance imaging (LGE-MRI). The anatomy is segmented from Cine MRIs, where the contours of the myocardium are more clearly visible compared to the LGE-MRI scans [6]. Most methods available consider a semi-automatic approach for scar segmentation [7, 8].

Currently, there are two methods for the visualization of scar transmurality. The first method is the mapping of scar information to a so-called bull's eye plot (BEP) (Fig. 1 (a)). Scar transmurality is presented as percentage for each segment of the BEP. The drawbacks of this approach are the non-anatomical visualization of the LV as a BEP and the missing information about the scar's location within the myocardium. Furthermore, no 3D guidance is possible. The second method is to visualize the scar as a 3D mesh (Fig. 1 (b)). The advantage of this approach is the 3D anatomical visualization. The disadvantage of this method is that there is no information about scar transmurality.

While Reiml et al. showed different scar visualization methods [9], in this work a novel method for 3D scar layer generation is presented. We propose an interactive 3D scar location and transmurality visualization method.

2   Scar layer generation

2.1   MRI segmentation

In the first step, the endocardium and epicardium are segmented from anatomical MRI scans. After the delineation of the myocardium, the anatomical scan is registered to the LGE-MRI, which is used for the segmentation of the scar tissue [7]. This tissue is segmented using a semi automatic approach [8]. Examples of Cine MRI and LGE-MRI are depicted in Fig. 1(c, d). The output of the segmentation is a mask containing the blood pool, the myocardium and the information about the myocardial scar, see Fig. 2 second box for a single slice.

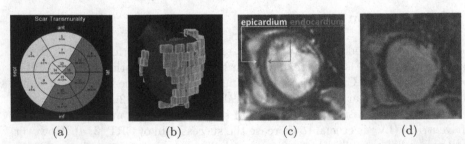

(a)   (b)   (c)   (d)

Fig. 1. (a) 2D visualization of the scar transmurality in a bull's eye plot. (b) 3D mesh visualization with the left ventricle's endocardium (dark red) and the 3D scar distribution (light purple). (c) 2D short axis Cine image of the LV for anatomy segmentation. (d) 2D short axis LGE image of the LV for scar tissue quantification.

2.2 Anatomy delineation

In the second step, the epicardium and the endocardium are extracted from each of the slices of the segmentation mask. The extraction is based on the marching squares algorithm, which finds the iso-surfaces in the segmentation mask [10]. The epicardial contour (yellow) and the endocardial contour (red) are visualized in Fig. 3 (a).

2.3 Layer computation

In the third step, the segmentation mask, as well as the endocardial and epicardial contour points are transformed into polar space (r, ρ) where r is the radius and ρ the angle (Fig. 4). Due to Cartesian coordinates (x, y), there are more epicardial points than endocardial points. Hence, it is more difficult to divide the area between the endocardium and the epicardium in multiple layers. There are

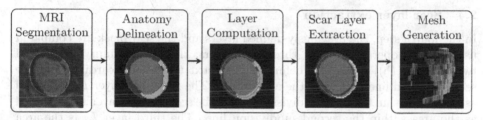

Fig. 2. Overview of the five steps for the 3D scar location and transmurality visualization. First, the left ventricle and the scar are segmented. Second, the epicardium and endocardium are delineated. Third, the layers are computed. Fourth, the scar layers are extracted. In the last step, the scar layer meshes are generated.

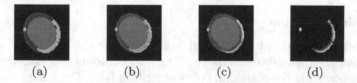

(a)   (b)   (c)   (d)

Fig. 3. Scar layer generation process illustrated in one slice. (a) Segmentation mask with detected epicardium (yellow) and endocardium (red). The blood pool is located inside of the endocardium and the myocardium is between the endocardium and epicardium. Within the myocardium, the scar is shown in a lighter shade of gray and white. (b) Calculated layers. (c) Scar layers. (d) Scar layer masks.

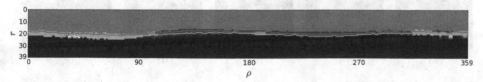

Fig. 4. Transformed mask image into polar space with computed layers (red and orange) between the endocardium and epicardium.

several advantages using polar coordinates instead of Cartesian coordinates. The epicardium and endocardium in Cartesian coordinates are roughly circular but do not have the same perimeter. In polar space, the transformed epicardium and endocardium outlines have the same length and run almost in parallel (Fig. 4). Afterwards, the endocardial and epicardial contour points are interpolated. From the interpolated contours, the layers between the endocardium and epicardium are computed (Fig. 4). The distance between the endocardium and the epicardium is calculated and then divided into multiple layers. For n layers, the myocardium needs to be divided $m = n - 1$ times. For each angle ρ, m values within the myocardium are calculated. After the delineation of the n layers in polar space, they are transformed back to Cartesian coordinates (Fig. 3 (b-d)). In this work, the number of layers is set to three. For the placement of the lead, it is useful to have an epicardial, a mid-myocardial and an endocardial layer to decide where the scar is located.

2.4   Scar layer extraction

In the fourth step, the previously defined layers and the scar mask are compared using logical operations. For three scar layers, the myocardium was divided twice (Fig. 3 (b)). The first defined line is next to the endocardium and the second defined line is close to the epicardium. The first filled layer L_1 is defined as the area within the first subdivision layer. The second filled layer L_2 is defined as the area within the second subdivision line. The third layer L_3 is the area within the epicardium. Then the filled layers are logically compared with the scar mask S and the three individual scar layer masks S_1, S_2 and S_3, where $S_1 = L_1 \wedge S$, $S_2 = \overline{L_1} \wedge L_2 \wedge S$ and $S_3 = \overline{L_1} \wedge \overline{L_2} \wedge L_3 \wedge S$ are obtained (Fig. 3 (c, d)).

2.5   Mesh generation

The final step is to extend the 3D scar mask with the slice thickness, as just a limited number of slices are available. The scar contours are extracted as 3D surface meshes using the marching cubes algorithm [10]. The image coordinates are transformed to patient coordinates to position the scar layers at the same position as the original scar mesh, Fig. 5.

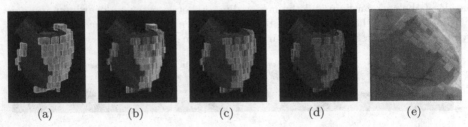

(a)   (b)   (c)   (d)   (e)

Fig. 5. (a) Endocardium (dark red) with one scar mesh in purple. (b) Endocardium with three scar layers. (c) Endocardium with two scar layers. (d) Endocardium with one scar layer. (e) Fluoroscopic image with overlaid endocardium and 3D scar layers.

3   Visualization

The subdivision of the scar mesh into several scar layers enables an interactive peeling of the scar in 3D. It can be scrolled from epicardium to endocardium and vice versa as depicted in Fig. 5 (b-d). The interactive adding and removing of the scar layers allows for a good localization, where the scar starts and ends, as well as an assessment of transmurality. If the scar is fully transmural, all scar layers are add up.

The 3D scar layers can be overlaid onto fluoroscopic images using manual 2D/3D registration, as depicted in Fig. 5 (e). This visualization method can be used during the intervention. For the overlay, the epicardial mesh of the LV is registered to the fluoroscopic image. Then, the epicardium, the endocardium, the scar mesh and the scar layers can be visualized in different colors. The colors and opacity can be adapted manually. Meshes, which the physician is not interested in, can be hidden. This supports the physician during the intervention, as only the required and important information is visible.

4   Evaluation and results

The scar layer visualization was evaluated using seven clinical data sets, acquired with a Siemens MAGNETOM Aera 1.5T scanner (Siemens Healthcare GmbH, Erlangen). For the evaluation, two tests are created. In the first test, nine physicians are shown four cases. For each case, two visualization methods are presented: the segmented LV overlaid with the 3D scar mesh and the segmented LV overlaid with the scar layer visualization. They are asked to decide which visualization method they would prefer. In 80.55 % cases, the clinical experts prefer the scar layer visualization, in 16.67 % cases they prefer the 3D scar mesh and in 2.78 % cases they do not have a preference.

In the second test, eight physicians are shown six 3D scar meshes and six scar layer meshes. For each visualization method, they should decide if the scar is epicardial or endocardial. The results are shown in Table 1. These two experiments show, that with the scar layer visualization, the clinicians can easily choose an optimal lead placement location as they can decide whether the scar is epicardial or endocardial.

5   Discussion and conclusion

In this paper, a novel method for interactive visualization of the scar information is presented. In CRT, the lead of the electrode is commonly placed on the epicardium. Precise information about the location and transmurality of the scar is needed, as it is electrically almost non-conductive. The results show that the clinicians could easier decide about the scar location. The precise control over how the scar transmurality is visualized in 3D allows the user to see the scar location to the extent of transmurality directly. An interactive scrolling through scar layers is realized, such that scar layers are added or removed from

Table 1. Evaluation with eight clinical experts and twelve scar meshes. They should decide for each mesh if the scar is epicardial, endocardial or they could not determine.

	3D Scar Mesh	Scar Layer Meshes
Correct	18.75 %	93.75 %
Wrong	6.25 %	6.25 %
No determination	75.00 %	0.00 %

the visualization. The epicardium and the scar meshes can be further overlaid onto fluoroscopic images. The overlay of the meshes can be used to guide an intervention.

Acknowledgement. The authors are grateful for the support from the Innovate UK grant 32684-234174. The research was supported by the National Institute for Health Research (NIHR) Biomedical Research Centre based at Guy's and St. Thomas' NHS Foundation Trust and King's College London. The views expressed are those of the authors and not necessarily those of the NHS, NIHR or the Department of Health. Concepts and information presented are based on research and are not commercially available.

References

1. Ponikowski P, Anker SD, AlHabib KF, et al. Heart failure: preventing disease and death worldwide. ESC Heart Fail. 2014;1(1):4–25.
2. Shea JB, Sweeney MO. Cardiac resynchronization therapy a patient 's guide. Circulation. 2003;108(9):64–6.
3. Kurzendorfer T, Brost A, Forman C, et al. Semi-automatic segmentation and scar quantification of the left ventricle in 3-D late gadolinium enhanced MRI. 32nd Annu Sci Meet ESMRMB. 2015; p. 318–9.
4. Cochet H, Denis A, Ploux S, et al. Pre-and intra-procedural predictors of reverse remodeling after cardiac resynchronization therapy: an MRI study. J Cardiovasc Electrophysiol. 2013;24(6):682–91.
5. Daubert JC, Saxon L, Adamson PB, et al. 2012 EHRA/HRS expert consensus statement on cardiac resynchronization therapy in heart failure: implant and follow-up recommendations and management. Europace. 2012;14(9):1236–86.
6. Tao Q, Piers SR, Lamb HJ, et al. Automated left ventricle segmentation in late gadolinium-enhanced MRI for objective myocardial scar assessment. J Cardiovasc Magn Reson. 2014;42(2):390–9.
7. Jolly MP, Xue H, Grady L, et al. Combining registration and minimum surfaces for the segmentation of the left ventricle in cardiac cine MR images. Proc MICCAI. 2009; p. 910–8.
8. Karim R, Bhagirath P, Claus P, et al. Evaluation of state-of-the-art segmentation algorithms for left ventricle infarct from late Gadolinium enhancement MR images. Med Image Anal. 2016;30:95–107.
9. Reiml S, Toth D, Panayiotou M, et al. Interactive visualization for scar transmurality in cardiac resynchronization therapy. Proc SPIE. 2016;9786:97862S–97862S–8.
10. Lorensen W, Cline H. Marching cubes: a high resolution 3D surface construction algorithm. CM Siggraph Computer Graph. 1987;21:163–9.

Analyzing Immunohistochemically Stained Whole-Slide Images of Ovarian Carcinoma

Daniel Bug[1], Anne Grote[2], Julia Schüler[3], Friedrich Feuerhake[2], Dorit Merhof[1]

[1]Institute of Imaging and Computer Vision, RWTH Aachen University, Germany
[2]Institute for Pathology, Hannover Medical School, Germany
[3]Oncotest GmbH, Germany
daniel.bug@lfb.rwth-aachen.de

Abstract. Digital pathology, driven by the increasing capabilities of modern computers, is an emerging field within medical research and diagnostics. A re-occurring task in pathology is the analysis of immuno-histochemical (IHC) stains, i.e. stains in which a specific type of immune cell is highlighted using corresponding antibodies. Automatic quantification of these images is a challenge due to large image sizes of up to 10 gigapixels, but provides a more objective and reproducible evaluation than the exhaustive task of manual analysis. In this context, we compare counting measures against area-based measures in the case of cytoplasmic and membrane-bound IHC stains. Our evaluation indicates a superior performance of the area-based method which reaches a Jaccard index of approximately 80%, while cell nuclei count-based approaches can be severely affected by variance due to masking effects when the cytoplasmic chromogenic staining covers the blue nuclear counterstain.

1 Introduction

In recent years, options for cancer treatment have been extended by immunotherapy, i.e. enabling the patients' immune system to effectively fight tumor growth by inhibiting immunosuppressive mechanisms that some tumors utilize to escape from elimination by immune cells. Due to these mechanisms in the tumor-micro-environment, the immune infiltration is an important measure to assess the activity or passivity of the immune system towards the tumor to quantify the success or failure of a medication. Immunohistochemical (IHC) stains visualize immune activity and can, in combination with modern whole-slide scanning systems, be used to enable computerized analysis of large tissue quantities and increase objectivity.

For the pathologist, preferred measures include cell or cell nuclei counts, morphological cell features and tissue or cell area based ratios. Related to this task, many algorithms can already be found in the literature, e.g. cell nuclei counting [1, 2], segmentation [1, 2, 3, 4] and area-related measures [4, 5, 6]. Furthermore, [7] provides a review listing additional methods for different stains.

Nearly all examples focusing on count- and segmentation-based measures propose their algorithms for nuclei-based markers, i.e. the antibody binding to

173

a protein expressed in the immune cells' nucleus (Fig. 2a). Depending on the medical task, another group of markers, coupling to proteins in the plasma surrounding the nucleus, are of interest, too. So far, the accurate evaluation of cytoplasmic (Fig. 2b) and membrane-bound (Fig. 2c) staining components have received less attention in literature than purely nuclear markers. For example, the cytoplasmic and membrane component have been treated by segmenting and evaluating subcellular components in [1]. This may be feasible for well separated cells, e.g. tumor cells, but is problematic for immune cells which are often small and do not show a clear separation of cytoplasmic and membrane-bound component, or in cases of large cell clusters with mixed staining components.

To address the need for an improved evaluation of these components, our contribution is a robust classification tool which provides a reliable area-based quantification. Moreover, we give a quantitative evaluation of counting measures based on common counting approaches.

2   Material and methods

In this work, a dataset of 21 images extracted from seven whole-slide images WSIs (three per slide) of ovarian carcinoma tissue is available for evaluation. The slides were immunohistochemically stained with Hematoxylin (HEM, blue color) and, using the membrane-bound and cytoplasmic CD45 marker, $3,3'$-Diaminobenzidine (DAB, brown color). An Aperio Scanner (At2, Leica Biosystems, Wetzlar, Germany) at 40× objective magnification was used to digitize the slides. These images were manually labeled and the annotations, comprising nuclei type (immune cell or not), nuclei position and a map of the stain-type, were verified by biomedical experts. Each extracted section contains approximately two megapixels and the dataset comprises 15.917 HEM-nuclei and 3.025 DAB-nuclei.

2.1   Method

Deconvolution methods, e.g. staining matrices, which are often applied in preprocessing steps, suffer from linear constraints or limited generalization properties. In order to circumvent these restrictions, we propose to learn the deconvolution

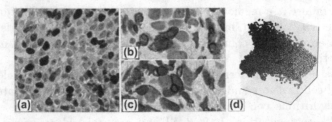

Fig. 1. Examples of different marker types and PCA-based custom color space: nucleus marker (a), marker with cytoplasmic (b) and cell-membrane-bound (c) signals in the image centers, first three principal components (d).

in a conventional machine-learning setting, based on a very limited amount of labeled training data. Although annotating a very small patch implies little manual effort, such a patch which covers most blue-brown variations is actually sufficient to train a robust classifier. While in many cases the generalization will be sufficient to work with, difficult slides can be treated separately by retraining with a labeling base as little as e.g. 250×250 pixels.

The initial step, prior to classification, is to augment the RGB representation of an image with the transformed color spaces LAB, HSV and a dedicated Hematoxylin-Eosin-DAB matrix decomposition [8]. By extending the color space, we include information from different linear and non-linear transformations which increases the chance to identify a mathematically simple, i.e. linear, function to separate the HEM and DAB channels. Additionally, a bilateral filter is used on each channel to remove noise.

Since the various color spaces encode the channels in very different intervals, each channel is normalized using mean-std scaling to balance the influence on the optimization while training the classifier. However, some of the information in the channels of the augmented representation is still correlated and therefore introduces redundancies which in practice prevents a successful training – usually showing an overly noisy classification output due to insufficient generalization.

Using a principal component analysis, we reduce redundancies and inherent noise, which decreases computational complexity and thus ensures the efficiency of the approach. In Fig. 2d the color space defined by the first three principal components is visualized, showing a strong separation of HEM and DAB stain.

As for the classification task itself, similar performance can be obtained using a linear Support-Vector Classifier (SVC) or a Gradient-Boosting Classifier (GBC) for the labeling of the colors. While the GBC proved to be insensitive to variations of its parameters, the SVC was optimized in terms of its penalty weight (i.e. C-parameter). Both classifiers achieve similar accuracies, but ultimately the SVC is preferred due to a notable advantage in computational speed.

Since the mapping is learned pixelwise, the resulting labeling will contain noise in edge regions, which is efficiently removed by applying morphological operations on each individual channel.

2.2 Evaluation

The performance of counting measures is illustrated by using a common type of seed detection (SD), which is a combination of morphological operators and local maximum detection in distance space on top of the classification output. In addition, we consider the cell nuclei counts from the free open-source software CellProfiler (CP), based on an adapted pipeline from [9], that incorporates Laplacian-of-Gaussian-based blob detection. Other methods could unfortunately not be included due to the inaccessibility of the code and differences in the computed metrics without access to intermediate results.

For evaluation, we measure the counted cell nuclei and the distances between detected nuclei and the nuclei labeled in the ground truth. All nuclei counts are quantified in terms of micro- and macro-averaged values. Micro-averaging

176   Bug et al.

Table 1. Results of the cell nuclei counts in terms of micro-average as well as mean accuracy and standard deviation. All values are in percent. SD: common seed detection. CP: CellProfiler.

	HEM-μavg.	HEM-mean	HEM-std	DAB-μavg.	DAB-mean	DAB-std
SD	113.15	115.30	10.07	128.30	118.87	88.99
CP	152.46	168.26	32.23	78.55	115.25	159.68

accumulates the predicted and ground truth nuclei counts from each image *before* computing the accuracy ratio, while the macroscopic version averages the accuracy ratios of each individual image.

For comparing the detected cell nuclei positions to the ground truth, we incorporate a Nearest-Neighbor classifier fitted to the ground truth positions of cell nuclei in the HEM and DAB channels, respectively. This metric is not exact, since it does not compute bidirectional correspondences, but rather has the characteristics of a precision measure.

While the comparison of the counts and distances is relatively straightforward, the Jaccard index $\mathcal{J} = (A \cap B)/(A \cup B)$, also known as intersection-over-union ratio, is used as area measure in order to quantify the agreement to the ground truth. Herein, A and B represent arbitrary sets, which can be interpreted as mask images by replacing $\cap$ with the Boolean *AND*, and $\cup$ with the Boolean *OR* operator. A value of 0 implies no overlap between the masks, while the maximum is achieved at Jaccard index 1. We prefer this measure over the commonly used Dice coefficient, since $\mathcal{J}$ satisfies the triangle equation and thus is a valid metric, while the Dice coefficient is semi-metric and tends to yield overly positive results.

3   Results

First, we present the results of the different cell-segmentation approaches for deriving cell nuclei counts in Table 1. For both investigated approaches, the number of cell nuclei tends to be over-predicted on average in the HEM channel with only little variance, while the DAB channel suffers from a very high variance in the predicted number, clearly showing some limitations of common cell nuclei counting strategies in case of cytoplasmic IHC stains, under the herein tested conditions.

However, in spite of the overly sensitive nuclei detection step, the resulting distribution of distances, shown as a boxplot in Fig. 2, indicates that the proposed positions in a vast majority of cases are very close to an actual cell-nucleus.

Fig. 2. Distances of each proposed nucleus to closest ground truth nucleus in pixels. A single cell-nucleus has an average diameter of approximately 32 pixels. SD: common seed detection. CP: CellProfiler.

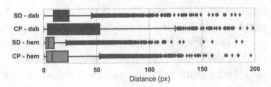

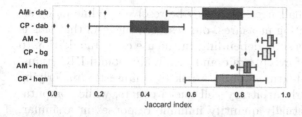

Fig. 3. Area estimates for DAB (dab), hematoxylin (hem) and background (bg). These measures are much more stable, given the large variance in the cell nuclei counts. AM: proposed area measure. CP: CellProfiler.

In this second part of the evaluation, the SD approach has a clear advantage over the CP pipeline. Given an average diameter of approximately 32 pixels, the SD estimates are usually within the reach of a ground truth nucleus, whereas the CP pipeline usually proposes far too many objects and thus predicts many of them in background areas far away from actual nuclei.

As a third quantity, the area measures are considered. Fig. 3 illustrates the Jaccard index for the areas associated with DAB, HEM and background. In the CP prediction, a high variance remains in both the HEM and DAB channel, with a median DAB Jaccard index of approximately 0.45. For the proposed area measure approach, the HEM channel is predicted with a median close to 0.85 at a very low variance, which indicates a reliable prediction, while the DAB channel remains slightly below 0.8 with moderate variance. Note that since the labels are mutually exclusive, no channel can achieve an optimal score of 1.0 exclusively. Since DAB stain and HEM stain are usually in direct pixel neighborhood, slight confusions inevitably happen between these two classes.

4   Discussion

As shown above, the measures based on the area contribution of a specific stain can be much more reliable than the computationally more demanding counting measures in case of the considered plasmatic IHC stains. This also makes sense from a perspective of error propagation, since the nuclei detection steps usually build on top of some form of initial segmentation. In the proposed solution, the classification results in lower variances than the Otsu-method incorporated in the CP pipeline, which fails if the channel statistics strongly deviate from expected values. Especially applying the Otsu-method in slides with low DAB content, the algorithm tends to over-predict objects in this channel, since the automatic threshold is set too low. Since a patch-wise approach is the obvious choice for the processing of entire WSIs, the local information will lead to very different statistics, even within a single WSI. Computing global statistics from subsampled levels of an image pyramid may help to compute robust thresholds in some cases, but it should be noted that, depending on the success of medication, it is not untypical to have slides with no immune activity at all, which drastically influences the DAB channel statistics on a global level. Classification is more robust in this situation, but its weakness – not considered in this work – will likely be variances in the model, i.e. differences in the image appearance due to varying staining protocols. However, with the small required amount of labeled data to train the color classifier, such challenges can easily be resolved. While many algorithms aim at providing counting measures, our research suggests that this is not always the most reliable measure, depending on the use case. In addition to the very different appearance of cytoplasmic and membrane-bound IHC stains, WSIs with strong background textures imply a risk to confuse the underlying detectors and may lead to nearly arbitrary cell nuclei counts, while computationally less expensive steps actually quantify immune responses in a similar, more reliable way, in cases where individual nucleus features are not of particular interest or cannot be computed due to difficult cell cluster configurations. In principle, are-based quantification approaches do not exclude combination with additional classification steps that could be implemented to further reduce false positives. However, a limiting factor herein would be the computational expense for scaling the processing to full WSIs.

In summary, the proposed method of classifying the stain components constitutes, with a Jaccard index of approximately 85% (HEM-channel) and 78% (DAB-channel), a fast and reliable measure for IHC quantification.

References

1. Di Cataldo S, Ficarra E, Acquaviva A, et al. Automated segmentation of tissue images for computerized IHC analysis. Comput Methods Programs Biomed. 2010;100(1):1–15.
2. Vink J, Van Leeuwen M, Van Deurzen C, et al. Efficient nucleus detector in histopathology images. J Microsc. 2013;249(2):124–35.
3. Jung C, Kim C, Chae SW, et al. Unsupervised segmentation of overlapped nuclei using bayesian classification. IEEE Trans Biomed Eng. 2010;57(12):2825–32.
4. Li X, Plataniotis K. Circular mixture modeling of color distribution for blind stain separation in pathology images. IEEE J Biomed Health Informatics. 2016;PP:10.1109/JBHI.2015.2503720.
5. Varghese F, Bukhari AB, Malhotra R, et al. IHC profiler: an open source plugin for the quantitative evaluation and automated scoring of immunohistochemistry images of human tissue samples. PloS One. 2014;9(5):e96801.
6. Tuominen VJ, Ruotoistenmäki S, Viitanen A, et al. ImmunoRatio: a publicly available web application for quantitative image analysis of estrogen receptor (ER), progesterone receptor (PR), and Ki-67. Breast Cancer Res. 2010;12(4):1.
7. Irshad H, Veillard A, Roux L, et al. Methods for nuclei detection, segmentation, and classification in digital histopathology: a review : current status and future potential. IEEE Rev Biomed Eng. 2014;7:97–114.
8. Ruifrok AC, Johnston DA. Quantification of histochemical staining by color deconvolution. Anal Quant Cytol Histol. 2001;23(4):291–9.
9. Du Z, Abedalthagafi M, Aizer AA, et al. Increased expression of the immune modulatory molecule PD-L1 (CD274) in anaplastic meningioma. Oncotarget. 2015;6(7):4704.

Efficient Epiphyses Localization Using Regression Tree Ensembles and a Conditional Random Field

Alexander O. Mader[1,2], Hauke Schramm[1,2], Carsten Meyer[1,2]

[1]Institute of Applied Computer Science, Kiel University of Applied Sciences
[2]Department of Computer Science, Faculty of Engineering, Kiel University (CAU)
alexander.o.mader@fh-kiel.de

Abstract. Accurate localization of sets of anatomical landmarks is a challenging task, yet often required in automatic analysis of medical images. Several groups – e.g., Donner et al. – have shown that it is beneficial to incorporate geometrical relations of landmarks into detection procedures for complex anatomical structures. In this paper, we present a two-step approach (compared to three steps as suggested by Donner et al.) combining regression tree ensembles with a Conditional Random Field (CRF), modeling spatial relations. The comparably simple combination achieves a localization rate of 99.6 % on a challenging hand radiograph dataset showing high age-related variability, which is slightly superior than state-of-the-art results achieved by Hahmann et al.

1 Introduction

Object localization is an important step in the automatic analysis of medical images. One common problem involving object localization is Bone Age Assessment (BAA). In order to evaluate the skeletal maturity, e.g., to diagnose growth disorders, the region of interest around an epiphyseal plate has to be extracted. However, localization of these epiphyses is difficult due to the (1) high ambiguity between single epiphyses and (2) large anatomical variability caused by different patient ages. Two recent approaches showed high performance on this task: Hahmann et al. [1] proposed to use a global hand model to perform a coarse localization of all epiphyses on a low resolution image, followed by a fine localization on a high resolution crop of the image. For both steps a combination of the Discriminative Generalized Hough Transform (DGHT) with the Shape Consistency Measure (SCM) is used. In contrast, Donner et al. [2] proposed a three step approach going from local to global context. First, a coarse pixel-wise epiphyses classification is performed using Random Forests (RF). Second, a refinement step aggregates all classifications using a Hough Forest (HF), resulting in multiple localization hypotheses per epiphysis. Finally, a Markov Random Field (MRF) is used to model the spatial relations between different epiphyses in order to infer the most likely selection of localization hypotheses over all landmarks.

In this paper, we show that a local-to-global strategy as followed by Donner et al. can be simplified while achieving similar results as the state of the art on a large hand radiograph dataset showing high anatomical variability. First, an ensemble of decision tree regressors [3] is used to generate localization hypotheses by focusing on local structures only. The idea is to generate – in a single step instead of two steps as done by Donner et al. [2] – a list of localization hypotheses that contains the true location as accurately as possible, but not necessarily as first best hypothesis (i.e., confusions between different epiphyses are tolerated since they will be resolved in the second step). Second, a Conditional Random Field (CRF) is used to model the global spatial relations between landmarks, similar to [2]. Simple geometric potentials in combination with a large search-space containing at least one good configuration allow for exceptional performance, given an efficient approximate inference strategy. Following this approach, a localization accuracy of 99.6 % over all images and landmarks is achieved on a hand radiograph dataset (provided by Prof. Deserno from Uniklinik RWTH Aachen), slightly superior than the previous state-of-the-art results by Hahmann et al.

2   Materials and methods

The proposed approach consists of two steps; an overview is given in Fig. 1. First, n localization hypotheses $\hat{\mathcal{X}}_i = \{\hat{\mathbf{x}}_{i,1}, \ldots, \hat{\mathbf{x}}_{i,n}\}$ are generated for each landmark $i \in \{1, \ldots, N\}$ by using landmark-specific ensembles of decision tree regressors rating the local environment in terms of image descriptors. Second, the obtained localization hypotheses in combination with spatial features, e.g., distance and orientation, are encoded in a CRF. Approximate inference is used to find the most likely set of hypotheses $\{\mathbf{c}_i \in \hat{\mathcal{X}}_i \mid i\}$ among all possible combinations.

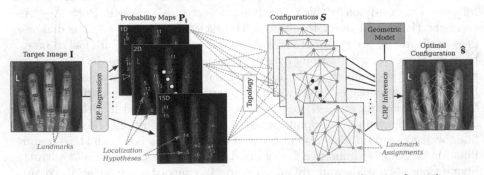

(a) Generating localization hypotheses   (b) Generating localization hypotheses

Fig. 1. Demonstration of our two-step approach on one cropped test image: (a) Generation of localization hypotheses by applying each landmark-specific regression tree ensemble and showing the target image overlayed by the probability map. (b) Inference is used in combination with a spatial model to find the most probable configuration out of all possible configurations using our CRF model with indicated topology.

2.1   Regression tree ensembles for accurate localization hypotheses

Goal of the first step is to predict (as accurately as possible) candidate positions for each landmark on local context only. At this stage we tolerate confusions of different landmarks, since they will be resolved in the second step. I.e., any (not necessarily the first) of the n best localization hypotheses should be as close as possible to the true position. The basic idea is to transform an image $\mathbf{I} : \mathbb{R}^2 \rightarrow \mathbb{R}$ into a pseudo (not normalized) probability map $\widetilde{\mathbf{P}}_i : \mathbb{R}^2 \rightarrow \mathbb{R}^+$ in which the location of the highest value $\hat{\mathbf{x}}_{i,1} = \arg\max_{\mathbf{x}} \widetilde{\mathbf{P}}_i(\mathbf{x})$ corresponds to the most likely predicted position of the target landmark i. For each landmark i an ensemble of $K = 128$ decision tree regressors [3] is used to transform feature vectors $\mathbf{f}_i^k(\mathbf{x})$, computed for a certain position $\mathbf{x}$ in image $\mathbf{I}$ for the k-th regression tree, into pseudo probabilities $\widetilde{p}_i^k(\mathbf{x})$. This is done for all pixels in the image and averaged over all trees k to form the pseudo probability map $\widetilde{\mathbf{P}}_i$, which is additionally smoothed with a Gaussian kernel $\mathcal{N}_i$ (see below). Finally, Non-Maximum Suppression (NMS) with a minimal distance between peaks of 15 pixel is applied to find local maxima. The n best local maxima are used as localization hypotheses $\hat{\mathcal{X}}_i = \{\hat{\mathbf{x}}_{i,1}, \ldots, \hat{\mathbf{x}}_{i,n}\}$ for each landmark i.

To extract the feature vector $\mathbf{f}_i^k(\mathbf{x})$ for a certain pixel $\mathbf{x}$ we use the same method as Donner et al. Each tree in the ensemble is associated with an individual sampling mask to extract $F = 128$ pixel intensity values from a local patch. The mask is obtained by sampling locations from $\mathbf{X} \sim$ i.i.d. $\mathcal{N}\left(\mathbf{0}, \frac{1}{25}\begin{pmatrix} s_1^2 & 0 \\ 0 & s_2^2 \end{pmatrix}\right)$ with $\mathbf{S} = (s_1\ s_2)$ being the patch size; in our experiments $\mathbf{S} = (50\ 80)$. Finally, the masks origin is placed at $\mathbf{x}$ and the intensity value at $\mathbf{x}$ is subtracted from the marked pixel intensities, resulting in our F-dimensional feature vector $\mathbf{f}_i^k(\mathbf{x})$.

Boostrapping is used to train the regression trees in a discriminative fashion by iteratively growing a set $\mathcal{O}_i^k \subseteq \mathbb{R}^F \times \mathbb{R}$ of feature vectors and corresponding target values over all training images. Starting with the first training image and $\mathcal{O}_i^k = \varnothing$, "positive" samples are generated by computing the feature vectors $\mathbf{f}_i^k(\mathbf{x})$ for all $M = 81$ pixel within a circle with radius $R = 5$ around the respective annotated landmark position $\mathbf{x}_i^*$. We allow for some ambiguity by introducing a Gaussian distribution $\mathcal{N}_i\left(\mathbf{x}_i^*, \frac{1}{9}R^2\begin{pmatrix} 1 & 0 \\ 0 & 1 \end{pmatrix}\right)$ around $\mathbf{x}_i^*$ such that $\sim 98.9\%$ of the probability mass is within radius R, and use the density values computed at position $\mathbf{x}$ as regression targets. These M samples (feature vectors and regression values) are added to the set of samples $\mathcal{O}_i^k$. An intermediate tree is trained in each iteration on all samples currently in $\mathcal{O}_i^k$ and used to generate "negative" samples by applying the intermediate tree to the training image. NMS is used to find the M pixel with the largest pseudo probabilities outside the circle located at $\mathbf{x}_i^*$. For those M "negative" pixel, feature vectors are computed and added – with a target regression value 0 – to the growing set of samples $\mathcal{O}_i^k$. This procedure is continued over all training images using a more discriminative newly trained intermediate tree in each iteration to find negative samples. At the end, a single, final regression tree is trained on the full set of samples $\mathcal{O}_i^k$ and added to the ensemble. We use variance reduction to train all regression trees without limiting the tree depth. In practice, samples are generated from batches of 10 images instead of single images to reduce the amount of intermediate regression trees and thus their training. The whole bootstrapping procedure is performed for each tree in each of the N ensembles individually. Fig. 1 a shows three pseudo probability maps created by applying ensembles trained on three different landmarks. Note the sharp peaks and the confusions between different epiphyses.

2.2 Modeling spatial relations in a CRF

To find the best global configuration, i.e., predicting the most probable location $c_i \in \hat{\mathcal{X}}_i$ for every landmark i, the spatial relations between individual landmarks are modeled in a CRF. We use $s_i \in \{1, \ldots, n\}$ to denote the assignment of $c_i = \hat{x}_{i,s_i}$ in order to define the pseudo probability distribution $\widetilde{P}(\mathbf{s} \mid \mathbf{I})$. This pseudo probability $\widetilde{P}(\mathbf{s} \mid \mathbf{I})$ is then subject to maximization, hence the missing normalization. Each landmark is assigned an unary term $U_{i,l}$, which depends on landmark i and judges how well the regressor ensemble assumes that the l-th candidate for the i-th landmark corresponds to the true position. We make use of the pseudo probability $\widetilde{\mathbf{P}}_i$ by normalizing over the set of all image pixels

$$U_{i,l} = \widetilde{\mathbf{P}}_i(\hat{\mathbf{x}}_{i,l}) \Big/ \sum_{\mathbf{x}} \widetilde{\mathbf{P}}_i(\mathbf{x}) \tag{1}$$

Three binary terms are used to capture the spatial relations between two different landmarks i and j, assuming a certain topology of the CRF. First, a Gaussian distribution is used to model the distance between i and j, with the parameters mean $\mu_{i,j}$ and variance $\sigma_{i,j}^2$ being estimated on the training set

$$L_{i,l,j,m} = f(\|\hat{\mathbf{x}}_{i,l} - \hat{\mathbf{x}}_{j,m}\| ; \mu_{i,j}, \sigma_{i,j}^2) \tag{2}$$

Second, a von Mises distribution is used to model the orientation of a line from i to j. The key parameters $\mu_{i,j}$ and $\kappa_{i,j}$ are estimated on the training annotations with g being the probability density function of a von Mises distribution and $\alpha(\mathbf{x})$ denoting the angle between $\mathbf{x}$ and the x-axis

$$O_{i,l,j,m} = g(\alpha(\hat{\mathbf{x}}_{i,l} - \hat{\mathbf{x}}_{j,m}); \mu_{i,j}, \kappa_{i,j}) \tag{3}$$

The third binary term is a hard constraint to exclude cases that are biologically impossible, which improves the accuracy of approximate inference strategies. To do this, we model the alignment of two neighboring landmarks in the xy-plane. Possible alignments of landmarks i and j are defined in $\mathcal{A}^{i,j}$ and derived from the anatomy, with $\mathbf{1} : \mathbb{Z}^2 \to \{0,1\}$ being the indicator function testing if the given alignment is contained in $\mathcal{A}^{i,j}$

$$A_{i,l,j,m} = \mathbf{1}_{\mathcal{A}^{i,j}}[\text{sgn}(\hat{\mathbf{x}}_{i,l} - \hat{\mathbf{x}}_{j,m})] \tag{4}$$

Finally, we combine unary and binary terms in a CRF represented by a graph $G = (V, E)$, where $V = \{1, \ldots, N\}$ is the set of nodes corresponding to the landmarks ($N = 12$ epiphyses) and $E \subseteq V^2$ is the set of edges between two nodes

$$\widetilde{P}(\mathbf{s} \mid \mathbf{I}) = \prod_{i \in V} U_{i,s_i} \cdot \prod_{i,j \in E} L_{i,s_i,j,s_j} \cdot O_{i,s_i,j,s_j} \cdot A_{i,s_i,j,s_j} \tag{5}$$

Table 1. Localization performance of our proposed method (RF + CRF) on the hand radiograph dataset in comparison to the results achieved by the method of Hahmann et al. (DGHT + SCM), listed as amount of correctly localized images in percent (%).

Landmark	1D	2D	3D	5D	6D	7D	9D	10D	11D	13D	14D	15D	Mean
DGHT + SCM	**99.5**	99.1	99.3	**99.7**	99.3	**99.3**	99.0	99.5	99.8	99.0	99.3	99.8	99.4
RF + CRF	98.8	**99.8**	**99.5**	98.8	**99.8**	99.0	**100.0**	**100.0**	**100.0**	99.3	**99.8**	**100.0**	**99.6**

This joint measure is then subject to maximization in order to find the most likely configuration $\hat{s} = \arg\max_{s \in S} \widetilde{P}(s \mid I)$ over all configurations S. Due to the large number of possible configurations $|S| = n^N$, an exact solution is intractable to compute if n is large (even for $n = 10$). Instead, we make use of an approximate inference algorithm called Lazy Flipper [4]. This is a move making strategy for discrete models, guaranteeing an optimal solution in a Hamming radius to a subgraph size (we use 3). This allows to balance the trade-off between runtime and accuracy. An appropriate starting configuration is crucial for good performance, thus we start with the first localization hypothesis for each landmark, which corresponds to the maximization of the unary terms only.

3 Results

We compared the proposed method against the state-of-the-art approach of Hahmann et al. [1] on a challenging corpus from Uniklinik RWTH Aachen featuring hand radiographs. The objective is to localize 12 well-defined landmarks, each being an epiphyseal plate, in a set of 412 images from patients in the age of 3 to 18 years given a training set of 400 images. As introduced by Fischer et al. [5] as human-like performance, a localization is considered successful if the predicted position is within a threshold of $t = \text{image\_height} \cdot \frac{6}{256}$ to the true position. The CRF topology was derived by using the 8-connected neighborhoods of all epiphyses treating them as a 4×3 grid resulting in 35 connections (Fig. 1b). We chose to use the $n = 15$ best localization hypotheses for each landmark, for which the localization performance is listed in Table 1 in comparison to the results of Hahmann et al. An average localization accuracy of 99.6 % over all 12 landmarks has been achieved. In 96.4 % of the 412 images, all epiphyses were correctly localized, while 1, 1, 1 and 12 images still contained 5, 3, 2 and 1 error, respectively. Examples of typical errors are shown in Fig. 2b. Our Python implementation (not yet optimized for runtime) needed ~ 11 hours total training time and required ~ 32 seconds for a single test image on $2 \times$ Intel XEON E5-2540 CPUs, which reduces the training time compared to [1] by an order of magnitude at comparable test time. An evaluation of the number of localization hypotheses n is illustrated in Fig. 2a. The localizer alone has an accuracy of 93.5 %, but was already improved by more than ~ 4 percent points using $n = 2$ hypotheses instead of 1. If n increases beyond ~ 10, the localization accuracy saturates at increasing runtime. Note that the CRF results are close to the upper bound, which is caused by the artificially limited number of localization hypotheses.

4 Discussion

In this paper, we described a simple two-step approach for localizing spatially correlated landmarks. First, we showed that it is not necessary to use a prior classification step to confine the candidate region for each landmark (first step in [2]). Instead, a local regression for candidate landmark positions in combination with non-maximum suppression is sufficient, since confusions of a landmark position with a different landmark can be resolved in the second step, if the number of candidate positions per landmark, used by the graphical model, is large enough. To train the regression tree ensemble and account for ambiguities in the ground truth annotations, we introduce a sharply peaked Gaussian distribution around the true position of a landmark, which accounts for the accuracy of the landmark candidates. To achieve this accuracy, Donner et al. [2] needed a Hough regression forest in addition to a binary classification step and Hahmann et al. [1] needed a second-level, local DGHT model.

Acknowledgement. This work has been financially supported by the Federal Ministry of Education and Research under the grant 03FH013IX5. The liability for the content of this work lies with the authors.

References

1. Hahmann F, Böer G, Gabriel E, et al. Classification of voting patterns to improve the generalized Hough transform for epiphyses localization. SPIE MI. 2016.
2. Donner R, Menze BH, Bischof H, et al. Global localization of 3D anatomical structures by pre-filtered Hough Forests and discrete optimization. Med Im Anal. 2013.
3. Criminisi A, Robertson D, et al. Regression forests for efficient anatomy detection and localization in computed tomography scans. Med Im Anal. 2013.
4. Andres B, Kappes JH, Beier T, et al. The lazy flipper: efficient depth-limited exhaustive search in discrete graphical models. ECCV. 2012.
5. Fischer B, Brosig A, Deserno TM, et al. Structural scene analysis and content-based image retrieval applied to bone age assessment. SPIE Med Imaging. 2009.

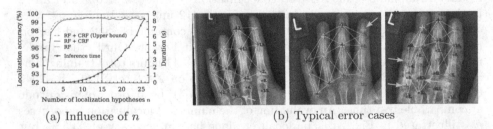

(a) Influence of n (b) Typical error cases

Fig. 2. (a) Localization performance of different settings shown over different numbers of localization hypotheses n as well as the average inference time. (b) Illustration of some error cases caused by (from left to right) anatomical aberration, localizer inaccuracy in combination with a too large NMS minimum distance and distorted images.

Real-Time-Capable GPU-Framework for Depth-Aware Rigid 2D/3D Registration

Matthias Utzschneider[1], Jian Wang[2], Roman Schaffert[1,2], Anja Borsdorf[2], Andreas Maier[1,3]

[1]Pattern Recognition Lab, FAU Erlangen-Nuremberg, Erlangen
[2]Siemens Healthineers, Forchheim
[3]Erlangen Graduate School in Advanced Optical Technologies, Erlangen
matthias.utzschneider@fau.de

Abstract. 2D/3D image fusion is used for a variety of interventional procedures. Overlays of 2D images with perspective-correctly rendered 3D images provide the physicians additional information during the interventions. In this work, a real-time capable 2D/3D registration framework is presented. An adapted parallelization using GPU is investigated for the depth-aware registration algorithm. The GPU hardware architecture is specially taken into account by optimizing memory access patterns and exploiting CUDA-texture memory. The real-time capability is achieved with a median runtime of one 2D/3D registration iteration of 86.1 ms with an median accuracy of up to 1.15 mm.

1 Introduction

Imaging gained more and more importance in interventional medicine over the last decades. In the family of diverse medical imaging modalities, X-ray fluoroscopy is the standard routine for many interventional procedures. The fluoroscopic images are acquired intra-operatively by the interventional C-arm system. Intra-operative images are often combined with pre-operative images acquired by Computed Tomography (CT) or Magnetic Resonance Tomography (MRT) to give the physicians information about the 3D position of interventional devices to provide guidance. The interventional fluoroscopies are combined with 3D images by rendering a perspective-correct view of the 3D image and superimpose it onto the 2D fluoroscopy. This procedure is called 2D/3D image fusion. For an accurate overlay of fluoroscopy and CT image, the application has to compensate for misalignments often introduced by patient movement. To maintain the accuracy of the overlay, 2D/3D registration algorithms are applied. Furthermore, any interventional application has to meet time constraints. These circumstances make it necessary for the implementations to be performance-oriented and adjusted to the processing architecture. In the recent years, the use of special hardware like Graphic Processing Units (GPUs) has been investigated for computationally intensive tasks in high performance computing. For example, rendering of Digitally Reconstructed Radiographs (DRRs) is an often used approach in 2D/3D

185

registration, which is well parallelizable and computational intensive. GPUs became very common for implementations of 2D/3D registration algorithms [1].

In this paper a real-time registration implementation of an algorithm [2] based on the point-to-plane correspondence (PPC) model [3] for rigid registration is presented. The proposed approach makes use of the high performance of GPUs for applications with a potential for high parallelism and exploits special hardware optimizations for GPUs. This paper is structured as follows. In Sec. 2, an overview of the registration algorithm is given and the parallelization method for the overall algorithm and for computationally intensive sub-steps is described. Runtime performance is evaluated and results are presented in Sec. 3. In Sec. 4, results are summarized and future development possibilities are outlined.

2   Materials and methods

2.1   Depth-aware registration algorithm

To correct the misalignments and preserve the accuracy of the 2D/3D overlay, a transformation $\mathbf{T}_{\mathrm{Reg}} \in \mathbb{R}^{4 \times 4}$ has to be estimated to compensate for the motion. $\mathbf{T}_{\mathrm{Reg}}$ is determined by the depth-aware registration based on the feature-based PPC model [3]. With this model, a linear system of equations is formulated using a set of feature points $\{\mathbf{w}\}_{\mathrm{corr}}$ for the observed volume and a set of corresponding 2D points $\{\mathbf{p}'\}_{\mathrm{corr}}$ on the fluoroscopic image I_0 [3]. For the proposed approach, an initial set of feature points with an high 3D image gradient, e.g. on bone surfaces $\{\mathbf{w}\}_{\mathrm{init}}$ is extracted from the volume using the 3D Canny filter [4]. In the preselection step, occluding contour points $\{\mathbf{w}\}_{\mathrm{sel}}$ are selected from the current viewing direction [3]. In the tracking step, correspondences for $\{\mathbf{w}\}_{\mathrm{sel}}$ are searched with Depth-layer-gradient Images (DLIs) [5] of the volume and gradient images of the fluoroscopy using a patch-matching approach. This patch-matching routine [2] determines the set of feature points and correspondences $\{\mathbf{w}, \mathbf{p}'\}_{\mathrm{corr}}$ for the estimation of $\mathbf{T}_{\mathrm{Reg}}$. The transformation $\mathbf{T}_{\mathrm{Reg}}$ is computed by solving the system of equations using iterative-reweighted least square optimization.

2.2   GPU-parallelization of the registration algorithm

The above algorithm offers the ease of parallelization to reduce the overall runtime of the approach. To harness the high parallel processing potential of GPUs, the algorithm is implemented in Nvidia CUDA for Nvidia GPUs. All sub-steps are implemented with the parallelization adapted to the sub-steps properties. The rendering of DLIs is similar to the DRR generation, which is well parallelizable for GPUs [1]. For the DLI-rendering, the volume is initially stored in a 3D CUDA-texture. The advantage of using CUDA-textures for sampling is the efficient hardware-implemented interpolation and 3D spatial caching. The preselection as well as the patch-matching routine are executable for every feature point independently. Therefore, the GPU-implementation yields great potential for a runtime improvement. The well parallelizable steps, i.e. preselection and patch-matching, are performed on the GPU for all initial feature points in parallel. Furthermore, all feature points are processed in the GPU memory to avoid CPU-GPU memory transfer latencies. The final estimation of $\mathbf{T}_{\text{Reg}}$ is performed on the CPU and is the sole step executed on the CPU. Therefore, only feature points with correspondences as well as the correspondences themselves are transferred from the VRAM to the processors main-memory. An overview of the implemented GPU registration framework is given in Fig. 1.

2.3   Patch-matching parallelization

To improve the performance of the patch-matching step, two approaches are investigated. The routine uses Gradient Correlation [6] on multiple patches in the vicinity of each feature point to find corresponding points between DLIs and the gradient image of the fluoroscopy. A feature-based and a patch-based parallelization is examined to achieve real-time performance. The feature-based method distributes all patch-matching computations necessary for one single feature point to one single CUDA-thread each. This approach increases the simultaneously executed computations significantly compared to a multi-core CPU implementation with at least 32 threads processing in parallel. In the patch-based routine, each patch processed for a feature point position is assigned to one CUDA-thread. Patches processed for one feature point overlap strongly and therefore GPU memory is accessed in close spatial vicinity. To benefit from caching and to coalesce memory accesses, all patches for one feature points are processed in parallel by concurrently working threads on the GPU. To further improve data access read-only data caching is used for DLI-images and fluoroscopy gradient images, which enables L1-caching of all accessed data.

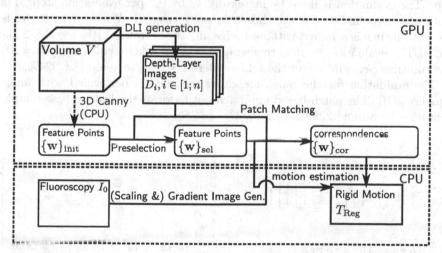

Fig. 1. Overview of the GPU-based registration Framework. All data and steps within the dashed lines reside respectively are executed on the denoted hardware architecture.

2.4 Depth-layer-image sampling

DLIs are used to find correspondences for feature points in a patch-matching routine. The DLI-rendering is implemented in a CUDA kernel using a ray-based parallelization. The memory access patterns of the kernel is adapted to the spatial caching of CUDA-textures. To further improve the runtime-performance of the kernel, the sampling step k_s is varied. By increasing k_s, the necessary number of volume-texture evaluations decreases, but it can worsen the accuracy due to lack of evaluated sampling points. The optimal sampling step is determined, which does not deteriorate the mean Target Registration Error (mTRE) [7] of the overall approach and yields the best runtime result for DLI-rendering.

3 Results

The evaluation of the runtime performance is done on a high performance test-system using a modern Nvidia GPU for professional rendering (Intel Xeon E4-1620v3@3.5GHz, 8GB DDR4-RAM, NVIDIA Quadro K2200 (640 CUDA-Cores, 1 GHz, 5 SMs). The evaluation setup from [3] with ten image sequences of a thorax phantom is used for the runtime evaluation. All runtime measurements are averaged over ten runs. The accuracy of the approach is indicated by the mTRE and the mean Projection Error (mPE) [3]. In the first evaluation, the different patch-matching methods are evaluated for the best runtime. The best volume sampling step for rendering DLIs is determined by an accuracy and runtime evaluation. The overall runtime-performance is evaluated using the determined sampling step and patch-matching approach.

The volume sampling step k_s is initially chosen as 1.0 voxel per sampling step. The evaluation is done by increasing k_s by 0.2 per evaluation step. The runtime and the mTRE for the chosen k_s are measured. With $k_s = 2.0$ voxels, the best runtime is achieved without increasing the overall mTRE, see Fig. 2 and Fig. 3. The evaluation results are averaged over all image sequences (#1-#10). The run-time performance of the DLI-rendering step is increased by 224%.

The evaluation for the patch-matching methods is performed with image sequence #10. The patch-based approach outperforms the feature-based implementation by around 228%, see Tab. 1.

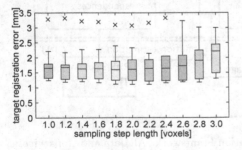 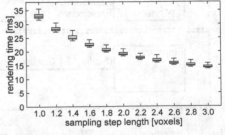

Fig. 2. Error evaluation for different k_s [sampling step length].

Fig. 3. Runtime evaluation for different k_s [sampling step length].

Table 1. Average and best runtimes of the patch-matching implementations.

Implementation	Average [ms]	Best [ms]	Speed-Up (Average)
GPU (feature-based):	92.11	84.82	-
GPU (patch-based):	40.31	34.53	×2.28

For the evaluation of the overall framework, the patch-based implementation and a sampling step of $k_s = 2.0$ voxels per sampling step is used. An average runtime of 86,1 ms and a best runtime of 73,1 ms is reached in the evaluation setup, which is considered real-time capable for dynamic 2D/3D registration [8]. In comparison with a single-core CPU implementation using an OpenGL DLI-rendering a speed-up of ×41.2 is achieved, see Tab. 3. The mTRE depending on the image sequence is 0.86 mm at best and 1.21 mm in average and does not exceed 2.0 mm for 8 out of 10 sequences, see Tab. 2. The mPE does not exceed 2.0 mm for all sequences and is 1.15 mm in average and 0.80 mm at best, see Tab. 2.

4   Discussion

In this paper, a GPU-based real-time 2D/3D registration framework is presented. A depth-aware registration approach using the PPC model is implemented for Nvidia GPUs. The framework makes use of the high parallelism of GPUs and is optimized for Nvidia GPU architecture exploiting CUDA-texture memory and read-only data-cached memory access. The implementation is adjusted for the special architectural demands of GPUs by coalescing GPU memory accesses and taking spatial caching-strategies of CUDA-texture memory into account. Real-time capability [8] and a runtime performance of 13 frames per second at best is achieved with the GPU-framework and an adapted volume sampling step. Only one approach for 2D/3D registration reaches a similar framerate and a higher runtime-performance is not reached by approaches reported in literature [9] to the best knowledge of the author.

Sequence	#frames	$mTRE$ [mm]	$mRPE$ [mm]
1	33	4.39 ± 0.35	1.18 ± 0.12
2	93	1.23 ± 0.40	1.03 ± 0.22
3	111	1.16 ± 0.20	1.13 ± 0.21
4	111	1.08 ± 0.28	1.06 ± 0.19
5	110	1.53 ± 0.24	1.17 ± 0.28
6	101	0.83 ± 0.23	0.80 ± 0.12
7	105	3.48 ± 2.92	1.27 + 0.47
8	117	1.77 ± 0.68	1.29 ± 0.14
9	114	0.86 ± 0.24	0.80 ± 0.16
10	121	1.19 ± 0.25	1.49 ± 0.23

Table 2. $mTRE$ and $mRPE$ and standard deviation of the implemented approach.

Table 3. Average and best runtimes of one registration iteration for the different implementations.

Implementation	Average [ms]	Best [ms]	Speed-Up (Average)
CPU (single-core$\|k_s = 1.0$)	3553.27	2633.44	-
GPU (feature-based$\|k_s = 1.0$)	174,36	171,93	$\times 20, 38$
GPU (patch-based$\|k_s = 2.0$)	86.11	73.47	$\times 41, 2$

For further development, the GPU framework is to be completed by implementing the final motion estimation step on the GPU. With the achieved real-time capability multi-start approaches similar to [10] are feasible to be investigated.

References

1. Abdellah M, Eldeib A, Owis MI. GPU acceleration for digitally reconstructed radiographs using bindless texture objects and CUDA/OpenGL interoperability. Conf Proc IEEE Eng Med Biol Soc. 2015; p. 4242–5.
2. Borsdorf A, Wang J. Verfahren zur 2D-3D-Registrierung, Recheneinrichtung und Computerprogramm. DE Patent 102015208929, May 13; 2016.
3. Wang J, Borsdorf A, Heigl B. Gradient-based differential approach for 3-D motion compensation in interventional 2-D/3-D image fusion. Proc Int Conf 3D Vis. 2014;1:293–300.
4. Canny J. A computational approach to edge detection. IEEE Trans Pattern Anal Mach Intell. 1986;8(6):679–98.
5. Wang J, Borsdorf A, Hornegger J. Depth-layer-based patient motion compensation for the overlay of 3D volumes onto x-ray sequences. Proc BVM. 2013;3(13):128–22.
6. Wein W, Roeper B, Navab N. 2D/3D registration based on volume gradients. Proc SPIE. 2005;5747:144–50.
7. van de Kraats E, Penney GB, Tomaževič D, et al. Standardized evaluation methodology for 2-D-3-D registration. IEEE Trans Med Imaging. 2005;24(9):1177–89.
8. Heimann T, Mountey T, John M, et al. Real-time ultrasound transducer localization in fluoroscopy images by transfer learning from synthetic training data. Med Image Anal. 2014;18(8):1320–8.
9. Liao R, Zhang L, Sun Y, et al. A review of recent advances in registration techniques applied to minimally invasive therapy. Med Image Anal. 2013;5(15):983–98.
10. Otake Y, Wang A, Stayman JW, et al. Robust 3D-2D image registration: application to spine interventions and vertebral labeling in the presence of anatomical deformation. Phys Med Biol. 2013;1(58):8535–53.

Defining Restrictions and Limits of Registration-Based Quantification of Geometric Deformation in Cerebral Blood Vessels

Daniel Schetelig[1], Jan Sedlacik[2], Felix Schmidt[3], Jens Fiehler[2], René Werner[1]

[1]Department of Computational Neuroscience,
University Medical Center Hamburg-Eppendorf
[2]Department of Diagnostic and Interventional Neuroradiology,
University Medical Center Hamburg-Eppendorf
[3]Department of Osteology and Biomechanics,
University Medical Center Hamburg-Eppendorf
d.schetelig@uke.de

Abstract. Hemodynamic and mechanical parameters are assumed to play an important role in explaining the initiation, growth and rupture of cerebral aneurysms. Pulsatile deformation of the vascular system due to the changes in pressure during the cardiac cycle are of high interest. Typical spatial and temporal resolution of the image data causes the quantification of geometric deformation to be challenging. In addition, flow velocity changes and the inflow of contrast agents cause vessel intensity variations. These variations in intensity can be mistaken as geometric deformations, leading to an overestimation of the true geometric deformation. In this work, a novel flow phantom is designed to generate ground-truth datasets, which are used to further investigate the relationship between intensity variations and the estimation of geometric deformation. The ground truth image data is used to investigate feasibility and limits of pulsatile deformation estimation using non-linear registration.

1 Introduction

Currently, the assessment of risk of rupture of aneurysms depends primarily on size and location of the investigated aneurysms [1]. However, using only size and location of the respective aneurysm omits hemodynamic and mechanical factors of the vascular system, which are thought to play an important role in the appearance and evolution of aneurysms [2]. Yet, these hemodynamic and mechanical factors are still to be incorporated into the risk assesment of aneurysms. This study focuses on the analysis of the pulsatile geometric deformation of the vascular system, specifically the quantification of geometric deformation of blood vessels. While some publications exist, which claim to detect and quantify geometrical changes of blood vessels, the subject remains challenging: Publications in this domain typically depend on temporally resolved magnetic resonance angiography (MRA) and/or computed tomography angiography (CTA) images.

Using these modalities, the image intensities are dependent on flow velocity and/or the inflow of a contrast agent. Thus, vessel intensities fluctuate across the cardiac cycle, which undermines the accuracy of, for instance, vessel segmentation methods and renders precise segmentation-based motion and deformation quantification challenging. This obstacle becomes even more prominent when analyzing cerebral blood vessels since these vessels are in the same order of magnitude as the spatial resolution of used imaging modalities, requiring the segmentation method to be sub-pixel accurate. This study focuses on MR as main image modality, as the spatial resolution for MR images is typically smaller than for CT images. It is plausible that a precise motion/deformation analysis algorithm for MR images would therefore also be applicable to CT data.

Since the evaluation of segmentation and motion/deformation analysis algorithms is problematic without ground truth knowledge of geometric properties of used data, a hardware flow phantom capable of generating pulsatile flow was designed to produce ground truth images. As the geometric properties of the flow phantom are known, the generated data set is well suited to serve as a testing base for segmentation and motion/deformation analysis algorithms.

The main contributions of our presentation will be: In line with the BVM workshop character, we report on our experiences during the process of designing the flow phantom. A current registration-based approach for pulsatile deformation analysis is reimplemented and evaluated using the generated phantom dataset. The goal of this study is to investigate whether current motion/deformation analysis approaches are suitable for this challenging problem.

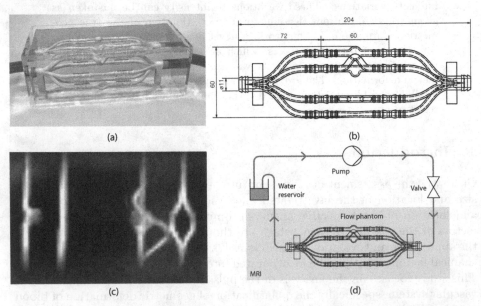

Fig. 1. Overview of the developed flow phantom prototype and the schematic experimental setup. (a) computer aided design, (b) technical drawing, (c) maximum intensity projection of MR scan, (d) measurement setup.

2 Materials and methods

2.1 Hardware flow phantom prototype

The measurement setup of the phantom is shown in Fig. 1(d). While the flow phantom itself is placed inside the MR, the remaining parts are arranged outside. The pump provides static pressure and therefore continuous flow, which can be interjected at a desired rate using the valve, simulating the mechanic action of the heart and generating a pulsatile flow profile. Computer-aided design and a technical drawing of the phantom are shown in Fig. 1 (a) and (b). While the intake and outtake of the flow phantom are fixed, the middle part is exchangeable. This allows for a variety of structures in different sizes to be used as a phantom. The current setup consists of six modular tube structures, which have been modeled in reference to anatomical structures (straight tube, stenosis, helix, bifurcation, double-sided aneurysm, one-sided aneurysm). All structures are 3D-printed, which allows for easy creation of new structures. To ensure that all 3D-printed structures are manufactured accurately, all structures of the flow phantom have been scanned using a HR-pQCT with a spatial resolution of 41 μm/px, which enabled us to replace inaccurate parts. The used material has a high Young's modulus relative to the applied pressure to ensure that the structures do not deform during the experiment. The setup exists for three inner diameters ($\varnothing_{i1}= 4$ mm, $\varnothing_{i2}= 3$ mm, $\varnothing_{i3}= 2$ mm, wall thickness of 1 mm), which allows for the evaluation of segmentation or motion/deformation analysis algorithms to be performed at different levels of precision and complexity. The flow phantom generates pulsatile flow with a plausible physiological flow velocity [3].

A possible objection to the flow phantom might be the use of water instead of blood. Furthermore, the generated pulse wave does not resemble an exact cardiac pulsation. While it is true that blood has a different viscosity than water, which might result in slightly different flow patterns, the differences in flow velocity fluctuations between blood and water would be negligible. The main objective of the flow phantom is to simulate the principles of varying flow velocity and the effects on measured intensities, which should, given the limits of the spatial and temporal resolution of MR sequences, not depend on the used fluid and the precise shape of the flow velocity profile. Therefore these aspects do not imply a fundamental lack in imitation of the mechanics of the cardiac cycle and the phantom seems viable to serve as a ground truth.

2.2 Image acquisition and data description

The phantom image datasets were acquired using TWIST [4] (time-resolved angiography with interleaved stochastic trajectories) and Flow [5] MR sequences with a magnetic flux density of 3T. The contrast-media enhanced TWIST sequence (4 ml GdDTPA-BMA [Omniscan], dilution 1:5) is used to study the effects of intensity variations due to contrast media inflow. The Flow sequence served as a basis to analyze the influence of flow velocity induced intensity variation. The spatial resolution for the TWIST-sequence is 1.3 mm/px and 1.0 mm/px (isotropically) for the Flow-sequence, respectively.

2.3 Registration-based deformation estimation

While most publications seem to use simple thresholding methods for vessel segmentation and subsequent analysis of pulsatile geometric deformation [6, 7], Oubel et al. proposed a registration-based algorithm for the estimation of wall motion, which promises to be an advancement in this field of study [8]. Their proposed algorithm uses non-linear registration with B-spline interpolation functions and mutual information as distance metric, which was assumed to be robust against intensity variations during the inflow of contrast agent or changes in flow velocity. The approach was reimplemented for our study using elastix [9]. A multi-resolution cubic B-spline registration with mutual information as metric was used. Every phase of the data sets is registered to the first phase, generating a set of transformations for every point in time and space relative to the first phase. Following Oubel et al., landmarks are automatically defined using the edge information of the phantom structures to analyze the temporal changes and quantify the assumed geometric deformations. These landmarks are propagated using the set of transformation generated by the registration approach. The displacement of the landmarks is then calculated by computing the Euclidean distance between each pair of points for every point in time.

3 Results

The MRI measurements of the flow phantom design provided ground truth data. An exemplary maximum intensity projection is shown in Fig. 2. When viewed closely, deformations and intensity variations appear visibly in the phantom dataset, although the physical flow phantom is static. This inevitably increases the difficulty of (semi-)manual segmentation and deformation analysis considerably since the image sequence seems to reproduce an actual deformation. Therefore the implementation of a (semi-)manual segmentation approach does not seem feasible.

Instead, the registration-based approach might provide more reliable results for the quantification of geometric deformation of the flow phantom. The results of the landmark motion for a TWIST- and a Flow-phantom-dataset (red: $\varnothing_i$

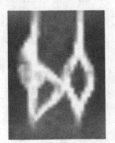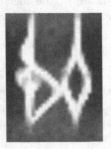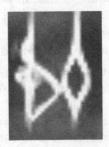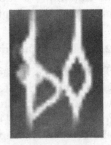

Fig. 2. Temporal maximum intensity projection of MRI image sequence of the phantom with 3 mm inner diameter.

= 4 mm, blue: $\emptyset_i = 3$ mm) are shown in Fig. 3. The registration-based approach detects nonzero motion. Especially the TWIST dataset (contrast-media enhanced) reflects the typical inflow curve of a contrast agent, represented in the determined deformations. The results of the Flow dataset depicts a smaller, yet still nonzero landmark motion and vessel deformation. Since the physical flow phantom exhibits no geometric deformation, the calculated deformation should be zero. However, the spatial resolution is at 1.3 mm / px (TWIST), respectively 1.0 (Flow), rendering the estimated deformation still in sub-pixel size. While the non-zero deformation is problematic, the current result could indicate that a geometric deformation could only be reliably quantified, if the deformation surpasses a minimum expansion. Therefore, instead of a precise quantification of geometric deformation, the results could be used to define a minimum threshold of geometric deformation, which must be apparent to quantify the geometric deformation reliably.

4   Discussion

We presented a newly developed modular flow phantom which provides a reliable ground truth for the evaluation of algorithms for blood vessel segmentation and deformation analysis. The focus of this work was to establish the flow phantom and evaluate the influence of intensity variations on the motion and deformation analysis of blood vessels. The flow phantom produces image data suitable to serve as ground truth. However, the produced data reveals effects in relationship with changes in flow velocity which are of high interest. The registration-based motion analysis and deformation approach provides promising, yet still improvable results. Although the deformation estimation is in very small bounds, it would be desirable to produce a zero value deformation estimation for the static flow phantom. Nonetheless, the current results of this study can be used to define a minimum limit for a vessel deformation, in order to be reliably quantifiable.

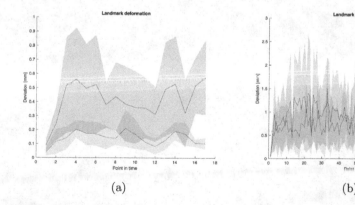

(a)   (b)

Fig. 3. Phantom data landmark deformation by a registration-based deformation estimation approach. (a) Twist: phantom data set (red: $\emptyset_i = 4$ mm, blue: $\emptyset_i = 3$ mm), (b) Flow: phantom data set (red: $\emptyset_i = 4$ mm, blue: $\emptyset_i = 3$ mm).

For the near future, we intend to further investigate the effects of flow velocity changes on intensities in MRI sequences. Therefore a flow phantom with a reproducible deformation is to be designed, to simulate the deformation of vessels in vivo more precise. In addition, a robust segmentation and motion/deformation analysis algorithm is to be developed respectively the current implementation tuned, aimed to compensate for the previously specified challenges, extending to reproducible deformations.

References

1. Wiebers DO, Whisnant JP, Huston J, et al. Unruptured intracranial aneurysms: natural history, clinical outcome, and risks of surgical and endovascular treatment. Lancet. 2003;362(9378):103–10.
2. Meyer FB, Huston J, Riederer SS. Pulsatile increases in aneurysm size determined by cine phase-contrast MR angiography. J Neurosurg. 1993;78(6):879–83.
3. Lindegaard KF, Lundar T, Wiberg J, et al. Variations in middle cerebral artery blood flow investigated with noninvasive transcranial blood velocity measurements. Stroke. 1987;18(6):1025–30.
4. Laub G, Randall K. syngo TWIST for dynamic time-resolved MR angiography. MAGNETOM Flash. 2006; p. 92–5.
5. Markl M, Frydrychowicz A, Kozerke S, et al. 4D flow MRI. J Magn Reson Imaging. 2012;36(5):1015–36.
6. Kuroda J, Kinoshita M, Tanaka H, et al. Cardiac cycle-related volume change in unruptured cerebral aneurysms: a detailed volume quantification study using 4-dimensional CT angiography. Stroke. 2012;43(1):61–6.
7. Nishida T, Kinoshita M, Tanaka H, et al. Quantification of cerebral artery motion during the cardiac cycle. AJNR. 2011;32(11):206–8.
8. Oubel E, Cebral JR, De Craene M, et al. Wall motion estimation in intracranial aneurysms. Physiol Meas. 2010;31(9):1119–35.
9. Klein S, Staring M, Murphy K, et al. Elastix: a toolbox for intensity-based medical image registration. IEEE Trans Med Imaging. 2010;29(1):196–205.

Dental Splint Fabrication for Prospective Motion Correction in Ultrahigh-Field MR Imaging

Gabriel Mistelbauer[1], Daniel Stucht[2], Yan L. Arnold[2], Oliver Speck[2], Bernhard Preim[1]

[1]Dept. Simulation and Graphics, Otto-von-Guericke University Magdeburg, Germany
[2]Dept. Biomed. Mag. Resonance, Otto-von-Guericke University Magdeburg, Germany
gmistelbauer@isg.cs.uni-magdeburg.de

Abstract. For prospective motion correction in ultrahigh-field magnetic resonance imaging, optical tracking is employed by fixating a tailored dental splint on the subject's upper jaw. However, producing such dental splints is cumbersome and exposes subjects to significant discomfort due to the required dental cast preparation. To catalyze the production of these custom-made splints, we propose a semi-automated workflow.By retrospectively digitizing dental casts of five subjects using a 3D laser scanner, we virtually graft the dental splints and, once visually analyzed and approved, they are fabricated by a 3D printer.This process increases subject comfort and reduces the preparation time.

1 Introduction

Magnetic resonance imaging (MRI) has become an important modality for medical diagnosis and neuroscientific research due to its non-invasive nature. The availability of enhanced contrast mechanisms and the increased signal-to-noise ratio (SNR) at higher field strengths promoted ultrahigh-field magnetic resonance imaging (UHF-MRI), enabling anatomical, vascular and functional imaging with much higher resolution [1]. Various problems arise from the relatively long scan time of typically several minutes for a single volume. Particularly at high resolution, data acquisition is sensitive to subject motion, which can induce artifacts and significantly degrade image quality. An effective correction of 3D rigid-body motion of the head can be achieved by using prospective motion correction (PMC) [2]. This method employs motion tracking to perform a real-time update of the MRI system's spatial encoding (gradients and frequencies) during data acquisition. In our current setup, 6 degrees of freedom (DOF) head movement is tracked with a single camera using a moiré pattern target.

Several fixation methods for the optical target, e.g. tape, clay or goggles, at different locations, e.g. between the eyes or on the forehead, have been analyzed. Even though PMC with these fixation methods might help to reduce strong motion artifacts and improve image quality, the stability and, thus, the accuracy is not suitable for ultrahigh resolution imaging [3]. As we attach the target to the subjects upper jaw using a custom-made dental splint, it is rigidly moving with the head. Hence, the tracked data represents the motion of the human brain, rendering these splints suitable for UHF-MRI [4]. The production of conventional dental splints (top image of Fig. 1(d)) takes several days. Consequently, subjects are invited a least twice: once for taking an imprint to form the dental cast and once to perform the actual study. If the dental splint does not perfectly fit, a third visit is necessary. This renders PMC impractical for studies with a large number of subjects. We suggest an optical scan to obtain a 3D model of the subjects teeth. The dental splint is created using an automated segmentation of the data and fabricated with a 3D printer at lower time effort and cost.

For this proof of concept study, we use digitized dental casts to graft dental splints. As intra-oral scanners are already available, we expect that the 3D information can be acquired directly from the subjects jaw for future studies, as described by Salmi et al. [5]. They create dental occlusal splints using surface extrusion of the acquired geometric mesh. Since computing offset surfaces is rather complicated, especially in highly curved regions as the teeth, artifacts might occur. Motivated by their approach, the contributions of this paper can be summarized as follows:

– a semi-automated approach for virtual dental splint identification,
– a volumetric method to graft artifact-free splints of arbitrary thickness, and
– a quick and cost-effective production of these dental splints.

2   Materials and methods

Since we aim to produce the splint and perform the actual MRI examination in only one visit, we simplify and catalyze the conventional process, i.e. make it less personnel-intensive, by proposing a new workflow (Fig. 1) that uses 3D printing. In the first step, we retrospectively digitize dental casts using a 3D laser scanner. Secondly, the region-of-interest (RoI) of the desired dental splint is determined and, thirdly, the digital model of the dental splint is generated and subject to quality assurance in form of visual inspection. Once approved, it is exported and, as fourth step, 3D printed. Each step of our workflow is subsequently detailed.

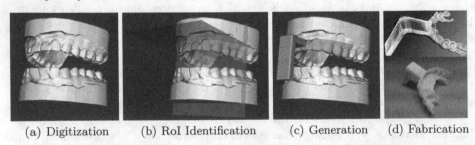

(a) Digitization   (b) RoI Identification   (c) Generation   (d) Fabrication

Fig. 1. Our proposed workflow. (a) shows the digitized dental cast of the upper jaw (yellow) and the mirrored (white) as context below. The RoI of the dental splint is determined in (b) and the splint is generated in (c). The conventional dental splint is shown in the top image of (d) and our fabricated splint in the bottom image.

2.1   Dental cast digitization

The physical dental casts of the subjects' upper jaws have been digitized with a Minolta Vivid 910 / VI-910 non-contact 3D digitizer. The casts have been placed on a computer-controlled turntable and twelve scans with an angular turn of 30° between each have been acquired. In total, we recorded 24 scans per dental cast of five subjects, two full rotations from two different viewing angles to capture all details of the physical casts and reduce post-processing.

The registration and merging has been accomplished with the Polygon Editing Tool software from Minolta. The resulting 3D mesh of the cast is then imported into Autodesk MeshMixer for post-processing, i.e. closing holes and merging double surfaces. After removing minor artifacts, such as falsely joint teeth, the mesh is re-meshed to obtain a uniform distribution of triangles. Finally, the mesh is properly aligned to determine the RoI of the dental splint.

2.2   Region-of-Interest identification

After digitizing the 3D dental cast to obtain a 3D triangular mesh $\mathcal{M}_\triangle$, the RoI enclosing the dental splint has to be determined. Motivated by Kronfeld et al. [6], we define the RoI by automatically estimating two clipping planes (Fig. 1(b)).

Since the dental splint should optimally cover only teeth and not the gum, the first clipping plane should separate teeth from gum. We compute the mean curvature at all vertices of $\mathcal{M}_\triangle$, since it captures local changes. Kronfeld et al. [6] suggest to fit a plane to the vertices with a mean curvature value below -0.3, i.e. concave regions, for a good separation. By computing the full 3×3 covariance matrix of all vertices around the geometric centroid of $\mathcal{M}_\triangle$, the plane $\mathcal{T}$, referred to as transverse plane, is defined by the centroid c_T and the direction with the largest eigenvalue. This plane splits the space into two half spaces $\mathcal{T}^+$ (superior) and $\mathcal{T}^-$ (inferior) according to the direction of its normal vector n_T (superior). As the splint might not cover all teeth, the RoI has to be constrained further.

The second clipping plane is specified parallel to the xz-plane and referred to as coronal plane, denoted with $\mathcal{C}$. Again, this plane splits the space into two half spaces $\mathcal{C}^+$ (anterior) and $\mathcal{C}^-$ (posterior) depending on the direction of its normal vector n_C (anterior). Initially, its centroid c_C is set to c_T.

The RoI $\mathcal{R}$ of the dental splint is then the intersection of the inferior and anterior half spaces, denoted by $\mathcal{R} = \mathcal{T}^- \cap \mathcal{C}^+$. The geometric preview $\mathcal{P}_\triangle$ of the dental splint is obtained as the intersection of $\mathcal{M}_\triangle$ with $\mathcal{R}$, denoted as $\mathcal{P}_\triangle = \mathcal{M}_\triangle \cap \mathcal{R}$. Both planes can be manually adjusted by moving their centroids along their normal vectors, while simultaneously updating $\mathcal{P}_\triangle$. This facilitates the user a visual assessment of the dental splint before generation and fabrication.

2.3   Dental splint generation

Once the RoI of the dental splint is specified, we compute the geometry of the splint by using the digitized dental cast $\mathcal{M}_\triangle$. Therefore, we voxelize $\mathcal{M}_\triangle$ and then, subsequently, apply several 3D image processing operations.

Voxelizing a mesh requires specifying the spacing, i.e. the number of voxels per millimeter, of the target volumetric dataset. Since the initial bounds of the volumetric dataset tightly fit $\mathcal{M}_\triangle$, we enlarge the dataset inferior and anterior. This prevents the dental splint from exceeding the dataset due to its thickness and attached tracking construction. As result, we obtain a volumetric representation $\mathcal{M}_\boxplus$ approximating the geometric representation $\mathcal{M}_\triangle$, denoted as $\mathcal{M}_\triangle \mapsto \mathcal{M}_\boxplus$. Within the volumetric dataset, the dental cast $\mathcal{M}_\boxplus$ is marked as foreground (value of 1) and all other voxels as background (value of 0).

We then attach, i.e. mark as foreground, an L-shaped volumetric tracking construction $\mathcal{L}_\boxplus$ (Fig. 1(c)) to $\mathcal{M}_\boxplus$ at the most anterior part of $\mathcal{R}$, leading to the volumetric input $\mathcal{I}_\boxplus = \mathcal{M}_\boxplus \cup \mathcal{L}_\boxplus$. Subsequently, we perform 3D morphologic dilation on the foreground with a spherical structuring element (SE) of such a radius in voxels that it represents the desired thickness of the splint in millimeters. Since all voxels, including the interior, of $\mathcal{I}_\boxplus$ are marked as foreground, this operation creates a thick layer around $\mathcal{I}_\boxplus$ denoted as $\mathcal{I}_\boxplus^\oplus = \mathcal{I}_\boxplus \oplus \mathrm{SE}$. We then subtract the original volumetric input from the dilated one, leaving only the outer shell behind, denoted as $\overline{\mathcal{I}}_\boxplus = \mathcal{I}_\boxplus^\oplus - \mathcal{I}_\boxplus$. The voxels of the dental splint are computed by the intersection of $\mathcal{R}$ with the volumetric outer shell $\overline{\mathcal{I}}_\boxplus$, denoted as $\mathcal{S}_\boxplus = \overline{\mathcal{I}}_\boxplus \cap \mathcal{R} = \{\forall \boldsymbol{v} \in \overline{\mathcal{I}}_\boxplus | (\boldsymbol{v} - \boldsymbol{c}_T) \cdot \boldsymbol{n}_T < 0 \wedge (\boldsymbol{v} - \boldsymbol{c}_C) \cdot \boldsymbol{n}_C > 0\}$. However, this leads to one-voxel thin parts that might be problematic for 3D printing. To remove these remnants and boundary noise, a morphological opening is applied on $\mathcal{S}_\boxplus$ using a spherical SE with a radius of one voxel, denoted as $\mathcal{S}_\boxplus^\circ = \mathcal{S}_\boxplus \circ \mathrm{SE}$.

To fabricate the volumetric dental splint, it is converted back to a geometric representation $\mathcal{S}_\boxplus^\circ \mapsto \mathcal{S}_\triangle$, using marching cubes. Finally, we smooth the obtained geometric representation using an algorithm that is based on the work of Taubin [7] and export the dental splint as STL file that is sent to the 3D printer.

2.4 Dental splint fabrication

The dental splint is additively manufactured by a Stratasys Mojo 3D printer using the FDM Thermoplastics ABSplus with soluble support material. Since the dental splints should accurately adapt to the teeth, we print them with their tracking constructions facing downward, as printing support material inside the splints might result in unwanted small remnants even after being washed out.

3 Results

We automatically manufactured dental splints for five subjects (Fig. 2), voxelized with a spacing of 0.2, i.e. five voxels per millimeter, and expanded 3 cm inferior and anterior. The splints and tracking constructions are 1 mm thick and the L-shaped tracker spans $10 \times 20 \times 3$ mm anterior and $10 \times 3 \times 30$ mm inferior. We present (Fig. 2) the digitized dental casts and splints as well as the fabricated dental cast and splints (two hours 3D printing time on average, excluding cast digitization). Our workflow is implemented in C++, using VTK and ITK, and executed on an Intel i7 at 4 GHz with 16 GB RAM and an Nvidia GTX 560 Ti. Our automated dental splint creation takes on average two minutes.

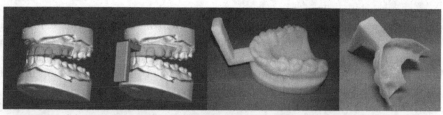

(a) Subject 1: Easy case. Transverse plane well estimated.

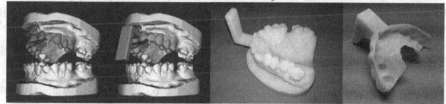

(b) Subject 2: Hard case. Highly varying teeth. Splint overflows to gum.

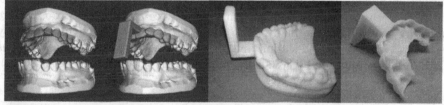

(c) Subject 3: Medium case. Teeth slightly varying. Splint overflows to gum.

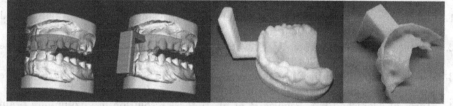

(d) Subject 4: Hard case. Damaged dental cast. Splint highly overflowing to gum.

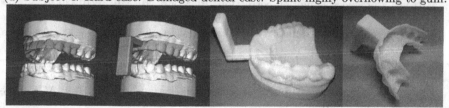

(e) Subject 5: Easy case. Transverse plane well estimated.

Fig. 2. Automatically generated results of our approach, without any user adjustments of the transverse and coronal planes. To serve as context, we display the upper jaw (yellow) transversely mirrored as lower jaw (white). For each subject, we present, from left to right, the digitized dental cast, the generated dental splint, the fabricated dental splint alone and attached to the fabricated cast.

4   Discussion

To conclude, we presented an approach for fabricating dental splint using digitized 3D dental casts. Our proposed workflow streamlines as well as standardizes the production of tracking constructions for PMC in UHF-MRI. This does not only facilitate a larger population to access this rather recent acquisition modality, but also catalyzes this process.

As future work, we plan to investigate more flexible materials, as described by Bickel et al. [8], compared to the stiff splints as currently fabricated. Combined with the teeth segmentation presented by Kronfeld et al. [6] or Wu et al. [9], this would create a dental splint that might snap to the teeth. The visual assessment of the splint geometry before the fabrication can be improved using visual analytics approaches such as proposed by Schmidt et al. [10].

Acknowledgement. The dental casts were created in the local department of oral and maxillofacial surgery for five subjects (three male and two female, between 26 and 43 years of age) from alginate impressions. The study was performed with the approval of the ethics committee of the Otto-von-Guericke University Magdeburg, Germany. The work of this paper is partly funded by the Federal Ministry of Education and Research within the Forschungscampus STIMULATE (grant no. 13GW0095A) and the NIH (grant no. R01DA021146).

References

1. Balchandani P, Naidich TP. Ultra-high-field MR neuro-imaging. AJNR Am J Neuroradiol. 2015;36(7):1204–15.
2. Godenschweger F, Kägebein U, Stucht D, et al. Motion correction in MRI of the brain. Phys Med Biol. 2016;61(5):32–56.
3. Herbst M, Lovell-Smith C, Haeublein B, et al. On the robustness of prospective motion correction for clinical routine. Proc 21st Sci Meet. 2013; p. 3766.
4. Stucht D, Danishad KA, Schulze P, et al. Highest resolution in vivo human brain MRI using prospective motion correction. PloS one. 2015;10(7):e0133921.
5. Salmi M, Paloheimo KS, Tuomi J, et al. A digital process for additive manufacturing of occlusal splints: a clinical pilot study. J R Society Interface. 2013;10(84):20130203.
6. Kronfeld T, Brunner D, Brunnett G. Snake-based segmentation of teeth from virtual dental casts. Comput Aided Des Appl. 2010;7(2):221–33.
7. Taubin G. A signal processing approach to fair surface design. Proc ACM SIGGRAPH. 1995; p. 351–8.
8. Bickel B, Bächer M, Otaduy MA, et al. Design and fabrication of materials with desired deformation behavior. ACM Trans Graph. 2013;29(4):63:1–10.
9. Wu K, Chen L, Li J, et al. Tooth segmentation on dental meshes using morphologic skeleton. Comput Graph. 2013;38(1):199–211.
10. Schmidt J, Preiner R, Auzinger T, et al. YMCA – Your mesh comparison application. Proc IEEE VAST. 2014; p. 153–62.

Reliable Estimation of the Number of Compartments in Diffusion MRI

Simon Koppers[1], Christoph Haarburger[1], J. Christopher Edgar[2], Dorit Merhof[1]

[1]Institute of Imaging & Computer Vision, RWTH Aachen University
[2]Children's Hospital of Philadelphia, University of Pennsylvania
simon.koppers@lfb.rwth-aachen.de

Abstract. A-priori knowledge of the number of fibers in a voxel is mandatory and crucial when reconstructing multi-fiber voxels in diffusion MRI. Especially for clinical purposes, this estimation needs to be stable, even when only few gradient directions are acquired. In this work, we propose a novel approach to address this problem based on a deep convolutional neural network (CNN), which is able to identify important gradient directions and can be directly trained on real data. To obtain a ground truth using real data, 100 uncorrelated Human Connectome Project datasets are utilized, with a state-of-the-art framework used for generating a relative ground truth. It is shown that this CNN approach outperforms other state-of-the-art machine learning approaches.

1 Introduction

Diffusion Imaging makes it possible to acquire information about the course and location of neuronal fibers in the human brain. In early stages, diffusion was assumed to be representable by a single Gaussian tensor. A disadvantage of this approach was that it was not possible to reconstruct complex fiber structures such as crossing, fanning or kissing fibers in a voxel. This is a problem as such complex fiber structures occur in up to 90% of voxels containing human white matter [1]. To address this issue, high angular resolution diffusion imaging (HARDI) and multi-compartment models were introduced, methods that require a multitude of diffusion images and a-priori knowledge of the number of fibers in a voxel [2]. First approaches were based on a simple threshold to divide the signals, with the threshold set manually for each dataset [3]. Due to the fact that this is not feasible for large group studies, a more common approach minimizes a generalization error starting with a single fiber and then increases in order to optimize the error function [4]. A general drawback of methods that minimize an error function is that they rely on their model, which often requires many acquired diffusion gradients.

Another model proposed in [5] introduced a support vector regression (SVR) approach, describing the number of compartments in a non-discrete manner. Utilizing this novel approach, the adequate number of compartments is estimated directly from the signal.

In the recent past, CNNs achieved very good results in the field of Diffusion Imaging outperforming current state-of-the-art methods [6, 7, 8]. It was shown that a CNN is able to identify important neighboring information between gradient directions in a voxel. In this work, the SVR approach is replaced utilizing a CNN in order to further improve performance. In the present study, evaluation is quantitatively performed on human data, utilizing data from the Human Connectome Project as ground truth.

2   Materials and methods

2.1   Material

The WU-Minn Human Connectome Project (HCP) dataset consists of diffusion MRI brain scans acquired with a 3T Siemens Connectome MRI scanner that recorded 145 axial slices with a resolution of $1.25 \times 1.25 \times 1.25 \, \text{mm}^3$. In total, data was acquired for 288 diffusion gradients, comprising 18 scans with no diffusion gradient (b = 0) and 3 shells comprising 90 scans each, at $b = 1000 \, \frac{s}{mm^2}$, $b = 2000 \, \frac{s}{mm^2}$, and $b = 3000 \, \frac{s}{mm^2}$. For this work, an arbitrary subset containing 100 scans from healthy subjects was chosen from the WU-Minn HCP dataset. Because of its high resolution, the HCP dataset is reduced such that for every subject, only a single axial slice (slice index 70) with a b-value of $b = 3000 \, \frac{s}{mm^2}$ was utilized (Fig. 1). In addition, this slice was resampled utilizing a spherical harmonic basis for 90, 45 and 15 gradient directions in order to have the same set of gradient directions across all subjects and to evaluate the effect of a decreased number of gradients.

To generate a reliable real data ground truth, DIAMOND [4], which minimizes a generalization error, was utilized using all three shells comprising 288 acquired gradients. It is openly available in CRKit and achieves an error rate below 1% on synthetic data at a SNR of ≥ 30 db. An example of the resulting ground truth can be seen in Fig. 1. It categorizes the voxels of the brain into four different types of voxels: single-fiber (red), two-fiber (yellow), three-fiber (green) and isotropic voxels (blue).

2.2   Signal projection

To estimate the number of compartments with a CNN, each dMRI signal vector was transformed into a 2D image by cyclic shifting it and adding it to its right side in order to generate an image as proposed in [7]. Using this image, the CNN can perform convolutions and learn features arising from correspondences between signal values in the dMRI gradient neighborhood. Utilizing this pre-processing, the CNN can be trained more easily in comparison to a normal fully-connected neural network. In addition, we improved the pre-processing proposed in [7], by shifting only $\frac{M}{2}$ times, where M represents the number of acquired diffusion gradients, as further shifting only adds redundant information, reducing the size of the generated image by 50%.

2.3   Neural network architecture

An overview of all layers and corresponding parameters is provided in Tab. 2.3. The input is first convolved with 32 kérnels with 5×5 shape each. Then, a recti-fied linear unit (ReLU) is employed for feature extraction, followed by a second convolutional layer with 64 3×3 convolution kernels. Utilizing a 5×5 kernel first results in a rough segmentation of important gradients, while the second convolutional kernel further identifies the most important information. After an additional ReLU nonlinearity, a max pooling layer extracts features translation invariantly. After that, a fully connected layer with 20% dropout probability reshapes the signal to 1024 neurons. The dropout can be interpreted as a reg-ularizer that forces the net to learn more robust features. After another ReLU, the output is transformed with a softmax function. When the softmax function is applied to the output of a neural network that solves a classification problem, it can be interpreted as a probability of the input belonging to a class. In this work, the cross entropy is used as loss function, which is minimized utilizing the stochastic gradient descend algorithm with a learning rate of $\eta = 0.005$. The whole network is build utilizing the open-source library TensorFlow.

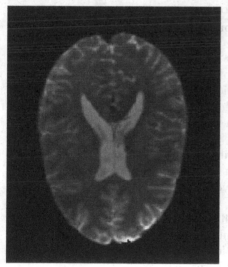

(a) HCP dataset

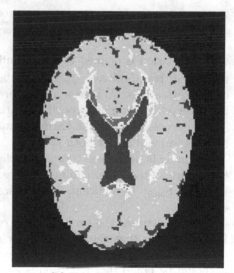
(b) Resulting relative GT

Fig. 1. Exemplary slice of the HCP dataset and its resulting ground truth (GT) based on DIAMOND. Red represents single-fiber voxels, yellow two-fiber voxels, green three-fiber voxels and blue isotropic voxels.

Table 1. Topology of the CNN for estimating the number of compartments N_c.

#	Type	Parameters
1	2D convolution	$32 \times 5 \times 5$
2	ReLU	-
3	2D convolution	$64 \times 3 \times 3$
4	ReLU	-
5	max pooling	2×2 pool size
6	fully-connected	1024 neurons
7	ReLU	-
8	fully-connected	4 neurons
9	softmax	-

3   Results

The performance of estimation the number of compartments is evaluated by their F1-score, which is defined as

$$F1 = 2 \cdot \frac{\text{precision} \cdot \text{recall}}{\text{precision} + \text{recall}} \tag{1}$$

where precision is defined by $\frac{t_p}{t_p+f_p}$ and recall by $\frac{t_p}{t_p+f_n}$, with t_p containing the number of true positives, f_p the number of false negatives and f_n the number of false negatives. Whereas a high precision rate denotes that there are only few false positives, a high recall indicates that there are only few false-negatives. The F1-score, which is the harmonic mean between precision and recall, results in a low value if one of both gets low.

Training is performed over 20 epochs with batches of 80 samples, and testing takes part on the 20 remaining samples. In addition, each signal S is divided by its mean $S_{b=0}$. In addition, a discretized version of the SVR proposed in [5] is evaluated.

Tab. 2 contains the precision, the recall as well as their resulting F1-scores. It can be seen that the SVR approach only provides a reasonable recall if 90 gradient directions are used, and achieves a lower value in all other cases. Overall, it should be noted that precision is always lower than recall.

Fig. 2 shows results on a slice. Both approaches achieve reasonable and homogeneous results. However, the SVR approach tends to label three-fiber voxels as isotropic voxels, whereas the CNN approach shows problems estimating isotropic voxels as three fiber voxels.

4   Discussion

The estimation of number of compartments achieves very good results and shows only a few weaknesses in the considered settings for both CNN and SVR. In both cases, classification benefits from a higher number of input gradients. However,

Table 2. Resulting precision, recall and the resulting F1-score for the CNN approach and the SVR approach.

Method	#Gradients	Precision	Recall	F1-score
	15	71.48%	81.08%	75.60%
CNN	45	74.63%	83.28%	78.37%
	90	79.21%	81.97%	80.30%
	15	66.79%	79.78%	71.57%
SVR	45	71.61%	82.60%	76.01%
	90	73.97%	85.15%	78.65%

it should be noted that the CNN outperforms the SVR approach in nearly every setting as shown in Tab. 2. Only at 90 gradient directions does the SVR method achieve a better recall score than the CNN method.

Fig. 2 shows the limitation of this work, as the CNN classifier may overestimate the number of compartments per voxel towards a three-fiber voxel, a bias likely due to an unbalanced class weighting in the training data. In comparison, the SVR seems to penalizes three-fiber voxels, resulting in a higher false-positive rate for two-fiber and isotropic voxels. The same trends can be seen in Tab. 2, as the precision seems to limit the F1-score for the SVR as well as for the CNN, due to a higher false-positive rate. We addressed this issue by resampling underrepresented classes. This did not result in an improvement, though. This issue should therefore be further investigated by adding a class weight factor in the loss function or truncating data from overrepresented classes in the training data.

Moreover, since the utilized dataset has high resolution versus common dMRI acquisitions, it contains a considerable level of noise and thus it is likely that the ground truth suffers from label noise that limits the classifier's performance. To address this issue and to make CNN applicable across different scanner types, individual synthetic data for training is required as shown in [5].

To conclude, the present study demonstrates how CNN can be utilized for estimating the number of gradients in a voxel, with present finding showing that CNN outperforms state-of-the-art machine learning algorithms. Furthermore, preprocessing was improved by removing redundant information, thus reducing the size of the generated input image by 50%.

Acknowledgement. Data were provided by the Human Connectome Project, WU-Minn Consortium (Principal Investigators: David Van Essen and Kamil Ugurbil; 1U54MH091657) funded by the 16 NIH Institutes and Centers that support the NIH Blueprint for Neuroscience Research; and by the McDonnell Center for Systems Neuroscience at Washington University. This work was supported by the International Research Training Group 2150 of the German Research Foundation (DFG).

Fig. 2. Exemplary labeled slice estimated using the CNN and the SVR approach with 45 gradient directions as input. Red represent single-fiber voxels, yellow two-fiber voxels, green three-fiber voxels and blue isotropic voxels.

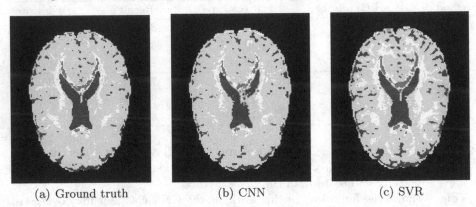

(a) Ground truth   (b) CNN   (c) SVR

References

1. Jeurissen B, Leemans A, Tournier J, et al. Investigating the prevalence of complex fiber configurations in white matter tissue with diffusion MRI. Hum Brain Mapp. 2013;34(11):2747–66.
2. Tuch D, Reese T, Wiegell M, et al. High angular resolution diffusion imaging reveals intravoxel whitematter fiber heterogeneity. Magn Reson Med. 2002;48(4):577–82.
3. Schultz T, Westin C, Kindlmann G. Multi-diffusion-tensor fitting via spherical deconvolution: a unifying framework. Proc MICCAI. 2010.
4. Scherrer B, Schwartzman A, Taquet M, et al. Characterizing brain tissue by assessment of the distribution of anisotropic microstructural environments in diffusion-compartment imaging (DIAMOND). Magn Reson Med. 2015.
5. Schultz T. Learning a reliable estimate of the number of fiber directions in diffusion MRI. Proc MICCAI. 2012.
6. Golkov V, Dosovitskiy A, Samann P, et al. q-space deep learning for twelve-fold shorter and model-free diffusion MRI scans. Proc MICCAI. 2015.
7. Koppers S, Merhof D. Direct estimation of fiber orientations using deep learning in diffusion imaging. Proc MLMI. 2016.
8. Koppers S, Haarburger C, Merhof D. Diffusion MRI signal augmentation. From single shell to multi shell with deep learning. Proc CDMRI. 2016.

Epipolar Consistency Conditions for Motion Correction in Weight-Bearing Imaging

Bastian Bier[1], André Aichert[1], Lina Felsner[1], Mathias Unberath[1],
Marc Levenston[2], Garry Gold[2], Rebecca Fahrig[2], Andreas Maier[1]

[1]Lehrstuhl für Mustererkennung, Friedrich-Alexander-Universität Erlangen-Nürnberg
[2]Department of Radiology, School of Medicine, Stanford University, USA
bastian.bier@fau.de

Abstract. Recent C-arm CT systems allow for the examination of a
patient's knees under weight-bearing conditions. The standing patient
tends to show involuntary motion, which introduces motion artifacts in
the reconstruction. The state-of-the-art motion correction approach uses
fiducial markers placed on the patients' skin to estimate rigid leg motion.
Marker placement is tedious, time consuming and associated with patient discomfort. Further, motion on the skin surface does not reflect the
internal bone motion. We propose a purely projection based motion estimation method using consistency conditions of X-ray projections. The
epipolar consistency between all pairs of projections is optimized over
various motion parameters. We validate our approach by simulating motion from a tracking system in forward projections of clinical data. We
visually and numerically assess reconstruction image quality and show
an improvement in Structural Similarity from 0.912 for the uncorrected
case to 0.943 using the proposed method with a 3D translational motion
model. Initial experiments showed promising results encouraging further
investigation of practical applicability.

1 Introduction

Recent C-arm cone-beam CT systems support flexible trajectories, including
horizontal scans of the knee joint in standing position under weight-bearing conditions [1]. These trajectories allow for the observation of knee kinematics under
load [2], which might lead to a better understanding of knee cartilage health.
A major problem of the acquisition is involuntary patient motion during the
scan. Different motion correction methods have been proposed to mitigate motion artifacts in reconstructed images. The state-of-the art method uses fiducial
markers and applies a 3D rigid motion to the estimated 3D marker positions,
aligning them with detected 2D marker positions on the detector [3, 4, 5]. However, marker placement is tedious, since they have to be placed such that they do
not overlap in the projection images. This leads to longer examination time and
patient discomfort. In addition, skin motion may not optimally represent the actual joint motion. Another approach by Berger et al. [6] uses bone segmentations
of a previously acquired supine acquisition and performs a 2D/3D registration of

the segmented bone with the projection images. However, a previously acquired motion free reconstruction is rarely available and the method is computationally highly expensive. Other approaches are purely image [7] or projection-based [8]. Sisniega et al. evaluate a sharpness measure to estimate sub-millimeter motion, but are restricted to a small region of interest [7]. Unberath et al. use maximum intensity projections from an initial reconstruction to align the bone outlines in 2D [8].

In this work, we investigate another purely projection-based motion correction method using Epipolar Consistency Conditions (ECC) [9]. ECC can be used to define a consistency metric on the relative geometry of any pair of X-ray images, which can be optimized for motion parameters. We tried 3 motion models: 2D detector shifts, 3D patient translation, and a rigid 3D patient motion. Experiments on a clinical supine acquisition were performed, where real patient motion is used to simulate motion corrupted projection images.

2   Materials and methods

2.1   Epipolar consistency conditions

Epipolar Consistency Conditions (ECC) are conditions on corresponding line integrals in two pre-processed X-ray projections I_0, I_1. Their respective source positions define a pencil of planes $\mathbf{E}^\kappa$ around the baseline, associated with an angle κ to the iso-center. By intersection with the detectors, any such plane defines two lines $\mathbf{l}_0^\kappa$, $\mathbf{l}_1^\kappa \in \mathbb{P}^2$ in oriented projective space of the images, which both contain information of the same plane $\mathbf{E}^\kappa$ through the object. ECC allow us to express a metric of inconsistency using integrals of such lines

$$\frac{\partial}{\partial t}\rho_{I_0}\left(\mathbf{l}_0^\kappa\right) - \frac{\partial}{\partial t}\rho_{I_1}\left(\mathbf{l}_1^\kappa\right) \approx 0 \tag{1}$$

where $\rho_I(\mathbf{l})$ denotes the integral over line $\mathbf{l} = (-\sin(\alpha), \cos(\alpha), -t)^\top \in \mathbb{P}^2$ of angle α and distance to the image origin t, in projective space of image I . The inconsistency metric for two projection indices i and j is

$$ECC_i^j = \int_{[-\frac{\pi}{2}, \frac{\pi}{2}]} \left(\frac{\partial}{\partial t}\rho_{I_j}\left(\mathbf{l}_j^\kappa\right) - \frac{\partial}{\partial t}\rho_{I_i}\left(\mathbf{l}_i^\kappa\right)\right)^2 d\kappa \tag{2}$$

2.2   Motion model

Given the geometry of the j-th image, defined by a projection matrix $\mathbf{P}_j \in \mathbb{R}^{3\times 4}$, $j \in \{1, \ldots, n\}$, we can model detector shifts and rigid patient motion simply by matrix-multiplication $\mathbf{P}_j' = \mathbf{H}_j \cdot \mathbf{P}_j' \cdot \mathbf{T}_j$ with

$$\mathbf{H}_j = \begin{pmatrix} 1 & 0 & d_u^j \\ 0 & 1 & d_v^j \\ 0 & 0 & 1 \end{pmatrix} \text{ and } \mathbf{T}_j = \begin{pmatrix} \mathbf{R}_j & \mathbf{t}_j \\ \mathbf{0} & 1 \end{pmatrix} \tag{3}$$

where d_u^j and d_v^j denote detector domain shifts and $\mathbf{T}_j$ is a rigid patient motion in 3D comprised of a translation vector $\mathbf{t}_j \in \mathbb{R}^3$ and a rotation about the iso-center $\mathbf{R}_j \in SO(3, \mathbb{R})$, defined by Euler-angles $\mathbf{r} = \left(r_x^j, r_y^j, r_z^j\right)^\top$.

2.3   Optimization

Let $M(\boldsymbol{\phi})$ denote the sum over ECC_i^j for all ordered pairs of projections $\{i, j\} \subset \{1, \ldots, n\}^2$, transformed according to Sec. 2.2, where the parameter vector $\boldsymbol{\phi}$ may contain only detector shifts $\boldsymbol{\phi}^{2D} = \left(d_u^1, d_v^1 \ldots d_u^n, d_v^n\right)^\top$, translation vectors $\boldsymbol{\phi}^{3D} = (\mathbf{t}_1, \ldots, \mathbf{t}_n)^\top$, or full 6D rigid transformations $\boldsymbol{\phi}^{6D} = (\mathbf{t}_1, \mathbf{r}_1 \ldots, \mathbf{t}_n \mathbf{r}_n)^\top$. We then minimize the inconsistencies

$$\boldsymbol{\phi}^\star = \underset{\boldsymbol{\phi}}{\arg\min}\, M(\boldsymbol{\phi}), \qquad (4)$$

using gradient-free numerical optimization. To reduce the total number of parameters, we run n successive optimizations of parameters for only one projection, and repeat this procedure until the solution has sufficiently converged.

2.4   Experiments

All experiments use the geometry of a real acquisition with 248 projections with a detector size of 1240×960. Reconstruction was performed using a standard FDK with a sharp kernel. We forward projected a high quality supine reconstruction of the knees under 3D rigid motion. The motion parameters are taken from a real patient measured with a motion capture system, while performing a squat with $60°$ flexion [3]. We compared the reconstructions using our novel approach (estimating either 2D detector shifts, 3D translation or 6D rigid motion) with the

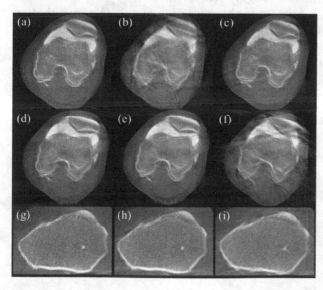

Fig. 1. Reconstructed images. Ground truth (a), no correction (b), Müller et al. [5] marker-based (c), proposed method optimized 2D shifts (d), 3D translation (e) and 6D rigid motion (f). The last row (g)-(i) shows detail views of (a), (c) and (e) at a different slice.

ground truth motion free reconstruction, the motion corrupted reconstruction, and the state-of-the-art marker-based approach [5]. We calculated the Structural Similarity (SSIM) and further analyzed the estimated parameters.

3 Results

Fig. 1 shows motion-compensated 3D reconstructions. Without any motion correction, streaks and blurring artifacts are present, compare Fig. 1b. ECC motion estimation with 2D detector shifts and 3D translation (Fig. 1d and Fig. 1e) considerably improved image quality, while results for 3D rigid motion were not as good (Fig. 1f). Using the state-of-the-art marker-based approach, only some motion induced streak artifacts remain, see Fig. 1c. A detail view in Fig. 1(g)-(i) shows that image quality for the state-of-the-art method is still slightly better.

Further, we registered all reconstructions to the ground truth result and computed the SSIM, shown in Table 1. Our method peaks at a SSIM of 0.943 and shows an improvement compared to the uncorrected case with an SSIM of 0.912. The best result is achieved by state-of-the-art with a SSIM of 0.987.

In the following, we only show the results of our best results, which has been the estimation of 3D tranlation. Fig. 2 shows a comparison to ground truth motion parameters. Note, that the ground truth and the state-of-the-art method are based on a rigid model with additional rotation, whereas our method only estimates translations. Generally, the motion is recovered well for both methods. Noticeable is the peak of the state-of-the-art method around projection 45. In these views, markers overlap in the projection images and thus motion estimation becomes inaccurate, which leads to the streaks in the reconstruction. Further, the proposed method reproduces high frequencies of the motion signal in the middle views and the beginning and the end of the Y-parameter very accurately, while the Z-parameter is generally roughly recovered.

We now focus on the X-parameter in the top row in Fig. 3. Observe, that an accurate estimation of the high frequencies is possible in areas, where the object motion is parallel to the detector. In other words, our method estimates motion along the viewing direction less accurately. Note however, that such motion can be observed in the images only as a small scaling and thus has less effect on the reconstruction than motion parallel to the detector. This fact is visualized in the bottom row in Fig. 3, where the translation vector is projected onto the detector plane.

Table 1. Structural similarity (SSIM) results.

Method	SSIM
Uncorrected	0.912
State-of-the-art [5]	0.987
2D shifts	0.933
3D translation	0.943
6D rigid motion	0.892

4   Discussion

We suggest a novel projection-based method to estimate patient motion during knee-scans under weight-bearing conditions. Our method exploits redundancies in projection domain to optimize the consistency over patient motion parameters, and unlike state-of-the-art methods requires neither a reference scan in supine

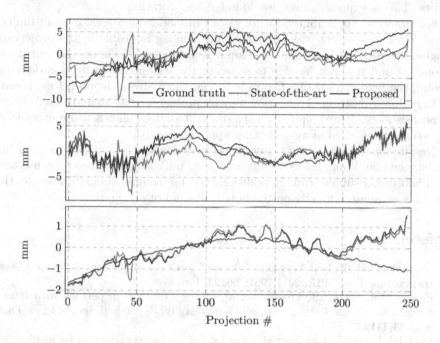

Fig. 2. Raw motion parameters x, y and z.

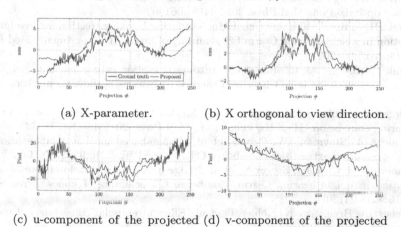

(a) X-parameter.   (b) X orthogonal to view direction.

(c) u-component of the projected (d) v-component of the projected
translation on detector.   translation on the detector.

Fig. 3. Analysis of the translation vector in view direction and detector projection.

position nor fiducial markers attached to the patient. We validate the approach on forward projections of real patient data under real patient motion.

In our experiments we compensate for 3D patient motion using 2D detector shifts, 3D translations and full 6D rigid motion. For 2D and 3D models, we are able to show considerable improvements when compared to no compensation, although state-of-the-art marker-based compensation yields slightly better results. This is expected, since we do not model rotations.

For practical applicability, future work must address several current limitations. First, we currently assume that only one leg is visible in the projection images. However, with our clinical setup it is not realistic to have a patient stand on one leg and it is not feasible to separate the legs in the projection domain. Second, the field-of-view of a C-arm is too small to always fit both legs, resulting in major truncation. Truncation may be problematic as an additional source of inconsistency. Third, epipolar consistency has been shown to be capable of correcting 6DOF rigid motion in other applications [10].

Despite current limitations, this paper presents the first step towards using consistency conditions for extremity imaging, mitigating the need for markers or an additional supine scan. In addition to being computationally feasible, the motion is estimated directly on the bones, instead of on the skin surface.

References

1. Maier A, Choi JH, Keil A, et al. Analysis of vertical and horizontal circular C-arm trajectories. Proc SPIE. 2011;7961:796123-1-8.
2. Powers CM, Ward SR, Fredericson M. Knee extension in persons with lateral subluxation of the Patella : a preliminary study. J Orthop Sports Phys Ther. 2013;33(11):677-85.
3. Choi JH, Fahrig R, Keil A, et al. Fiducial marker-based correction for involuntary motion in weight-bearing C-arm CT scanning of knees. Part I. Numerical model-based optimization. Med Phys. 2014;41(6):061902.
4. Choi JH, Maier A, Keil A, et al. Fiducial marker-based correction for involuntary motion in weight-bearing C-arm CT scanning of knees. II. Experiment. Med Phys. 2014;41(6):061902.
5. Müller K, Berger M, Choi J, et al. Automatic motion estimation and compensation framework for weight-bearing C-arm CT scans using fiducial markers. Proc IFMBE. 2015; p. 58-61.
6. Berger M, Müller K, Aichert A, et al. Marker-free motion correction in weight-bearing cone-beam CT of the knee joint. Med Phys. 2016;43(3):1235-48.
7. Sisniega A, Stayman JW, Cao Q, et al. Image-based motion compensation for high-resolution extremities cone-beam CT. Proc SPIE. 2016;9783:97830K.
8. Unberath M, Choi JH, Berger M, et al. Image-based compensation for involuntary motion in weight-bearing C-arm cone-beam CT scanning of knees. Proc SPIE. 2015;9413:94130D.
9. Aichert A, Breininger K, Köhler T, et al. Efficient epipolar consistency. Proc CT Meeting. 2016; p. 259-62.
10. Aichert A, Wang J, Schaffert R, et al. Epipolar consistency in fluoroscopy for image-based tracking. Proc BMVC. 2015; p. 82.1-82.10.

Abstract: Patch-Based Learning of Shape, Appearance, and Motion Models from Few Training Samples by Low-Rank Matrix Completion

Matthias Wilms, Heinz Handels, Jan Ehrhardt

Institute of Medical Informatics, University of Lübeck
wilms@imi.uni-luebeck.de

Statistical shape, appearance, and motion models are widely used as priors in medical image analysis to, for example, constrain image segmentation [1] and motion estimation results [2]. These models try to learn a compact parameterization of the space of plausible object instances from a population of observed samples using low-rank matrix approximation methods (SVD or PCA). The quality of these models heavily depends on the quantity and quality of the training population. As it is usually quite challenging to collect large and representative training populations, models used in practice often suffer from a limited expressiveness.

Recently, we presented a novel approach for building statistical shape, appearance, and motion models with increased flexibility from few training samples [3]. Central to our approach is the assumption of locality: We assume that local shape, intensity, or motion variations have limited effects in distant areas. Based on this assumption, we propose to combine local information observed in different (real) samples of the small training population to generate a very large number of so-called virtual samples. This is done by partitioning real samples into patches and fusing distant patches of different samples into virtual ones. We circumvent the problem of inconsistencies at borders of patches originating from different objects by performing a sparse sampling. Given these sparse virtual samples, model training is set-up as an efficiently solvable low-rank matrix completion problem. By doing so, the assumed low-rank structure will automatically lead to consistent transitions between patches.

We evaluate models generated from these virtual samples for different shape and motion modeling applications and show that our approach leads to consistent models with increased flexibility and improved generalization ability.

Acknowledgement. This work is funded by the DFG (EH 224/6-1).

References

1. Cootes TF, Taylor CJ, Cooper DH, et al. Active shape models-their training and application. Comput Vis Image Underst. 1995;61(1):38–59.

2. Wilms M, Ha IY, Handels H, et al. Model-based regularisation for respiratory motion estimation with sparse features in image-guided interventions. Proc MICCAI. 2016; p. 89–97.
3. Ehrhardt J, Wilms M, Handels H. Patch-based low-rank matrix completion for learning of shape and motion models from few training samples. Proc ECCV. 2016; p. 712–27.

Abstract: Detektion des tibiotalaren Gelenkspaltes in intraoperativen C-Bogen Projektionen

Sarina Thomas[1], Marc Schnetzke[2], Jochen Franke[2], Sven Vetter[2], Benedict Swartman[2], Paul A. Grützner[2], Hans-Peter Meinzer[1], Marco Nolden[1]

[1]Abteilung für Medizinische und Biologische Informatik, DKFZ Heidelberg
[2]MINTOS, BG Unfallklinik, Ludwigshafen
s.thomas@dkfz.de

Bei circa 11% aller Frakturen des oberen Sprunggelenks (OSG) treten akute Verletzungen der Syndesmose auf, die aufgrund ihrer Instabilität einen operativen Eingriff erfordern [1]. Dabei kann die Stabilisierung mittels Stellschraube zu einer Fehlstellung der Fibula führen, welche ohne Korrektur mit einer Verschlechterung der Lebensqualität des Patienten einhergehen kann. Der Einsatz mobiler 3D C-Bogen ermöglicht eine räumliche Interpretation der Anatomie bei der Verifikation des Repositionsergebnisses. Gleichzeitig stellt die variable Ausrichtung des Scanners zum Patienten eine große Herausforderung beim Vergleich mit anderen Datensätzen dar. Bei der Beurteilung von OSG Frakturen mit Beteiligung der Syndesmose kann ein Vergleich mit der gesunden Gegenseite sinnvoll sein. Da ein weiterer Scan jedoch zusätzliche Strahlenbelastung sowie eine Erhöhung der Operationsdauer bedeutet, sollen stattdessen Einzelprojektionen der gesunden Gegenseite analysiert werden. In der vorliegenden Arbeit wird die Ausrichtung des Datensatzes durch die Detektion des tibiotalaren Gelenkspaltes bestimmt [2]. Ein Quadtree-basierter hierarchischer Varianzvergleich identifiziert potentielle Konturpunkte. Aus diesen werden dann mit Hilfe von Hough Transformationen Schaftkonturen und der Gelenkspalt extrahiert. Die Methode wurde auf 13 C-Bogen Datensätzen mit jeweils 100 Einzelprojektionen angewandt. Dazu wurden die anatomischen Sichtebenen von jeweils drei Unfallchirurgen manuell eingestellt, auf die Einzelprojektionen projiziert und mit den berechneten Ebenen verglichen. Die resultierende Korrelation zwischen Winkelabweichung und korrespondierendem Winkel gibt Aufschluss über bevorzugte Aufnahmerichtungen und dient als Basis für weiterführende klinische Experimente.

Literaturverzeichnis

1. Franke J, von Recum J, Suda AJ, et al. Intraoperative three-dimensional imaging in the treatment of acute unstable syndesmotic injuries. J Bone Joint Surg Am. 2012;94(15):1386–90.
2. Thomas S, Brehler M, Schnetzke M, et al. Intraoperative upper ankle joint space detection on inhomogeneous low contrast fluoroscopic C-arm projections; Procs SPIE, 2017 (angenommen).

A Feasibility Study of Automatic Multi-Organ Segmentation Using Probabilistic Atlas

Shuqing Chen[1], Jürgen Endres[1], Sabrina Dorn[2], Joscha Maier[2], Michael Lell[3], Marc Kachelrieß[2], Andreas Maier[1]

[1]Pattern Recognition Lab, Friedrich-Alexander-Universität Erlangen-Nürnberg
[2]Department of Medical Physics in Radiotherapy, German Cancer Research Center
[3]Institute of Radiology, University Hospital Erlangen
shuqing.chen@fau.de

Abstract. Thoracic and abdominal multi-organ segmentation has been a challenging problem due to the inter-subject variance of human thoraxes and abdomens as well as the complex 3D intra-subject variance among organs. In this paper, we present a preliminary method for automatically segmenting multiple organs using non-enhanced CT data. The method is based on a simple framework using generic tools and requires no organ-specific prior knowledge. Specifically, we constructed a grayscale CT volume along with a probabilistic atlas consisting of six thoracic and abdominal organs: lungs (left and right), liver, kidneys (left and right) and spleen. A non-rigid mapping between the grayscale CT volume and a new test volume provided the deformation information for mapping the probabilistic atlas to the test CT volume. The evaluation with the 20 VISCERAL non-enhanced CT dataset showed that the proposed method yielded an average Dice coefficient of over 95% for the lungs, over 90% for the liver, as well as around 80% and 70% for the spleen and the kidneys respectively.

1 Introduction

Automatic thoracic and abdominal multi-organ segmentation on clinically acquired computed tomography (CT) has been a challenging problem due to the inter-subject variance of human thoraxes and abdomens as well as complex 3-D relationship among organs. On CT images, the inter-subject variability (e.g., age, gender, stature, normal anatomical variants, and disease status) can be observed in terms of the size, shape, and appearance of each organ. Soft anatomy deformation (e.g., pose, respiratory cycle, edema, digestive status) complicates the segmentation problem even more.

To solve this problem, Toro et al. [1] proposed a method using anatomical hierarchy guided by spatial correlations. Kahl et al. [2] presented a method using feature-based registration. He et al. [3] introduced a method using multi-boost learning and statistical shape model. All of these methods use organ-specific prior knowledge. Therefore, a complicated preprocessing is necessary to obtain

218

organ-specific prior knowledge. Moreover, expanding the atlas becomes computationally expensive if more organs should be involved in the segmentation.

A probabilistic atlas-based approach [4] was proposed for the automatic segmentation of abdominal organs and revealed the benefit of probabilistic atlas. However, it only focused on the abdominal organs but didn't involve the organs in the thorax.

In this paper, we present a generic framework for automatic multi-organ segmentation using a probabilistic atlas with extension to the thorax. The atlas includes two lungs, liver, spleen, and two kidneys. The segmentation is then performed based on an atlas registration approach. No organ-specific prior knowledge is required in the proposed method.

2   Materials and methods

2.1   Overview of the proposed framework

Fig. 1 presents the flowchart of the proposed framework, which consists of two steps: the atlas construction and the multi-organ segmentation.

In the step of the atlas construction, all grayscale CT volumes of a training dataset are mapped onto one individual volume using affine transform at first. Subsequently, the alignments are improved by using non-rigid B-spline transform. After the alignments, an average CT volume is calculated. In order to generate a probabilistic atlas in the space of the reference volume, the ground truth segmentations of the training set are warped onto the reference space by using the results of the B-spline transform computed from their CT volumes. The presence of each voxel is then counted for each organ. The probability of a voxel belonging to a certain organ is then calculated by dividing the counts by the volume amount. The probabilities of all target organs build a vector-valued probabilistic atlas finally.

In the step of the segmentation, the coarse alignment of the new CT volume and the average volume is calculated by using affine transformation at first. The alignment is further improved with B-spline transformation. The probabilistic atlas is subsequently projected into the space of the test volume. In the vector-valued probabilistic atlas, one voxel can be labeled as different organ, we decide the organ type by taking the organ with the highest probability. The boundaries are estimated by a simple probabilistic threshold with 0.30.

2.2   Registration methods

As described previously, registration is an important part of the proposed framework, it is used in both atlas construction and segmentation steps. We used a Gaussian image pyramid approach in all registration steps to achieve better results and more reasonable processing time. Four resolutions (8,4,2,1) are applied for the affine transformation while two resolutions (8,2) are applied for the B-spline part. Similarity is measured by the Mattes' mutual information method [5], which is obtained by double summing over the discrete PDF (probability density function) values. The PDF is estimated using Parzen histograms. Furthermore, the B-spline transformation is constrained by using bending energy penalty term [6]. The cost function of the non-rigid B-spline registration in the proposed framework is summarized as

$$\arg\min_{\mathbf{T}}(S(\mathbf{T}) + \alpha R(\mathbf{T})) \tag{1}$$

where $\mathbf{T}$ is the transformation between the reference and the test image.

$S(\mathbf{T})$ is the negative of mutual information between the reference image and the transformed test image based on Parzen histograms [5]

$$S(\mathbf{T}) = -\sum_l \sum_k p(l, k \mid \mathbf{T}) \log \frac{p(l, k \mid \mathbf{T})}{p_{\text{Test}}(l \mid \mathbf{T}) p_{\text{Ref}}(k)} \tag{2}$$

where p is the joint probability distribution of the pair of registered images. p_{Ref} and p_{Test} are the marginal probability distribution of the reference image and the test image respectively. k and l indicate the histogram bins of the reference image and the test image.

$R(\mathbf{T})$ in Eq. 1 regularizes the transformation [6], is defined as

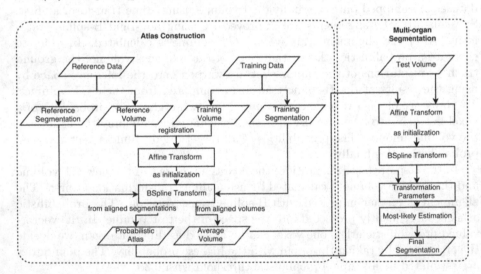

Fig. 1. Flowchart of the proposed method.

$$R(\mathbf{T}) = \frac{1}{V} \sum_x \sum_y \sum_z$$

$$\left[\left(\frac{\partial^2 \mathbf{T}}{\partial x^2} \right)^2 + \left(\frac{\partial^2 \mathbf{T}}{\partial y^2} \right)^2 + \left(\frac{\partial^2 \mathbf{T}}{\partial z^2} \right)^2 \right.$$

$$\left. +2 \left(\frac{\partial^2 \mathbf{T}}{\partial xy} \right)^2 + 2 \left(\frac{\partial^2 \mathbf{T}}{\partial xz} \right)^2 + 2 \left(\frac{\partial^2 \mathbf{T}}{\partial yz} \right)^2 \right]$$

where V denotes the number of voxels.

The α in Eq. 1 determines the weight of the regularization with respect to the similarity measure.

To solve the optimization problem, CMA-ES [7] and ASGD (adaptive stochastic gradient descent) [8] are employed for affine transformation and B-spline transformation respectively. The registration is implemented using the open source image registration toolbox Elastix [9].

3   Results

The proposed method is evaluated with the 20 unenhanced whole body CT data from VISCERAL [10]. 0.30 was taken as the threshold for the boundary estimation. The evaluation tool of VISCERAL was used to compare the segmentation result and the ground truth.

The dataset included 12 male image volumes and 8 female image volumes, so the test was divided into 2 gender groups at first. Leave-one-out cross validation was performed for each gender group. Fig. 2 presents one slice of an average volume and a probabilistic atlas. Fig. 3 plots the Dice coefficients of the segmentation results of the cross validation.

Furthermore, the proposed method was compared with the state-of-the-art methods. The lines 1-3 of Tab. 1 display the average Dice coefficients from other state-of-the-art methods [1, 2, 3]. The line 4 of Tab. 1 list the average Dice coefficients of our tests with a total of 23 cases including male, female and unisex cases. Note that the training and test data setup of these three methods are different from ours. The average Dice of our tests is above 95% for both lungs, around 90% for liver, and between 70% and 80% for other three organs.

4   Discussion

We proposed a generic framework for an automatic segmentation of multiple organs in abdomen and thorax using probabilistic atlas and registration. We constructed probabilistic atlases and segmented the target organs successfully. The cross validation showed the feasibility and the strong robustness of the method. However, the male group had the higher accuracy for kidneys and spleen

Table 1. Comparison of the Dice coefficients with other methods. '*' means that the methods use other test data. '-' means that no segmentation was provided.

Line		Right Lung	Left Lung	Right Kidney	Left Kidney	Liver	Spleen
1	*Toro et al. [1]	97.5%	97.2%	79.0%	78.4%	86.6%	70.3%
2	*Kahl et al. [2]	97.5%	97.2%	91.5%	93.4%	92.1%	87.0%
3	*He et al. [3]	95.7%	95.2%	-	-	92.3%	87.4%
4	Proposed	96.0%	95.7%	79.4%	73.1%	90.0%	81.3%

than the female group. The reasons for this observations could be: 1. the male group had more samples; 2. the non-rigid tissue variation of the female group was higher. In addition, lungs and liver were more accurate in our registration due to the metric mutual information.

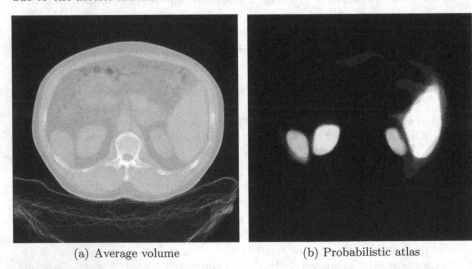

(a) Average volume   (b) Probabilistic atlas

Fig. 2. Example of an average volume (left) and a probabilistic atlas (right).

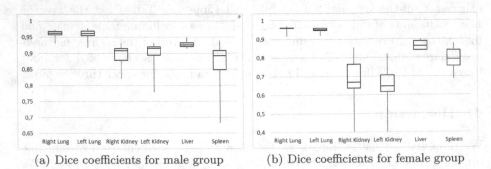

(a) Dice coefficients for male group   (b) Dice coefficients for female group

Fig. 3. Results of the cross validation. Left and right figures plot the Dice coefficients for each organ of the male group and the female group respectively.

Compared to the existing methods, our method provided competitive results. The comparison showed that the proposed method is promising and potential. These state-of-the-art methods used organ-specific prior knowledge such as anatomical spatial correlation, organ specific features, boundary profiles and shape variation information. Our method didn't employ any organ-specific prior knowledge. Our process is therefore compact and uncomplicated. Furthermore, it is easy to expand our atlas to incorporate more structures and organs.

To reduce the bias due to the reference selection, better solution for reference selection is required. In addition, using an automatic method [11] to detect the volume-of-interest can also improve the accuracy. Moreover, the decision of the organ type and the estimation of the boundary can be improved in the future work.

Acknowledgement. The authors gratefully acknowledge funding of the German Research Foundation (DFG), research grant No. MA 4898/5-1 and KA 1678/20.

Disclaimer. The concepts and information presented in this paper are based on research and are not commercially available.

References

1. Jiménez-del Toro OA, Dicente Cid Y, Depeursinge A, et al. Hierarchic anatomical structure segmentation guided by spatial correlations (AnatSeg–Gspac): VISCERAL Anatomy3. Proc Visc Chall ISBI. 2015; p. 22–6.
2. Kahl F, Ulén J, Alvén J, et al. Good features for reliable registration in multi-atlas segmentation. Proc Visc Chall ISBI. 2015; p. 12–7.
3. He B, Huang C, Jia F. Fully Automatic Multi-organ segmentation based on multi-boost learning and statistical shape model search. Proc Visc Chall ISBI. 2015; p. 18–21.
4. Park H, Bland PH, Meyer CR. Construction of an abdominal probabilistic atlas and its application in segmentation. IEEE Trans Med Imaging. 2003;22(4):483–92.
5. Mattes D, Haynor DR, Vesselle H, et al. PET-CT image registration in the chest using free-form deformations. IEEE Trans Med Imaging. 2003;22(1):120–8.
6. Rueckert D, Sonoda LI, Hayes C, et al. Nonrigid registration using free-form deformations: application to breast MR images. IEEE Trans Med Imaging. 1999;18(8):712–21.
7. Igel C, Hansen N, Roth S. Covariance matrix adaptation for multi-objective optimization. Evol Comput. 2007;15(1):1–28.
8. Klein S, Pluim JPW, Staring M, et al. Adaptive stochastic gradient descent optimisation for image registration. Int J Comput Vis. 2009;81(3):227–39.
9. Klein S, Staring M, Murphy K, et al. elastix: A Toolbox for intensity-based medical image registration. IEEE Trans Med Imaging. 2010;29(1):196–205.
10. Langs G, Müller H, Menze BH, et al. VISCERAL: towards large data in medical Imaging - challenges and directions. Proc MICCAI. 2013;7723:92–8.
11. Maier AK, Jiang Z, Jordan J, et al. Atlas-based linear volume-of-interest (ABL-VOI) image correction. Proc SPIE. 2013;8668:8668–83.

Assessing the Benefits of Interactive Patient-Specific Visualisations for Patient Information

Georg Hille[1], Nico Merten[1], Steffen Serowy[2], Sylvia Glaßer[1], Klaus Tönnies[1], Bernhard Preim[1]

[1]Department of Simulation and Graphics, University of Magdeburg, Germany
[2]Department of Neuroradiology, University Hospital of Magdeburg, Germany
georg.hille@ovgu.de

Abstract. Every surgical intervention results in physical injuries. There-fore, the patient's consent is required to avoid liability in case of bodily harm. In a lot of countries a stepwise clarification process is common, combining written and verbal clarification, the latter in form of a con-versation between patient and surgeon. However, many studies have shown that the quality of patient information is a weak spot in surgical treatment processes. Our approach, exemplary displayed for minimally invasive spine interventions, supports the clarification conversation by displaying intuitive, comprehensible and interactive 2D and 3D visuali-sations of both, the patient-specific anatomy and pathologies. Further-more, information about surgical plans in minimally invasive interven-tions, like radiofrequency or microwave ablation, could be demonstrated by virtually placing applicators within the patient-customized 3D scene. Visualisation and medical application experts evaluated the contribution and usability of this tool.

1 Introduction

Every medical intervention, minimally invasive procedures included, results in physical injuries the patient's consent is required to avoid liability in case of bodily harm. The patient's approval towards interventions is crucial for any medical treatment and must always have preceded a clarification conversation between patient and surgeon.

Due to the psychological burden of patients, their ability of fully understand-ing the interventional plan and treatment strategy might be impaired. Though, a well-informed and therefore more independent and responsible patient con-tributes to a higher satisfaction regarding medical treatments [1].

In a lot of countries a stepwise clarification process is common: a combination of written information in form of leaflets and a verbal clarification by the doctor. High-quality clarification could help to overcome fear of the treatment [2] and enhance awareness and compliance [3]. As an example of use we chose therefore spine surgery as a frequent type of surgery with a high risk of severe complica-tions depending on patient-specific spatial relations. Besides, medical specialists

224

like surgeons and neuroradiologists consider patient information as an integral part of their profession [4], but too often doubt their success in clarification, while tending to stick to ineffective information strategies [5]. Many studies have shown that the quality, communication and presentation, respectively of patient information is a crucial point during surgical treatment processes [3, 6]. Therefore, improvements of patient information methods may also enhance the satisfaction of doctors in terms of transferring medical informations towards the patient [6].

Studies showed that multimedia contents increased patient satisfaction [7, 8]. Most of them were examining the impact of multimedial patient information by films shown before the clarification conversation [7]. Their major drawback could be seen in presenting only generic, pre-recorded surgical information with no interaction possibilities and no further patient-specific information. Our approach is to improve the quality of the clarification conversation directly by involving patient-specific information in an interactive multimedia tool.

In this work, we present a 3D spine visualisation application including segmented vertebral bodies and metastases regarding pre-surgical patient information before neuroradiological interventions. Our prototypal tool, called "3D-SpineVis" should support the doctor to explain the surgical plan and treatment strategy to the patient by displaying patient-costumized anatomy and pathologies, gained e.g. through MR imaging, as well as illustrating minimally invasive instrument placing used during interventions like radiofrequency or microwave ablations. The purpose of this work was to examine whether our interactive and patient-specific tool gains benefits towards communicating and illustrating pre-surgical information during a patient-doctor conversation.

2   Materials and methods

Our prototypal "3D-SpineVis" tool was implemented in the medical image processing and visualisation environment MeVisLab[1]. It combines original pre-interventional image data, such as MR or CT images and segmentations of anatomical structures or tissues like bones and metastasis (Fig. 2).

In this paper, we exemplary demonstrate our approach for a pre-surgical clarification support before radiofrequency ablation of vertebral metastases. Therefore, we combined pre-interventionally acquired MR images of the spine with a semi-automatical vertebral body segmentation according to the method presented by Hille et al. [9] and a manual metastases segmentation. These information were jointly aligned to display both the original MR images, as a 3D volume with freely selectable and orientable clip planes, the vertebral body and metastases segmentations as 3D volumes and contour overlays within the MRI data. The visualisation can be adjusted by opacity and illumination and, therefore, different foci of attention could be represented. Next to the 3D visualisation a second image viewer is placed, displaying the MRI data slice by sclice. With one

---

[1] http://www.mevislab.de

click within a browseable 2D MRI data set with overlayed vertebral body and metastases segmentation contours, one can initially place an abstracted model of a minimally invasive intervention applicator. The user can rotate the applicator with the needle tip orientated towards the clicked voxel within the 3D scene to demonstrate potential patient-customized intervention plans (Fig. 2).

We asked five visualisation and medical application field experts to evaluate our tool. Since it should primarily gain benefits towards patients, it makes sense to ask non-medical persons. We asked them to assess the following eight statements, while ranking their agreeing or disagreeing in a five-point Likert scale from strongly disagree (- -) to stronlgy agree (++):

Q1) Multimedia-supported patient information enhance the quality of the clarification process.
Q2) Presenting patient-customized information constitutes a gain towards comprehension and clarification.
Q3) Presenting interactive information constitutes a gain towards comprehension and clarification.

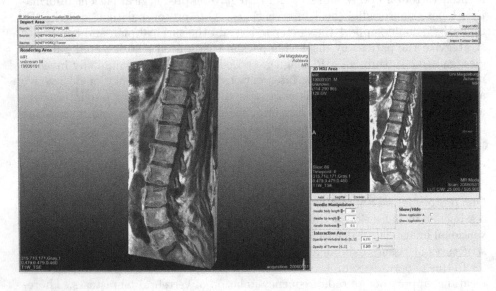

Fig. 1. The GUI of our prototypal "3D-SpineVis" application. On the top one can import the MRI or CT scans and the corresponding vertebral body and tumor/metastases segmentations (red box). The large viewer on the left is for spatially exploring the volume-rendered scene (blue box). Herein, a clinical expert could comprehensibly explain patient-specific spatial relations and give insight how to perform an ablative intervention with interactive models of minimally invasive applicators. On the upper right, both the original image data with super-imposed segmentation contours could be explored and the applicator models could be placed here per one-click (green box). In the yellow box in the lower right corner opacities of the segmented 3D objects could be adjusted (vertebral bodies in white, metastases in red), and it offers the option to show or hide the applicator models.

Q4) The presented prototypal tool is intuitive to use to display image-based information, like anatomical structures and pathologies.

Q5) The presented prototypal tool displays image based information, like anatomical structures and pathologies comprehensible.

Q6) In case that patients see generic multimedia material like pre-recorded videos prior to the patient-doctor conversation,

    a) presenting patient-customized and interactive information in the patient-doctor conversation has a benefit over generic media.

    b) presenting patient-customized and interactive information in the patient-doctor conversation is a suitable addition to generic media.

Q7) The presented prototypal tool is an contribution regarding information communication and visualisation within a patient clarification conversation.

3 Results

Fig. 3 shows the results of our evaluation. They show the opinions of our evaluatees as visualisation and medical application field experts, as well as potential patients. Exceptionless, every evaluatee considers multimedia support a quality enhancement towards the clarification process (Q1). The majority of the surveyed persons strongly agree that including interactively explorable and patient-specific information improves comprehension and clarification (Q2 and Q3). Regarding the intuitivity and comprehensibility of the presented "3D-SpineVis" tool (Q4 and Q5), only one evaluatee stated it as not intuitive, but comprehensible.

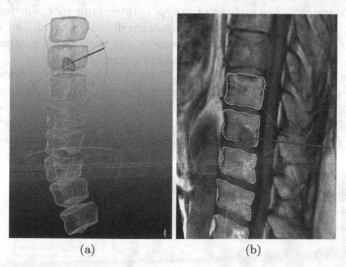

         (a)   (b)

Fig. 2. Details of the volume-rendered scene with applicator model tips placed within the metastases. It is possible to display only the segmented 3D objects with the placed applicator models (a), as well as to add further anatomical and structural information by displaying also the original MRI data (b). Therefore, the user could balance between simplified and more complex visualisations.

Besides, the remaining evaluatees agreed with both statements. Furthermore, the evaluatees assessed our tool as a suitable addition to generic media (Q6b), like pre-conversational shown videos, or even as superior (Q6a). Overall, our presented tool was evaluated from all surveyed persons as a possible contribution during a patient information conversation (Q7).

4 Discussion

The desire for a visual support during the clarification conversation reflects the contemporary trend towards technical assistance, to enhance vividness and comprehensibility of medical informations [8]. This assessment was also confirmed by our evaluatees, who unanimously stated that multimedia support would qualitatively improve patient information procedures. Furthermore, it was evaluated that both patient-specific and interactive visual information would increase the communication quality. While examining potential benefits of media support in research, so far, mostly films shown before the clarification conversation were discussed [7, 8]. Possible drawbacks of such films could be seen in their generic and non-interactive features. Hence, our evaluatees evaluated patient-customized and interactive information as a suitable addition to generic video material or even superior to it. To become a reasonable support for the patient-doctor conversation, both the operability of every multimedia tool and the presentation of information have to be intuitive and comprehensible. Our prototypal "3D-SpineVis" tool was largely assessed to be intuitive to handle, except from one evaluatee who disagreed. However, one must consider that user expertise increases with practise time and the prototypal state of our tool. Furthermore, it was found comprehensible regarding information display. Overall, our approach was evaluated as a possible contribution concerning information communication and visualisation within a patient information conversation.

The prototypal "3D-SpineVis" tool that we presented in this work was evaluated from all surveyed persons as a contribution towards communication and comprehensibility of patient information by supporting the patient-doctor conversation with specific and interactional visualisations of patient anatomy and pathology. Additionally, the surgeon could provide an insight into the patient-

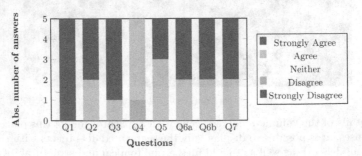

Fig. 3. The results of our survey.

specific surgical plan by placing models of minimally invasive interventional instruments.

Our approach offers different links to future work, e.g. simulation of treatment methods, like heatmaps of ablation procedures or further improvements of the 3D visualisation. Reasonable attempts like adaptive cutaways of volume render scenes, presented by Li et al. [10], could enhance the illustration of details, like metastases and medical applicator placement, while maintaining the overview and orientation within comprehensive anatomical models.

Acknowledgement. This work was supported by the German Ministry of Education and Research (13GW0095A) within the STIMULATE research campus.

References

1. Sechrest R, Henry D. Computer-based patient education: observations on effective communication in the clinical setting. J Biocommunication. 1995;23(1):8–12.
2. Anzenberger P, Jedinger O, Zarhuber K. Design and Development of a multilingual multimedia based presurgical Information and Clarification System for Tablet Computers. In: Proceedings of the (IADIS), International Conference on e-Health; 2012.
3. Ha JF, Longnecker N. Doctor-patient communication: a review. Ochsner J. 2010;10(1):38–43.
4. Keulers B, Scheltinga M, Houterman S, et al. Surgeons underestimate their patients' desire for preoperative information. World J Surg. 2008;32(6):964–70.
5. Keulers BJ, Welters CF, Spauwen PH, et al. Can face-to-face patient education be replaced by computer-based patient education? A randomised trial. Patient Educ Couns. 2007;67(1):176–82.
6. Ong LM, De Haes JC, Hoos AM, et al. Doctor-patient communication: a review of the literature. Soc Sci Med. 1995;40(7):903–18.
7. Evrard S, Mathoulin-Pelissier S, Larrue C, et al. Evaluation of a preoperative multimedia information program in surgical oncology. Eur J Surg Oncol. 2005;31(1):106–10.
8. Eggers C, Obliers R, Koerfer A, et al. A Multimedia Tool for the Informed Consent of Patients prior to Gastric Banding. Obesity. 2007;15(11):2866–73.
9. Hille G, Glaßer S, Tönnies K. Hybrid level-sets for vertebral body segmentation in Clinical Spine MRI. Procedia Computer Science. 2016;90:22–7
10. Li W, Ritter L, Agrawala M, et al. Interactive Cutaway Illustrations of Complex 3D Models. ACM Trans Graph. 2007;26(3):31.

Abstract: Effiziente Visualisierung von Vektorfeldern in der Strahlentherapie

Jan Meis[1,2], Hendrik Teske[1,2], Kristina Giske[1,2]

[1]Division of Medical Physics in Radiation Oncology, DKFZ Heidelberg
[2]National Center for Radiation Research in Oncology (NCRO),
Heidelberg Institute for Radiation Oncology (HIRO), Heidelberg
j.meis@dkfz.de

Bewegungsdaten in der Strahlentherapie werden als zeitabhängige, dreidimensionale, diskretisierte Vektorfelder beschrieben. Deren Visualisierung stellt eine Herausforderung in den Bereichen Speichermanagement und Berechnungszeit dar. Die Darstellung eines typischen 3D-Vektorfelds mithilfe 3D Pfeil-Glyphen in jedem Voxel bei einer typischen Auflösung würde ∼ 10 GB Speicher und ∼ 30 s CPU Berechnungszeit benötigen. Soll ein Vektorfeld nun auch mittels anderer Darstellungsarten wie z.B. Flusstrajektorien darstellt werden um die Übersichtlichkeit zu erhöhen, so vervielfacht sich auch die benötigte Berechnungszeit trotz der Reduktion der Glyphenanzahl. Um zukünftig 4D Lungenatmung animiert darzustellen, müssen Methoden entwickelt werden um Informationen aus einem Vektorfeld zu extrahieren ohne die Balance zwischen Ressourcenaufwand und vollständiger Darstellung zu verlieren.

Wir benutzen Particle-Tracing Methoden um animierte Strömungslinien im 3D Raum zu erzeugen. Die Strömungslinien werden als Bahnen zufällig im Raum verteilter Punkte erzeugt, die dann entlang des Vektorfeldes integriert werden. Die Glyphen werden entlang der Strömungslinien animiert dargestellt. Um Überschneidungen zu verringern und plötzliches Auftauchen und Verschwinden von Glyphen zu maskieren, wurde ein Verfahren für 2D Vektorfelder [1] auf 3D erweitert. Die Methode wurde bisher single-threaded auf der CPU realisiert. Der Rechenaufwand hierfür beträgt mehrere Minuten.

Unser aktueller Fokus ist es, diesen Prozess durch GPU-Parallelisierung zu beschleunigen. Im ersten Schritt wurde die Berechnung der Darstellung der Glyphen über CUDA realisiert. Der Vorteil ist, dass hierbei die CUDA-OpenGL Interoperabilität die langsamen Transfers zwischen GPU und CPU minimiert. Die aktuelle Implementierung führte zu einer Beschleunigung in der Berechnung der Pfeil-Glyphen um 200%.

Im nächsten Schritt soll auch die Strömungslinienberechnung parallelisiert und die Darstellung auf 4D Daten erweitert werden, um eine übersichtliche und schnelle Darstellung von z.B. Atembewegungen mittels Glyphen zu ermöglichen.

Literaturverzeichnis

1. Jobard B, Ray N, Sokolov D. Visualizing 2D flows with animated arrow plots. Compute Res Repository. 2012;abs/1205.5204. Available from: http://arxiv.org/abs/1205.5204.

Quantification of Guidance Strategies in Online Interactive Semantic Segmentation of Glioblastoma MRI

Jens Petersen[1,2], Sabine Heiland[1], Martin Bendszus[1], Jürgen Debus[3,4,5,6], Klaus H. Maier-Hein[2]

[1]Dept. of Neuroradiology, Heidelberg University Hospital, Heidelberg, Germany
[2]Junior Group Medical Image Computing, German Cancer Research Center, Heidelberg, Germany
[3]Dept. of Radiation Oncology, Heidelberg University Hospital, Heidelberg, Germany
[4]Heidelberg Institute of Radiation Oncology, Heidelberg, Germany
[5]Heidelberg Ion-Beam Therapy Center, Heidelberg, Germany
[6]Clinical Cooperation Unit Radiation Oncology, German Cancer Research Center, Heidelberg, Germany
jens.petersen@dkfz.de

Abstract. Interactive segmentation promises to combine the speed of automatic approaches with the reliability of manual techniques. Its performance, however, depends largely on live iterative inputs by a human supervisor. For the task of glioblastoma segmentation in MRI data using a Random Forest pixel classifier we quantify the benefit in terms of speed and segmentation quality of user inputs in falsely classified regions as opposed to guided annotations in regions of high classifier uncertainty. The former results in a significantly higher area under the curve of the Dice score over time in all tumor categories. Exponential fits reveal a significantly higher final Dice score for larger tumor regions (gross tumor volume and edema) but not for smaller regions (necrotic core, non-enhancing abnormalities and contrast-enhancing tumor). Time constants of the exponential fits do not differ significantly.

1 Introduction

Interactive semi-automatic segmentation strikes a much needed balance between fully automatic and fully manual segmentation techniques in that it employs an automatic approach in a manner that allows a human supervisor to provide training data interactively (online) to adjust the output of the classifier to their preference. Ideally this will allow the segmentation task to be fulfilled in a very short time with the reliability of expert supervision, a key factor for acceptance in a clinical environment. An added benefit is that interactive methods typically don't require previously available training data and can in turn be used to generate such data for automated methods to be applied on a larger scale.

Numerous interactive segmentation techniques exists, for example variants of active contours [1] or based on seed points [2, 3].

231

Another common approach is to let users annotate pixels in an image and to use these annotations to predict tissue types on the remaining image pixels [4, 5]. The result is presented to the user along with the original image so that they can make additional annotations for a new, improved prediction. The process is repeated until the user is satisfied with their segmentation. The speed with which a satisfactory result is obtained depends on where the user places their annotations and thus on which data (e.g. which slice of an image volume) is presented to the user in what way. Simpler approaches just display an overlay of prediction probabilities [4] or a semi-transparent segmentation, while others try to guide the user to specific regions, for example those where the classifier is uncertain [5].

For glioblastoma segmentation it has been shown that if a user annotates falsely classified regions instead of those regions that are most uncertain, a significantly better segmentation results after a small number of interaction cycles [6]. In this work we aim to quantify the performance over time of three different approaches.

2   Materials and methods

We simulate a human user in an interactive online learning environment. In an iterative fashion we let the simulated user annotate 10 connected pixels (a *scribble* or *stroke*) of a single tissue class in an image volume in each step. The cumulative annotated pixels are used to train a Random Forest classifier [7] (50 trees, maximum depth of 10, Gini impurity splits, majority voting) to make class predictions on the entire image volume. We compare the following three annotation methods:

- *UR*: Annotate within the region of highest classifier uncertainty as proposed in [6].
- *FR*: Annotate randomly in the falsely classified region.
- *FB*: Annotate randomly in the falsely classified region for a randomly selected class. This ensures an equal distribution of annotations among classes.

We evaluate the Dice score over 50 interaction cycles. Any measurement was repeated 5 times and averaged because of the random nature of the process. As a combined measure of segmentation quality and speed we use the normalized area under the curve AUC of the Dice score across the interaction cycles (which in this case is just the mean Dice score). Additionally we perform an exponential fit for the time dependent Dice score

$$d(t) = d_\infty \cdot \left(1 - \exp^{-t/\tau}\right) \tag{1}$$

where t is the normalized interaction cycle and d_∞ and τ represent separate measures of segmentation quality and speed of convergence, respectively. Such fits are only performed for the gross tumor volume, the edema region and the enhancing tumor region. The approach does not lend itself to the low classifier performance for the other tissues (necrotic core and non-enhancing abnormalities). Fig. 2 shows an overlay of all measurements for the whole tumor region, indicating that this approach is appropriate.

We use the 20 high grade glioma patients from the 2013 BraTS challenge [8] dataset for evaluation. In addition to the four contrasts T1, T1ce, T2 and FLAIR, the classifier utilizes the following features ($\sigma = 0.7$ and $\sigma = 1.6$): Gaussian smoothing, Gaussian gradient magnitude, Laplacian of Gaussian, Hessian of Gaussian eigenvalues, structure tensor eigenvalues.

A paired, two-sided Student's t-test is used to check how likely it is that two sets of measurements originate from the same population. We say that two sets differ significantly if $p < 0.01$. Because we test 38 separate combinations, we expect to find 0.38 significant differences by chance, which we consider acceptable.

3   Results

Tab. 1 shows the performance comparison of uncertainty-guided (UG) annotations and random corrections (FR). FR displays significantly higher AUC and d_∞ in the larger tumor regions (whole tumor and edema), while the AUC for the other regions is not only not significantly different, but in fact rather similar with $p \geq 0.480$. UG has a significantly higher d_∞ in the contrast-enhancing region. Time constants τ do not differ significantly.

The comparison of uncertainty-guided (UG) and class-balanced corrections (FB) in Tab. 2 reveals that FB has a significantly higher AUC than UG in almost all regions except for the edema, where p is just slightly higher than our

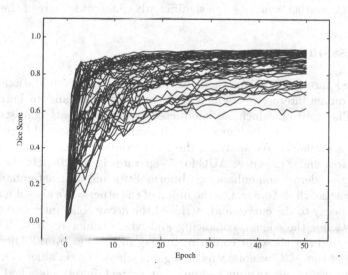

Fig. 1. Overlay of all measured Dice scores over time (i.e. interaction cycle) for the whole tumor region.

Table 1. Results of paired two-sample t-test comparing uncertainty-guided annotations (UG) and annotations in random falsely classified regions (FR) for *area under curve* AUC, exp-fit τ, exp-fit d_∞, showing mean sample difference (Δ), t-statistic (t) and probability of true null-hypothesis (p). 1σ standard deviation is displayed in parentheses. Regions are whole tumor (GTV – gross tumor volume), necrotic core (Core), edema (Edema), non-enhancing abnormalities (Non-Enhanc.) and contrast-enhancing abnormalities (Enhanc.). Significant differences are highlighted in bold.

		GTV	Core	Edema	Non-Enhanc.	Enhanc.
	Δ	**−0.056(56)**	0.014(118)	**−0.078(87)**	−0.014(87)	−0.004(99)
AUC	t	**−4.476**	0.508	**−3.922**	−0.720	−0.194
	p	**< 0.001**	0.617	**< 0.001**	0.480	0.848
	Δ	−0.002(39)		−0.016(41)		0.028(92)
τ	t	−0.195		−1.598		1.170
	p	0.848		0.130		0.262
	Δ	**−0.040(89)**		**−0.065(69)**		**0.015(27)**
d_∞	t	**−4.018**		**−3.805**		**2.144**
	p	**0.002**		**0.002**		**0.006**

significance threshold. UG also has a significantly higher d_∞ in the whole tumor and edema regions, with very similar d_∞ in the contrast-enhancing region. Again there is no significant difference in τ.

Finally, Tab. 3 lists the comparison of random corrections (FR) and class-balanced corrections (FB). While FB shows significantly higher AUC in the smaller tumor regions (necrotic core, non-enhancing and enhancing), FR performs significantly better in the larger two regions (whole tumor and edema) in terms of AUC. Neither τ nor d_∞ are significantly different for any of the classes.

4   Discussion

We compared three different methods of querying scribble annotations from a user for an online interactive segmentation task using a Random Forest pixel classifier. The data on which we conducted our experiments consisted of 20 glioblastoma patients for which groundtruth segmentation merged from 4 different experts is available. We analyzed the Dice score over time by means of the normalized area under the curve AUC for 5 separate classes, namely the necrotic tumor core, the edema, non-enhancing abnormalities and contrast-enhancing tumor as well as the whole tumor, i.e. the union of the others. We also fit a negative exponential decay to the curves and retrieved the decay constant τ and the limit Dice score d_∞ for the edema, enhancing and whole tumor regions. The other tissue classes did not allow for confident fits because of low overall Dice scores.

In terms of the AUC annotations in regions where the classifier is uncertain are significantly inferior to annotations that correct falsely classified regions. Random correcting annotations yield a significantly higher AUC in the larger regions edema and whole tumor. The fact that for these regions d_∞ is also sig-

Table 2. Results of paired two-sample t-test comparing uncertainty-guided annotations (UG) and class-balanced annotations in falsely classified regions (FB) for *area under curve* AUC, exp-fit τ, exp-fit d_∞, showing mean sample difference (Δ), t-statistic (t) and probability of true null-hypothesis (p). 1σ standard deviation is displayed in parentheses. Regions are whole tumor (GTV – gross tumor volume), necrotic core (Core), edema (Edema), non-enhancing abnormalities (Non-Enhanc.) and contrast-enhancing abnormalities (Enhanc.). Significant differences are highlighted in bold.

		GTV	Core	Edema	Non-Enhanc.	Enhanc.
AUC	Δ	**−0.045(62)**	**−0.105(67)**	**−0.057(88)**	**−0.094(72)**	**−0.076(107)**
	t	**−3.179**	**−6.806**	**−2.833**	**−5.718**	**−3.130**
	p	**0.005**	**< 0.001**	**0.011**	**< 0.001**	**0.006**
τ	Δ	−0.010(37)		−0.024(35)		0.040(89)
	t	−1.081		−2.723		1.185
	p	0.297		0.016		0.089
d_∞	Δ	**−0.034(26)**		**−0.048(49)**		−0.001(18)
	t	**−5.095**		**−3.971**		−0.142
	p	**< 0.001**		**0.002**		0.889

nificantly higher while there is no significant difference in τ indicates that the high AUC is mainly due to a higher final Dice score rather than a faster increase of Dice. The final Dice for uncertainty guided annotations in the enhancing region is significantly higher than for random corrections, likely because this region is usually small so that random annotations, even those limited to error regions, seldom fall within its bounds. Fewer training data consequently result in a poorer performance. This notion is supported by the comparison of balanced and random corrections. Measured by the AUC, balanced corrections, i.e. training data distributed evenly among classes, yield a significantly better performance in the three smaller regions, while random corrections do so in the two larger regions. Note that glioblastoma, especially when the edema is included, typically occupies a large protion of the brain. Since there is no significant difference in either d_∞ or τ it can be assumed that the differences in AUC come from both a higher overall Dice and a faster convergence towards it. Finally, and as a logical consequence, class-balanced corrections also significantly outperform uncertainty-guided annotations in terms of AUC in the smaller tumor regions. They do so for the whole tumor as well, while the difference for the edema region is not quite significant.

In summary, it is advantageous to perform an online interactive segmentation task such that the inputs correct the classifier instead of supplying information at points where it is uncertain. Our experiments also show that these regions need not be identical. Depending on whether the classes to be segmented in an image make up rather large or rather small portions, one should supply random corrections or corrections that treat different regions equally often.

Either way, our results support the findings in [6] that applications that wish to realize such an annotation model should present raw image data and current

Table 3. Results of paired two-sample t-test comparing annotations in random falsely classified regions (FR) and class-balanced annotations in falsely classified regions (FB) for *area under curve* AUC, exp-fit τ, exp-fit d_∞, showing mean sample difference (Δ), t-statistic (t) and probability of true null-hypothesis (p). 1σ standard deviation is displayed in parentheses. Regions are whole tumor (GTV – gross tumor volume), necrotic core (Core), edema (Edema), non-enhancing abnormalities (Non-Enhanc.) and contrast-enhancing abnormalities (Enhanc.). Significant differences are highlighted in bold.

		GTV	Core	Edema	Non-Enhanc.	Enhanc.
	Δ	**0.012(15)**	**−0.118(116)**	**0.022(17)**	**−0.080(57)**	**−0.072(85)**
AUC	t	**3.509**	**−4.447**	**5.773**	**−6.150**	**−3.701**
	p	**0.003**	**< 0.001**	**< 0.001**	**< 0.001**	**0.002**
	Δ	−0.012(40)		−0.015(43)		0.032(67)
τ	t	−1.216		−1.551		1.858
	p	0.241		0.137		0.083
	Δ	0.005(19)		0.010(29)		−0.013(23)
d_∞	t	1.143		1.595		−2.346
	p	0.269		0.127		0.033

segmentation in a manner that allows the user to easily identify falsely classified regions.

References

1. Kass M, Witkin A, Terzopoulos D. Snakes: active contour models. Int J Comput Vis. 1988;1(4):321–31.
2. Grady L. Random walks for image segmentation. IEEE Trans Pattern Anal Mach Intell. 2006;28(11):1768–83.
3. Rupprecht C, Peter L, Navab N. Image segmentation in twenty questions. Proc IEEE CVPR. 2015; p. 3314–22.
4. Sommer C, Straehle C, Koethe U, et al. ilastik: Interactive learning and segmentation toolkit. Proc IEEE ISBI. 2011; p. 230–3.
5. Petersen J, Bendszus M, Debus J, et al. A software application for interactive medical image segmentation with active user guidance. Proc MICCAI. 2016.
6. Petersen J, Bendszus M, Debus J, et al. Effective user guidance in an online interactive semantic segmentation. Proc SPIE Med Imaging. 2017; p. to appear.
7. Breiman L. Random forests. Mach Learn. 2001;45(1):5–32.
8. Menze BH, Jakab A, Bauer S, et al. The multimodal brain tumor image segmentation benchmark (BRATS). IEEE Trans Med Imaging. 2015;34(10):1993–2024.

Training mit positiven und unannotierten Daten für automatische Voxelklassifikation

Michael Goetz, Klaus H. Maier-Hein

Medical Image Computing, DKFZ Heidelberg
m.goetz@dkfz-heidelberg.de

Kurzfassung. Das Erstellen einer Trainingsbasis für lernbasierte Methoden zur Gewebecharakterisierung ist häufig fehleranfällig und zeitaufwendig. Sparse and Unambigious (SUR)-Annotationen können hier den Aufwand reduzieren, aber die Annotation mehrerer Gewebeklassen sind dennoch aufwendig. Wir stellen einen Ansatz vor, der das Training ermöglicht, wenn lediglich eine Gewebeklasse annotiert wurde. Diese als positive and unlabeled Learning"(PU-Learning) bezeichnete Methode reduziert den manuellen Annotationsaufwand. In unserer Arbeit zeigen wir zudem, dass die erzielten Segmentierungen sich nicht statistisch signifikante vom Stand der Forschung unterscheiden.

1 Einleitung

Das Segmentieren von pathologisch auffälligen Gebieten ist eine häufige Fragestellung in der medizinischen Bildverarbeitung. Typische und häufig beachtete Beispiele dafür sind zum Beispiel die Segmentierung von Gehirntumoren oder -blutungen. Voxelbasierte Klassifikation ist dabei in den letzten Jahren zu einem Quasi-Standard für die automatische Bearbeitung solcher Fragen geworden. Da die benutzten Modelle anhand vorher annotierter Trainingsdaten gelernt werden, können solche Verfahren gut auf neue Problemstellung angepasst werden, und liefern meist gute bis sehr gute Ergebnisse.

Eine Herausforderung bei dem Einsatz lernbasierter Methoden stellt vielfach die Bereitstellung der notwendigen Trainingsdaten dar. Die Annotation dieser Daten ist häufig umständlich und fehleranfällig. Bei Gehirntumoren werden mehrere Stunden benötigt um einen Patienten für die Trainingsbasis zu annotieren, wobei gleichzeitig eine große Unsicherheit innerhalb eines Bildes bleibt [1, 2]. Das ist vor allem für Bildgebung mit Magnetresonanz (MR) schwierig, da die Bildgebung sowohl vom Aufnahmegerät als auch der verwendeten Sequenz abhängt.

Ein typischer Ansatz um die Annotation zu vermeiden ist es auf bereits annotierte Wettbewerbsdaten, z.B. der BraTS Challenge [1], zurückzugreifen. Allerdings erlaubt das keine Anpassung an örtliche Gegebenheiten (Scanner, gefahrene Protokolle) oder an andere Fragestellungen. Auch der Einsatz von problemspezifische Informationen, z.B. Gehirnatlanten, kann den Bedarf an annotierten Trainingsdaten reduziern [3]. Dies erhöht zwar die Flexibilität im Bezug auf unterschiedliche Bildgebung, nicht aber für unterschiedliche Fragestellungen. Verma et al. umgingen dieses Problem, indem sie nur partielle Annotationen verwenden, untersuchten aber nicht den dadurch induzierten Fehler [4]. Der Ansatz einer partiellen Annotation wurde in [2] aufgegriffen. Dort wurde ein Algorithmus vorgestellt, der ohne signifikante Reduktion der Segmentationsleistung anhand spärlicher Annotationen trainieren kann. Allerdings müssen die spärlichen Annotation in allen Gewebeklassen vorgenommen werden, was bei einer vollständigen Annotation automatisch geschieht. Gerade bei umfangreichen Klasse, wie z.B. gesundem Gehirngewebe, kann dies sehr Zeitaufwendig sein. Auch für eine Annotation über Crowdsourcing ist dies negativ, da mehrere Klassen einen Wechsel des Werkzeuges erfordern und eine zusätzliche Fehlerquelle beinhalten.

Wir stellen einen neuen Algorithmus vor, der von spärliche Annotationen einer Klasse sowie unannotierte Daten um einen Klassifikator zur Gewebecharakterisierung trainieren kann. Wir zeigen dabei erstmalig a) den Einsatz von Positive and Unlabeled (PU)-learning Methoden zur Tumorsegmentierung, b) das PU-learning für Mehrklassen-Probleme genutzt werden kann, c) die bildweise Berechnung der Gewichte, und d) einen verbesserten Algorithmus zur Größenschätzung von Tumore.

2 Methoden

Um den notwendigen Annotationsaufwand zu reduzieren basiert unser Algorithmus auf der Annotation mithilfe weniger und eindeutiger Regionen (Sparse and Unambigious Region, SUR) wie sie auch in [2] benutzt werden. Eine Annotation des Hintergrunds bzw. von gesundem Gewebe ist im Gegensatz zu diesem Ansatz allerdings nicht nötig, so muss lediglich eine Gewebeklasse annotiert werden. Für das Training der Klassifikatoren liegen dann sowohl annotierte Beispiele von Tumorvoxel (positive Beispiele, $y = 1$), wie auch unannotierte Voxel, die sowohl Tumor wie auch gesundes Gewebe beinhalten (negative Beispiele, $y = 0$), vor.

Um mit diesen Trainingsdaten einen Klassifikator trainieren zu können benutzen wir einen Ansatz von Elkan und Noto [5]. Der zugrunde liegende Ansatz ist es, einen Klassifikator zu trainieren der zwischen annotierten und nicht annotierten Voxel unterscheiden kann. Werden diese Gruppen während des Trainings korrekt gewichtet, prädiziert der resultierende Klassifikator nicht den Annotationsstatus sondern das ursprünglich gesuchte Merkmal, in unserem Fall Tumor vs. Gesund.

Die korrekte Gewichte hängen von der Annotationsrate $\eta = \frac{n}{n+n'}$ ab, wobei n und n' die Anzahl der annotierten bzw. nicht annotierten Voxel sind. Zusätzlich wird das Verhältnis zwischen positiven und negativen Beispielen in den nicht annotierten Trainingsdaten U benötigt. Dieses entspricht der Wahrscheinlichkeit $P(\cdot)$ für positive Daten: $\pi = P(y = 1 \mid U)$. Die Gewichte sind dann $c_P = \frac{4 \cdot \pi}{\eta}$ und $c_U = \frac{1}{1-\eta}$ für die annotierten bzw. nicht annotierten Trainingsdaten, wobei wir die in [6] ermittelten Gewichte an die lokale Optimierung von Random Decision Forests (RDFs) angepasst haben.

Ist das Tumorvolumen bekannt, kann es genutzt werden um π direkt zu berechnet. Wenn nicht ist es möglich π automatisch zu schätzen und zusätzlichen Annotationsaufwand zu vermeiden. Eine Möglichkeit ist es den Unterschied zwischen den Verteilungen der annotierten Daten und den nicht annotierten Daten zu minimieren [6]. Da dieses Verfahren die Ähnlichkeit zwischen den Verteilungen über die Pearson Divergence bestimmt wird, bezeichnen wir es als Pearson Divergence Prior Estimation (PEPE). Allerdings setzt dieses Verfahren voraus das die annotierten Daten zufällig gezogen sind. Da dies bei einer manuellen Annotation nicht gewährleistet werden kann schlagen wir vor, die annotierten Daten vorher gemäß ihrer Auftrittswahrscheinlichkeit zu gewichten, wobei jede Observation $\mathbf{x}$ einzeln mit $w(\mathbf{x}) = \frac{P_{\mathrm{P}}(\mathbf{x})}{P_{\mathrm{U}}(\mathbf{x})}$ gewichtet wird (Abb. 2). Dabei bezeichnen P_{P} und P_{U} die Dichtefunktion der annotierten bzw. nicht annotierten Daten. Die dabei benutze "Domain AdaptationTechnik ist die gleiche wie in [2], wir bezeichnen das resultierende Verfahren als DA-PEPE. Da die Bilddaten eine natürliche Gruppierung der Voxel darstellen, berechnen wir Θ für jedes Bild und nicht, wie sonst üblich, für alle Beobachtungen individuell.

3   Daten und Experimente

Für die Validierung des vorgestellten Ansatzes werden zwei Kollektive von Patienten mit Glioblastomen und MR-Bildgebung mit vorhandenem Goldstandard benutzt. Das erste Kollektiv, DS-1, umfasst 19 Patienten mit jeweils 4 unterschiedlichen Kontrasten pro Patienten. Eine genaue Beschreibung dieses Kollektivs, der Vorverarbeitung der Daten, und der Klassifikationsmerkmalen die wir benutzen, findet sich in [2]. Ergänzend dazu werden die Trainingsdaten des 2014 MICCAI BraTS Wettbewerbs (DS-2) benutzt um die Funktion des PU-Ansatzes für Mehrklassenprobleme zu überprüfen. Die Daten sind auf der Wettebwerbsseite genauer beschrieben [1]. Wir verwenden für diese Daten die Vorverarbeitung und Merkmale des besten Random Forest-basierten Ansatz von 2014.

Die Annotation von DS-1 mit SURs wurde von einem erfahrenen Radiologen durchgeführt und sowohl Tumor wie auch gesundes Gewebe annotiert. Um den Ansatz zu evaluieren wurden nur die Tumorannotationen verwendet. Für DS-2 wurde die vorhandene, vollständige Segmentierung als Grundlage benutzt und darauf basierend PU-SUR-Annotationen erzeugt, da die Klasseneinteilung in

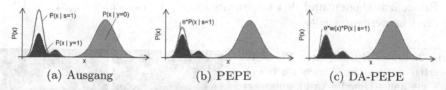

| (a) Ausgang | (b) PEPE | (c) DA-PEPE |

Abb. 1. Darstellung der Schätzung von π. (a) Die Flächen entsprechen der Verteilung von positiven ($y = 1$, blau) und negativer ($y = 0$, grau) Daten; die rote Linie entsprechend für die Verteilung der Annotationen ($s = 1$). (b) Die rote Linie wird durch Faktor Θ gewichtet, eine komplette Anpassung ist nicht möglich. (c) Durch die Funktion $w(x)$ kann der Faktor Θ genauer bestimmt werden. π kann aus Θ berechnet werden [6].

den Trainingsdaten zumindest teilweise automatisch vorgenommen wurde. Auf beiden Datensätzen wird das tatsächliche π aus den vorhandenen Goldstandard-Segmentierungen berechnet. Für DS-1 wird zusätzlich eine Schätzung mit PEPE und DA-PEPE berechnet. Aufgrund der semiautomatischen Generierung des Goldstandards haben wir bei DS-2 auf die Schätzung von π verzichtet.

Mit den unterschiedlichen Schätzungen für π werden anschließend Klassifikatoren für DS-1 trainiert. Neben den unterschiedlichen π zusätzlich noch Klassifikatoren mit zufällig gezogenen Voxel aus dem Goldstandard sowie gemäß des Ansatzes in [2] trainiert um mit dem Stand der Forschung vergleichen zu können. Zusätzlich wird in einer Versuchsreihe das tatsächliche π prozentual verändert um zu erfassen wie Sensitiv der Algorithmus auf eine Falschschätzung reagiert.

Für DS-2 wird ein Klassifikator mit dem bekannten π trainiert. Dabei wird der Klassifikator für alle vorhandenen Klassen trainiert, für die Klasse "Gesund"wurden keine annotierten Beispiele benutzt.

4   Ergebnisse

– *Annotations-Aufwand:* Die vollständige, manuelle Segmentierung eines Patienten von DS-1 und DS-2 dauerte mehr wie 4 Stunden [1, 2]. Eine SUR-basierte Annotation aller Klassen benötigt weniger als 5 Minuten. In DS-1 umfasste diese $0,25\,\%\pm0,15\,\%$ des gesamten Gehirnvolumen und $2,6\,\%\pm1,5\,\%$ des Tumorvolumen. Nur $55,1\,\%\pm16,5\,\%$ der SUR-Annotation umfassen Tumorgewebe.
– *Evaluation des PU-Ansatzes:* Auf DS-2 wird ein durchschnittlicher Dice-Score von $78,7\,\%\pm15,7\,\%$ für die kombinierten Tumorklassen erreicht. Abb. 2 (Rechts) zeigt Beispielergebnisse der erhaltenen Mehrklassen-Segmentierung.
– *Einfluss von π:* Abb. 3 zeigt den Verlauf des Dice-Scores, wenn die tatsächliche Tumorgröße prozentual verändert wird.
– *Schätzung des Tumorvolumens:* In DS-1 beträgt das mittlere Verhältnis von Tumor zu Gesamtgewebe $10,5\,\%$ (Berechnet aus der Goldstandard-Segmentierung). Der selbe Wert beträgt $7,6\,\%$ wenn PEPE, bzw. $8,5\,\%$ wenn DA-PEPE zur Schätzung des Volumens benutzt wird. Während die Schätzungen des Tumorvolumens vor allem bei geringeren Volumina mit PEPE besser sind, führt DA-PEPE bei größeren Volumina zu geringeren Abweichungen.
– *Evaluation des Komplettansatzes:* Abb. 4 gibt die Dice-Scores, die mit den Referenzmethoden und den unterschiedlichen Tumorschätzungen auf DS-1 erreicht werden, wieder.

Abb. 2. Links: Beispiel einer PU-SUR-basierten Annotation. Anders als bei [2] muss gesundes Gewebe nicht annotiert werden. Rechts: Beispiel eines Ergebnis auf den BraTS Testdaten. Der Algorithmus ist auch für ein Mehrklassenproblem geeignet. Gelb: Ödem, Rot: Aktiver Tumor, Blau: Nekrose.

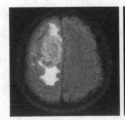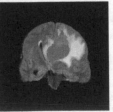

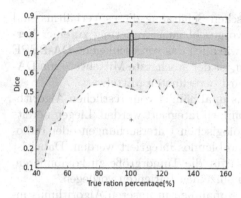

Abb. 3. Entwicklung des Dice Scores aufgetragen über die prozentuale Veränderung des tatsächlichen Tumorverhalten. Für die Versuche wurde auf DS-1 das aus den Goldstandards berechnete π prozentual verändert.

5   Diskussion

Wir haben gezeigt, dass spärliche Annotationen in einer einzelnen Gewebeklasse die Erstellung der Trainingsdaten deutlich vereinfacht. Gleichzeitig erzielt der von uns vorgestellte Ansatz Ergebnisse, die sich nicht signifikant von denen anderer State-of-the-Art Methoden abweichen.

Bereits in [2] wird gezeigt, dass SUR-Annotation eine deutlich schnellere Erstellung der Trainingsdaten für voxelbasierte Klassifikation ermöglichen. Da für unseren Ansatz nur die Annotation einer einzelnen Klasse vorgenommen werden muss, kann der Aufwand weiter reduziert werden. So haben wir in unseren Experimenten mehr als 40% der Annotationen einsparen können. Das reduziert nicht nur den notwendigen Zeitbedarf, sondern senkt gleichzeitig die Komplexität der Aufgabe. Statt zwei Aufgaben („Markiere Tumor" und „Markiere gesundes Gewebe") muss nur noch eine Aufgabe gelöst werden, was z.B. für Crowdsourcing das eine Halbierung der Tasks und somit der Kosten bedeutet.

Der vorgestellte Algorithmus ist robust gegenüber Fehleinschätzungen des Verhältnis von Tumor zu gesundem Gewebe. Erst größere Fehler in der Schätzung von π führen zu einer deutlichen Verringerung der Leistung (Abb. 3). Die

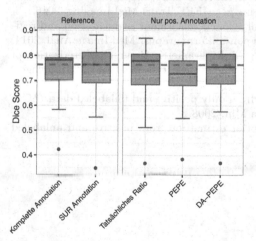

Abb. 4. Dice-Scores der Leave-one-out Experimente auf DS-1. Die Klassifikatoren für die komplette Annotation und SUR Annotation wurden gemäß [2] trainiert. Lediglich DA-PEPE – der von uns vorgeschlagene Algorithmus – ist signifikant besser als PEPE (p=.001, Wilcoxon signed-rank test), ansonsten gibt es keine signifikanten Unterschiede.

242   Goetz & Maier-Hein

vorgestellten Algorithmen zur automatischen Schätzung dieses Verhältnis sind ausreichend genaue, wobei die von uns vorgeschlagene Änderung zu einer Verbesserung führen. Obwohl sowohl PEPE wie auch das vorgeschlagene DA-PEPE die Tumorgröße tendenziell unterschätzen, ist der geschätzte Mittelwert von DA-PEPE näher an dem aus den Goldstandard berechneten Mittelwert.

Da die Schätzung des Tumorvolumens unabhängig vom restlichen Algorithmus ist, können bestehende Messungen einfach integriert werden. Liegen bereits Daten über das Tumorvolumen aus histologischen Untersuchungen oder radiologischen Messungen vor, können diese problemlos integriert werden. Dabei ist es auch möglich, unterschiedliche Quellen für die Tumorgröße zu kombinieren, je nachdem welche Information für einen einzelnen Patienten vorliegen.

Generell werden keine anatomischen Annahmen in unseren Algorithmus integriert. Anders als z.B. Atlas-basierte Verfahren ist das vorgestellte Verfahren unabhängig vom Zielorgan. Es kann ohne große Anpassungsprobleme auf andere Modalitäten oder Organe übertragen werden. Da die wesentliche Anpassung des Lernalgorithmus durch eine Gewichtung der Beobachtungen vorgenommen wird kann dieser Ansatz auch einfach in bestehende Algorithmen integriert werden.

Unsere Versuche haben gezeigt, dass die resultierenden Klassifikatoren eine ähnliche Erkennungsleistung bieten wie traditionell trainierte Klassifikatoren und auch für Mehrklassenprobleme geeignet ist (Abb. 4 und 3). Wird der vorgeschlagene Algorithmus verwendet, ist in unseren Experimenten kein signifikanter Unterschied zum Training von kompletten Annotationen oder dem Ansatz in [2] vorhanden. Gerade gegenüber [2] bedeutet das, dass unser Ansatz zwar den Annotationsaufwand reduziert, nicht aber die resultierende Genauigkeit.

Literaturverzeichnis

1. Menze BH, Jakab A, Bauer S, et al. The multimodal brain tumor image segmentation benchmark (BRATS). IEEE Trans Med Imaging. 2015.
2. Goetz M, Weber C, Binczyk F, et al. DALSA: domain adaptation for supervised learning from sparsely annotated MR images. IEEE Trans Med Imaging. 2016.
3. Parisot S, Wells W, Chemouny S, et al. Concurrent tumor segmentation and registration with uncertainty-based sparse non-uniform graphs. Med Image Anal. 2014.
4. Verma R, Zacharaki EI, Ou Y, et al. Multiparametric tissue characterization of brain neoplasms and their recurrence using pattern classification of MR images. Acad Radiol. 2008.
5. Elkan C, Noto K. Learning classifiers from only positive and unlabeled data. ACM SIGKDD Int Conf Knowl Discov Data Min. 2008.
6. du Plessis MC, Sugiyama M. Class prior estimation from positive and unlabeled data. IEICE Trans Inf Syst. 2014.

Lesion Ground Truth Estimation for a Physical Breast Phantom

Suneeza Hanif[1], Frank Schebesch[1], Anna Jerebko[2], Ludwig Ritschl[2],
Thomas Mertelmeier[2], Andreas Maier[1]

[1]Pattern Recognition Lab, FAU Erlangen-Nürnberg, Erlangen, Germany
[2]Siemens Healthineers, Erlangen, Germany
suneezahanif02@gmail.com

Abstract. The extraction of microstructures (like microcalcifications or masses) from a DBT phantom can be used for image quality assessment. A complete specification includes exact positions and dimensions of the microstructures, which is not always available. We propose a technique to estimate the required ground truth data from a set of multiple acquisitions. A 3D registration algorithm for DBT data is used to identify different breast phantom components and to perfectly align microstructures within the phantom. The registered data, showing variations of the same ground truth structures, is then combined to an estimate of the microstructures. This approach could be shown to improve the registration result itself, and to enable the determination of the actual parameters of the microstructures.

1   Introduction

Breast cancer is the most common cancer in women, and it is the second cause of cancer death in more developed regions [1]. Early diagnosis has higher chances of cure or can help to slow down the progress of the cancer.

Digital breast tomosynthesis (DBT) employs information from multiple images of a breast, scanned at different view angles, to allow readers to extract the 3D features in the breast tissue.

Due to the similarity of the elemental composition of normal and abnormal tissue, the optimization of image quality in DBT imaging is a critical factor, and optimal detection of masses and microcalcifications [2] is crucial. The extraction of such features from the images can be used for image quality assessment and can be carried out using physical phantoms and the knowledge about certain test objects in the phantom designed to meet specific requirements [3].

Although phantom images do not completely resemble clinical images, they have some advantages over clinical data as their complete structure is known by construction which usually delivers the ground truth in medical imaging. However, the generation of a proper testing breast phantom is still an ongoing research [4]. Several phantoms have been produced and while some of them mock up general tissue properties quite well, the specification is not necessarily accurate enough to determine the exact parameters of its contents.

To estimate the ground truth within the CIRS 20 breast phantom [5], we propose an image registration method to align its components and successively computate an approximation of the ground truth.

2 Methods

The computerized imaging reference system (CIRS) model 020 BR3D breast imaging phantom is distributed as a batch of six heterogeneous slabs. These include a single slab (we denote it as target slab) which contains an assortment of microcalcifications, fibers and masses of different sizes. The slabs can be rearranged to generate different DBT data ($6! \times 2^6 = 46080$ combinations) implying a variation of the local background structure as well as a repositioning of the target structures. Thereby, numerical errors in the reconstruction process affect result image structures differently. In our method, we want to take advantage of the partially rigid properties of the different compositions by aligning the target slab from different acquisitions, varying both the dose level and the reconstruction method.

2.1 Slab registration

In a first step, we try to align the corresponding inserts in the target slabs of different acquisitions and phantom compositions. In order to deal with the large image data sets (approximate volume size is $1300 \times 2400 \times 60$) and to improve convergence properties of the algorithm, a rigid registration algorithm with multistage scheme and multiresolution approach is used. As an initialization we use a reference image which is supposed to have an equal or better image quality than the images to be registered (for example from a high dose acquisition). The registration is first performed at the coarsest scale level. The transform parameters determined by the registration are then used to initialize the registration at the next finer level. This process is repeated till the finest level. In this way, large misalignments can be recovered early at a low scale and more detailed ones are accounted at increasingly fine resolutions.

With a 3-stage registration algorithm we were able to avoid significant misalignments. It is based on the idea of using simpler transforms and more aggressive optimization parameters at early stages. The 3D Euler transform (contains six degrees of freedom) is used for initial coarse registration levels and upgraded to an affine transform by incorporating more degrees of freedom at the finer levels.

Due to the indistinct texture of the simulated anatomical background, feature tracking, as it is often used for rigid motion problems [6], was replaced with the idea of using abstract texture information. In the first stages, normalized cross-correlation is used to avoid large misregistrations in the first iterations of the registration algorithm, while in later stages mutual information is used to remove small misalignments. The similarity measures are evaluated on image subsets containing the inserts regions. The intermediate and output images are evaluated by linear interpolation.

The registration problem can be formulated as a minimization problem

$$\hat{\boldsymbol{\mu}} = \underset{\boldsymbol{\mu}}{\text{argmin}} \; \mathcal{F}(\boldsymbol{\mu}, I_f, I_m) \tag{1}$$

where the staged cost function $\mathcal{F}$ represents the respective similarity measures that are minimized. I_f and I_m are the fixed and moving images respectively. $\boldsymbol{\mu}$ contains the external transform parameters and $\hat{\boldsymbol{\mu}}$ represents the best transform parameters that align the images.

To optimize the cost function in stage 1 and 2, regular step gradient descent optimizer is used [7]

$$\boldsymbol{\mu}_{k+1} = \boldsymbol{\mu}_k - a_k \kappa \nabla_{\boldsymbol{\mu}} \mathcal{F}, \quad \text{for } k = 1, 2... \tag{2}$$

where a_k is the step size, κ is a relaxation factor that can be varied between 0 and 1, and $\nabla_{\boldsymbol{\mu}}\mathcal{F}$ is the gradient of the cost function w.r.t $\boldsymbol{\mu}$. In the final registration stage, conjugate gradient descent line search optimizer is used for fine tuning. Here the update is a combination of the local gradient $\nabla_{\boldsymbol{\mu}}\mathcal{F}$ and the search direction $\boldsymbol{d}_{k-1}$ of the previous iteration

$$\boldsymbol{\mu}_{k+1} = \boldsymbol{\mu}_k + a_k \boldsymbol{d}_k, \quad \boldsymbol{d}_k = -\nabla_{\boldsymbol{\mu}}\mathcal{F} + \beta_k \boldsymbol{d}_{k-1}, \quad \text{for } k = 1, 2... \tag{3}$$

where β_k is determined by Polak-Ribiere conjugate gradient and a Golden section line search is used to find the best value for the step size a_k.

2.2   Ground truth estimation

The described registration allows an accurate positioning of the phantom details with respect to the reference or fixed image. We assume that in a set of registered images $\{I_i\}_{i=1,...,N}$, each image I_i contains a different part of the ground truth in a sense that it is overlayed by noise but always showing the same objects.

Image data obtained from different acquisition dose levels, slab combinations and reconstruction schemes contains different noise levels and variations in the spatial alignment of the microstructures. However, if depicting all these images as a (small) variation of the actual ground truth object, by minimizing the sum of squared distances the ground truth image can be estimated

$$\text{SSD}\left(\hat{I}\right) = \sum_{i=1}^{N} \left(I_i - \hat{I}\right)^2 \rightarrow \min \tag{4}$$

which is solved by

$$\hat{I} = \frac{1}{N} \sum_{i=1}^{N} I_i \tag{5}$$

The reliability of this estimate depends on the amount and variety reconstruction images and the degree of misalignment per image which is why the efforts for the registration were made.

The schematic in Fig. 1 illustrates the proposed idea of the CIRS 20 ground truth estimation using multiple reconstructed DBT data.

3   Experiments and results

The image dataset consisted of images from 10 random slab phantom compositions which were acquired at three dose levels: half of, equal to, and two times
reference radiation dose (determined by automatic exposure control). For reconstruction we used two DBT reconstruction schemes: filtered back projection
(FBP) and super resolution statistical artifact reduction (SRSAR) [8].

We tested if the proposed method allows improved ground truth estimation
from images of the same dose level and a single reconstruction scheme. The
images are registered to a reference from the set and the estimated image is
computed by (5), see Fig. 3 for the result images. For initial registration stage,
the optimizer parameters are set to $\kappa = 0.5$ and $a_k = 2.72$. Similarly the
minimum step size is set to large value, then, at each subsequent stages and
resolution levels, the minimum step size is reduced by a factor in order to allow
the optimizer to focus on progressively smaller regions.

The microstructure properties of both estimated and non-estimated reference
images were compared to the values specified in the datasheet of CIRS phantom
(Tab. 1).

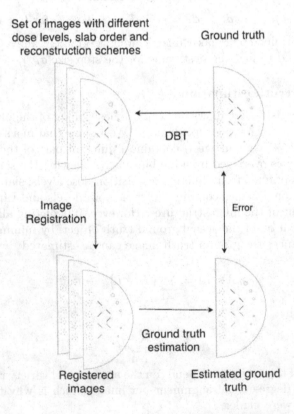

Fig. 1. Flow diagram for ground truth estimation from multiple reconstruction data.

Table 1. Ground truth estimation comparison with FBP reconstruction.

Microstructure	⊘ Datasheet	⊘ Single	⊘ Estimated
Microcalcification (1)	0.40 mm	0.30 ±0.11 mm	0.36 ±0.05 mm
Fiber (7)	0.60 mm	0.48 ±0.04 mm	0.58 ±0.02 mm
Mass (14)	6.30 mm	6.05 ±0.10 mm	6.26 ±0.07 mm
Mass (19)	1.80 mm	1.59 ±0.03 mm	1.63 ±0.02 mm

The average differences in diameter with respect to the specifications of the selected microstructures (microcalcification, fiber, largest mass and smallest mass) are 0.04 mm, 0.02 mm, 0.04 mm, and 0.17 mm in the estimated image, whereas for the single reference they are 0.1 mm, 0.12 mm, 0.25 mm and 0.21 mm, respectively. This means that the dimensions of the microstructures in the estimated image are closer to the actual values as compared to the single image.

In a second experiment the estimated image itself is then used as a reference image to study the improvements in overall image registration process as compared to the image taken from data set. Tab. 2 illustrates the average outcome in terms of mutual information for the target slab evaluated at the end of the registration process.

4   Conclusion

The implemented registration algorithm is tested on a large number of physically varied sample set and the results showed that the microstructures are perfectly registered with only differences occurring because of the different microstructures sizes, resulted from different dose levels and reconstruction schemes. Although the estimation from registered data is not able to acquire all possible noisy image

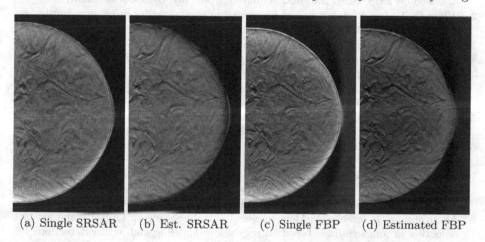

(a) Single SRSAR   (b) Est. SRSAR   (c) Single FBP   (d) Estimated FBP

Fig. 2. Single vs. estimated reference images for SRSAR and FBP reconstruction schemes.

Table 2. Mutual information after registration.

MI	FBP	Estimated FBP	SRSAR	Estimated SRSAR
Target slab	0.689 ± 0.221	0.844 ± 0.240	0.635 ± 0.342	0.801 ± 0.181

variations, the results indicate that we can still find a reasonable estimate in which the overall noise structure seems to cancel out sufficiently using a subset.

In terms of actual improvement, the computed diameters of the CIRS 20 phantom microstructures in the estimated image show values in a closer range to the specification values. This behaviour seems to be independent of the reconstruction scheme, however, the general idea allows a mixed set composed of images from different reconstruction schemes, as long as the alignment of details by the underlying registration aligns is working.

The estimation accuracy using the proposed approach is limited by the data nonetheless, so in consideration of an automated image quality assessment a sufficient variety of reconstruction data must be available. In future work it would also be interesting to see a validation of the proposed method using high resolution acquisition techniques like micro-CT.

Acknowledgement. The authors gratefully acknowledge funding by Siemens Healthineers. The concepts and information presented in this paper are based on research and are not commercially available.

References

1. Ferlay J, Soerjomataram I, Ervik M, et al.. GLOBOCAN 2012 v1.0, Cancer incidence and mortality worldwide: IARC cancerbase No. 11. Lyon, France; 2013. Accessed on 24/8/2016. Internet. Available from: http://globocan.iarc.fr.
2. White D, Tucker A. A test object for assessing image quality in mammography. Br J Radiol. 1980;53(628):331–5.
3. Suryanarayanan S, Karellas A, Vedantham S, et al. Comparison of tomosynthesis methods used with digital mammography. Acad Radiol. 2000;7(12):1085–97.
4. Cockmartin L, Bosmans H, Marshall NW. Comparative power law analysis of structured breast phantom and patient images in digital mammography and breast tomosynthesis. Med Phys. 2013;40(8):081920–1–17.
5. BR3D Breast Imaging Phantom - Model 020 - Data Sheet. Available from: http://www.cirsinc.com/file/Products/020/020%20DS%20102915.pdf.
6. Klüppel M, Wang J, Bernecker D, et al. On feature tracking in x-ray images. Proc BVM. 2014; p. 132–7.
7. Van der Bom I, Klein S, Staring M, et al.; International Society for Optics; Photonics. Evaluation of optimization methods for intensity-based 2D 3D registration in x-ray guided interventions. SPIE Med Imaging. 2011; p. 796223.
8. Abdurahman S, Jerebko A, Mertelmeier T, et al.; Springer. Out-of-plane artifact reduction in tomosynthesis based on regression modeling and outlier detection. Int Workshop Digit Mammography. 2012; p. 729–36.

Automatic Grading of Breast Cancer Whole-Slide Histopathology Images

Thomas Wollmann, Karl Rohr

University of Heidelberg, BIOQUANT, IPMB, and DKFZ Heidelberg,
Dept. Bioinformatics and Functional Genomics, Biomedical Computer Vision Group,
Im Neuenheimer Feld 267, 69120 Heidelberg, Germany
thomas.wollmann@bioquant.uni-heidelberg.de

Abstract. Grading of tissue based on microscopic images is a common and challenging task. We propose a new method for grading of whole-slide histology images of invasive breast carcinoma, which is based on mitotic cell detection. The method combines a threshold-based attention mechanism and a deep neural network for mitotic cell detection and grading. Our mitotic cell detector is learned from scratch using object centroids. We achieved competitive results in the recent MICCAI TU-PAC16 challenge.

1 Introduction

Tumor growth is an important indicator for determining the prognosis of breast cancer patients. A higher proliferation rate is generally related to a worse prognosis. Therefore, the quantification of the proliferation rate is an important biomarker to determine a suitable therapy. Currently, pathologists manually count mitotic cells in hematoxylin and eosin (H&E) stained histological slide preparations. Automation of this process is important and involves the detection of mitotic cells.

Several approaches for cell detection in tissue microscopy images exist (e.g., [1, 2, 3]). Especially for mitosis detection several challenges have been conducted to compare available methods using image sections [4, 5, 6], but complete whole-slide images (WSI) were not used.

In this work, we describe a new approach which combines a threshold-based attention mechanism with a deep neural network (DNN) for mitotic cell detection and grading of WSIs. Compared to previous approaches, our method conducts fast feature extraction, multi-scale factor disentangling, and voting in a DNN. Training of the mitotic cell detection method uses only ground truth centroids and corresponding original images. Detection of mitotic cells is performed on automatically determined regions of interest (ROIs) of WSIs. The detections are summarized over a selection of subregions within the ROI and classified into a proliferation score by a shallow decision tree. An additional dataset with annotated tumor grades is used to train the decision tree.

2   Methods

Our method uses a threshold-based attention mechanism to select a ROI with subregions of size $2\,\text{mm}^2$ from a whole-slide image (WSI). A machine learning method is used to predict the centroids of mitotic cells within each subregion. Using a shallow decision tree a tumour classification is obtained for the WSI.

2.1   ROI selection

For selecting an appropriate region of interest (ROI), we use a multi-scale pre-processing approach. Preprocessing is performed on the highest image scale to remove artefacts like ink or non-flat tissue on the slide. In the first step, for removing ink artefacts, thresholding is applied to a ratio image (intensities of the red channel divided by the intensities of the green channel) which yields a mask. Within this mask the intensities are set to the maximum intensity in each of the three color channels of a WSI. Since the maximum intensity corresponds to background, the masked pixels are not considered in the subsequent analysis (Fig. 1).

The second step of the preprocessing removes black structures. To this end, the intensities of the red and blue channel are added, and each pixel with an intensity below the 1% percentile of the intensity histogram is replaced by the maximum intensity of the original image. This step removes black structures like flipped tissue. Afterwards the image is thresholded based on the mean intensity of the red and blue channel. For determining the threshold, the 2% percentile of the histogram is used. The resulting image is smoothed with a Gaussian filter and downscaled so that $\sim$1.5 pixels represent $2\,\text{mm}^2$ (high power field) (Fig. 2). For this lower scale image, ten pixels with the highest intensities are selected and the corresponding $2\,\text{mm}^2$ subregions are extracted from the original high-resolution image. With this scheme the subregions have an overlap of up to 50%.

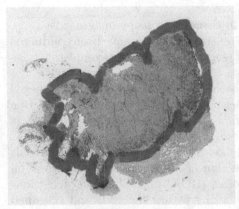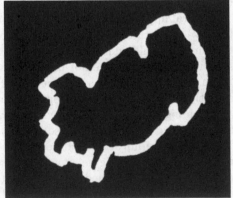

(a) Original WSI   (b) Detected artefacts (white)

Fig. 1. Example image demonstrating the artefact detection mechanism.

Finally, the subregions are rescaled to the pixel size the mitotic cell detector was trained on.

2.2 Mitotic cell detection and counting

Mitotic cell detection is conducted using a neural network. The network consists of a downsampling section, a factor disentangling section, and a pixelwise classification section with two branches. Fast feature extraction is achieved by strided convolutions. In our method, we use a formulation of the Hough transform in polar coordinates, which includes a voting procedure that exploits the predicted relative vote coordinates for each pixel. The optimization is formulated as a two task regression problem. The model is trained using the Adam optimizer [7].

2.3 Mitotic cell count thresholding

To determine the final score for the whole slide we calculated the 95% percentile of the cell counts of the analysed subregions. This feature is used within a shallow decision tree with two thresholds to obtain a score between 1 and 3. The lower threshold turned out to be 6 and the upper was 10. These thresholds match the guideline for grading tumors of [8], which gives a score of 1 for a cell count below 6 cells per high power field and a score of 3 for a cell count above 10 cells per high power field. The selection of the 95% percentile was determined by performing a grid search over different percentiles (70%-95%), mean, median, and maximum of the detected mitotic cell counts per image using the ground truth from the training dataset. Corresponding thresholds were determined by a grid search between 0 and 30.

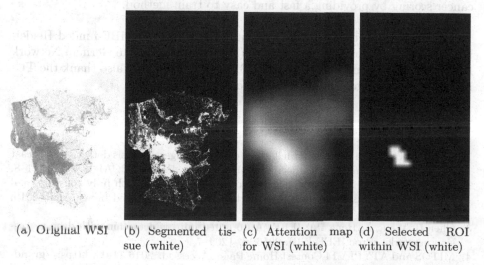

(a) Original WSI   (b) Segmented tissue (white)   (c) Attention map for WSI (white)   (d) Selected ROI within WSI (white)

Fig. 2. Example demonstrating the attention mechanism.

3   Results

Our method was applied to histology images of invasive breast carcinoma and achieved competitive results in the recent MICCAI TUPAC16 challenge [8]. The method was used to predict the proliferation score based on mitosis counting. Mitotic cell positions in images of 73 breast cancer cases were provided to train the mitotic cell detector. In addition, 500 WSIs with annotated proliferation scores were available. For testing, WSIs of 321 breast cancer cases were provided. To quantify the performance, the quadratic weighted Cohen's kappa value between the predicted and ground truth proliferation scores was used. Our method achieved a Cohen's kappa of 0.42 using cross-validation on the training dataset. Twelve different automatic methods that only used the provided training dataset were compared in the challenge, and our method was among the top-3 methods.

4   Discussion and conclusion

We presented an automatic method for breast cancer scoring based on whole-slide images (WSIs). Our method utilises a neural network for detecting mitotic cells. Detected mitotic cells are aggregated and used in a shallow decision tree to score the tumor. The algorithm can process WSIs in approximately five minutes on a standard workstation by using an attention mechanism and by classifying large image regions at once. The trade-off between statistical power and speed can be optimized by varying the number of regions in WSIs, where mitotic cells are counted. Our mitotic cell detection method is trained on centroids, which are relatively easy to acquire. The method achieved competitive results in the recent MICCAI TUPAC16 challenge. Our work contributes to the field of breast cancer scoring by providing a fast and easy to train method.

Acknowledgement. This work was supported by the BMBF-funded Heidelberg Center for Human Bioinformatics (HD-HuB) within the German Network for Bioinformatics Infrastructure (de.NBI) #031A537C. We also thank the TUPAC16 team for organising the challenge.

References

1. Cireşan DC, Giusti A, Gambardella LM, et al.; Springer. Mitosis detection in breast cancer histology images with deep neural networks. Proc MICCAI. 2013; p. 411–8.
2. Xie W, Noble JA, Zisserman A. Microscopy cell counting with fully convolutional regression networks. Proc MICCAI Workshop Deep Learn Med Image Anal. 2015; p. 1–10.
3. Chen H, Wang X, Heng PA; IEEE. Automated mitosis detection with deep regression networks. Proc IEEE ISBI. 2016; p. 1204–7.
4. MITOS and ATYPIA 14 Contest Home Page. Accessed: 2016-11-03. https://grand-challenge.org/site/mitos-atypia-14/.
5. Aptoula E, Courty N, Lefèvre S; IEEE. Mitosis detection in breast cancer histological images with mathematical morphology. Proc IEEE SIU. 2013; p. 1–4.

6. Veta M, Van Diest PJ, Willems SM, et al. Assessment of algorithms for mitosis detection in breast cancer histopathology images. Med Image Anal. 2015;20(1):237–48.

7. Kingma D, Ba J. Adam: A method for stochastic optimization. CoRR. 2014;abs/1412.6980.

8. TUPAC16 Contest Home Page. Accessed: 2016-11-03. http://tupac.tue-image.nl/.

Multi-Object Segmentation in Chest X-Ray Using Cascaded Regression Ferns

In Young Ha, Matthias Wilms, Mattias P. Heinrich

Institute of Medical Informatics, University of Lübeck
ha@imi.uni-luebeck.de

Abstract. Active shape and appearance models that are commonly employed for fast, regularized organ segmentation have several limitations. Here, we adapt the explicit shape regression framework popularized for deformable face alignment to the simultaneous segmentation of lungs, heart and clavicles in X-ray scans. ESR uses data-driven feature learning and combines multiple non-linear regressors in a cascaded manner. We performed extensive experiments and devised appropriate feature ranges, a suitable data augmentation scheme and representative shapes for multi-initialization. With these extensions we obtained new state-of-the-art results for X-ray segmentation outperforming all previous approaches applied to the same dataset and approaching human observer variability with sub-second computation times.

1 Introduction

Chest radiography is the most commonly used diagnostic X-ray examination, which helps detect abnormalities in the lungs, heart and chest wall. However, due to the overlay of anatomical structures in X-ray projections combined with the prevailing imaging noise, boundaries of structures are often ambiguous or occluded. These problems are difficult to deal with using automatic image segmentation tools. To aid clinical workflow in diagnosis and for automatic detection/tracking of contours during image-guided interventions, automatic multi-organ image segmentation algorithms are necessary.

Shape model based approaches such as active shape models (ASMs) and active appearance models (AAMs) are widely adopted [1], where the use of a shape prior enables robust segmentation (see overview in [2] for segmentation of chest X-ray images). These approaches can deal with shape occlusion and are robust against image noise. A disadvantage of statistical models is their limited ability to handle complex shape deformation in particular for small training datasets. This is due to their limitation to linear combinations of a number of eigenvectors of a statistical shape model and the use of a separate, disjoint model adaptation algorithm.

Recently, various shape alignment approaches based on non-linear regression algorithms have been pursued in the field of computer vision (e.g. [3, 4]). Cao et al. proposed an explicit shape regression (ESR), which unifies model formation and adaptation in a single framework [3]. The algorithm learns shape increments directly without relying on a parametric model. Multiple weak regressors called random ferns are combined to generate strong regressors, which yielded both robust and accurate results when applied to face landmark regression. The authors have shown improvements in accuracy compared to statistical shape models and exemplar-based face alignment techniques. The ESR was also successfully adopted in medical image processing for segmentation of a single structure, such as the prostate [5].

In this work, ESR is adapted for simultaneous segmentation of multiple anatomical structures in chest X-ray images. Segmentation of multiple structures is a complicated task for classical active shape models, since it requires a separate model adaptation for each structure. However, ESR has no such limitations and a wider range of variations can be implicitly explored, which makes it appropriate for multi-structure segmentation.

2   Materials and methods

In this section, the essential concepts of the ESR framework will be explained, followed by a description of our proposed adaptation for chest X-ray data as well as experimental design and its evaluation.

2.1   Explicit shape regression (ESR)

As illustrated in Fig. 1, ESR trains multiple regressors for the estimation of a final shape. Given a number of input features extracted from each image, the regressors learn a non-linear mapping between the feature and shape output spaces. Each feature is a gray-value difference between two pixels with certain offsets (pixel comparison features), with respect to the input shapes. These *shape indexed features* enable us to effectively describe the image context and they are robust against deformations and contrast changes. Pixel comparison features have also been successfully employed in medical 3D segmentation [6]. The outputs of the regressors are displacement vectors for all landmarks of a shape, which are used to iteratively deform the initial shapes to fit the structure in the image.

Two-level boosted regression. The regressors of ESR are combined in a cascaded manner as in [7], however, in ESR the cascaded regression method is extended into a two-level boosted regression for alignment of shapes. Given an image I_i and a 2D shape $S_i = [x_1, y_1, \ldots, x_N, y_N]^T$ consisting of N landmarks, the goal of shape alignment is to approximate the ground truth shape $\hat{S}_i$ by minimizing the shape alignment error $\|S_i - \hat{S}_i\|_2$. This requires a simultaneous regression of all landmarks within one shape, which makes it difficult to be handled by a weak regressor (e.g. a single fern as used in [7]) in each stage.

To deal with this problem, a boosting algorithm is used to generate a strong regressor, which can provide a reliable shape estimation. M weak regressors r_m^t

$(m = 1...M)$ referred to as *primitive regressors* are combined to form a *stage regressor* R^t in each stage t $(t = 1...T)$. An input (or previous) shape S_i^{t-1} of stage $t-1$ is updated to S_i^t during the stage using the output of R^t as follows

$$S_i^t = S_i^{t-1} + M_{S_i^{t-1}}^{-1} \circ R^t(I_i, S_i^{t-1}) \tag{1}$$

where $M_{S_i^{t-1}}^{-1}$ denotes the transformation of the ith shape from the reference frame into its original image frame.

In ESR, random ferns [8] are used as primitive regressors. They are similar to random forests with binary decision trees, where a series of binary tests are performed on each input data. However, they have a non-hierarchical structure, i.e. all binary tests can be performed in parallel. For each fern, S features are selected together with a random threshold to define the binary tests and therefore 2^S bins (leaf nodes). Feature selection is performed using a correlation-based feature selection method, which chooses the features that have a high correlation with the regression target and low correlation to each other [3].

The output of each fern is computed based on the regression targets y_i of training shapes, which are the difference vectors of the ground truth and input shapes. During training, samples are mapped into a certain bin of a fern based on their feature response, where the regression targets are accumulated. The accumulated regression targets are averaged at the end, and a shrinkage parameter controlling the magnitude of estimation from each fern is multiplied, which prevents over-fitting in training. The regression output of R^t is a set of displacement vectors, which are simply summed over all ferns when applying stage t during testing.

Data augmentation and multiple initialization. Each training sample consists of an image I_i, a training shape $\hat{S}_i$ and an arbitrary initial shape S_j. By selecting different initial shapes for the same image and training shape, a new training sample can be augmented. Data augmentation for training samples increases accuracy and robustness of shape alignment results without the need for image warping.

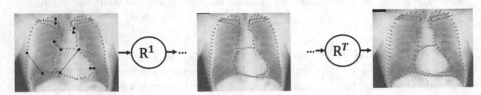

Fig. 1. Explicit shape regression trains multiple stage regressors, which learn the mapping between input features and displacement vectors for all landmarks of a shape. Left image: pixel comparison features are marked as two squares connected by a solid line. Center image: updated shape with output displacement vectors obtained using the first trained regressor. Right image: final shape estimation with accumulated displacement vectors of all stages.

During testing, regression is performed using multiple initial shapes. The final shape estimation is made by computing median values of each landmark coordinate. After exploiting different types of multiple initial shapes, we have obtained the best result using representative shapes generated by k-means clustering on the training shapes.

2.2 Experiment

Dataset. A publicly available chest X-ray image database [9] is used for segmentation of anatomical structures by ESR. The database consists of 247 images (1024x1024 pixels), which are divided into two folds; odd numbered images for training and even numbered images for testing. Manual segmentations are provided by [2], which include 166 corresponding landmarks for five structures in each image: left and right lungs, heart and left and right clavicles.

Experimental setup. Mean point-to-surface errors are computed for each shape. For a result comparison with other methods in [2], results of left and right lungs and left and right clavicles are combined. The images are smoothed using a Gauss filter with $\sigma = 2$ in both training and testing, which proved to be an important modification to the original ESR method.

For the experiments, the fern depth $S = 5$, number of ferns in a stage $M = 500$, number of stages $T = 10$, number of candidate pixels $P = 400$ and the shrinkage parameter $\beta = 1000$ are used. Different numbers of initial shapes for data augmentation as well as different range of local coordinates are tested to find optimal values for the given task. In test, 5 representative shapes of the training population computed using k-means clustering are used for shape initialization.

After the segmentation using the optimal parameters, the results are compared with the results using the following methods provided in [2], including the inter-observer differences (human observer). For comparison with shape model based approaches, the results using ASM with parameters tuned for the dataset (ASM tuned) as well as AAM with whiskers (AAM whiskers) are considered. In addition, results using pixel classification are compared, where segmentation is performed by classifying pixels using k-Nearest Neighbor classifiers and the results are post-processed to obtain a single connected structure (PC post-processed).

3 Results

Mean point-to-surface errors of segmentation results of lungs, heart and clavicles using various segmentation methods are given in Table 1. For each test image, the segmentation of all five structures using one initial shape took ≈ 30.6 ms using a 2.67 GHz CPU. The result shows that ESR outperforms the other compared approaches (in particular for the heart) and is close to the accuracy of the human observer. The maximum segmentation errors of the heart and clavicles using our

Table 1. Segmentation errors of lungs, heart and clavicles given in millimeter (mm). Mean point-to-surface distance is used for error computation.

	Lungs		Heart		Clavicles		Total
	$\mu \pm \sigma$	Max	$\mu \pm \sigma$	Max	$\mu \pm \sigma$	Max	μ
Human observer	1.64 ± 0.69	9.11	3.78 ± 1.82	16.26	0.68 ± 0.26	2.02	1.71
ESR	1.73 ± 1.12	8.49	$\mathbf{3.79 \pm 1.75}$	9.21	$\mathbf{1.68 \pm 0.78}$	4.41	$\mathbf{2.04}$
ASM tuned	2.30 ± 1.03	7.67	5.96 ± 2.73	16.55	2.04 ± 1.36	9.13	2.80
AAM whiskers	2.70 ± 1.10	8.74	6.01 ± 2.88	19.38	3.38 ± 3.71	41.27	3.38
PC post-processed	$\mathbf{1.61 \pm 0.80}$	8.34	5.20 ± 2.59	18.72	2.90 ± 1.54	12.55	2.52

approach are the lowest of all compared methods. Segmentation of clavicles is difficult for automatic segmentation methods, due to their low bone density and large variations in their orientation and position.

In training, increasing the number of training data augmentations and selecting features using pixel comparisons near the shape boundaries have substantially improved the accuracy of our segmentation. The results are obtained using the range of local coordinates $\kappa = 0.05$, which was selected via cross validation and for each training image and shape, the rest of the training shapes (123 shapes) are used as initial shapes for data augmentation. In testing, the accuracy of segmentation can be further improved by performing regression using a set of representative shapes and combining the results for final segmentation.

In Fig. 2, the two best and two worst results are shown. The best results have a total error of ≈ 1 mm and are almost identical to the ground truth. As shown in the worst results, non-visible edges under the left lungs caused by air in the colon (left) and due to shadows of nearby structures (right) can lead to larger errors in segmentation.

4 Discussion

In this work, the segmentation of multiple anatomical structures in medical X-ray images has been addressed using a cascaded shape regression approach. Unlike classical model based approaches, where permissive shape variations are

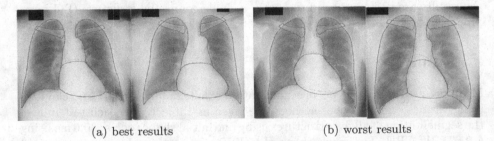

(a) best results   (b) worst results

Fig. 2. The two best results and two worst result of segmentation is shown. The ground truth shapes are shown in cyan for comparison.

limited by a parametric statistical shape model, our approach can approximate complex shape variations using multiple stages of non-linear regression. Four key extensions have been made to adapt the original explicit shape regression (ESR) framework from face alignment [3] to medical X-ray segmentation: (1) a Gaussian smoothing was employed to enhance the applicability of simple pixel comparison features; (2) an appropriate feature offset range close to anatomical boundaries was found to improve accuracy; (3) extensive data augmentation to encounter the small number of training images; and (4) a k-means clustering approach for multi-shape initialization was included. The result demonstrates that this extended ESR framework outperforms all previous approaches applied to the same X-ray dataset of [2] and produces segmentation results close to inter-observer accuracy in 150 milliseconds (with five initial shapes). Future work includes integration of ESR for tracking of organ boundaries in image-guided radiation therapy [10].

Acknowledgement. This work is funded by the German Research Foundation DFG (HE 7364/1)

References

1. Cootes TF, Roberts MG, Babalola KO, et al. 1. In: Paragios N, Duncan J, Ayache N, editors. Active Shape and Appearance Models. Boston, MA: Springer US; 2015. p. 105–22.
2. van Ginneken B, Stegmann MB, Loog M. Segmentation of anatomical structures in chest radiographs using supervised methods: a comparative study on a public database. Med Image Anal. 2006;10(1):19–40.
3. Cao X, Wei Y, Wen F, et al. Face alignment by explicit shape regression. Int J Comput Vis. 2013;107(2):177–90.
4. Lindner C, Thiagarajah S, Wilkinson JM, et al. Fully automatic segmentation of the proximal femur using random forest regression voting. IEEE Trans Med Imaging. 2013;32(8):1462–72.
5. Cheng J, Xiong W, Gu Y, et al. Cascaded shape regression for automatic prostate segmentation from extracorporeal ultrasound images. Proc MICCAI. 2013; p. 65–74.
6. Heinrich MP, Blendowski M; Springer. Multi-organ segmentation using vantage point forests and binary context features. Proc MICCAI. 2016; p. 598–606.
7. Dollar P, Welinder P, Perona P. Cascaded pose regression. Proc IEEE Comput Soc Conf Comput Vis Pattern Recognit. 2010; p. 1078–85.
8. Özuysal M, Calonder M, Lepetit V, et al. Fast keypoint recognition using random ferns. IEEE Trans Pattern Anal Mach Intell. 2010;32(3):448–61.
9. Shiraishi J, Katsuragawa S, Ikezoe J, et al. Development of a digital image database for chest radiographs with and without a lung nodule: receiver operating characteristic analysis of radiologists' detection of pulmonary nodules. Am J Roentgenol. 2000;174(1):71–4.
10. Wilms M, Ha IY, Handels H, et al.; Springer. Model-based regularisation for respiratory motion estimation with sparse features in image-guided interventions. Proc MICCAI. 2016; p. 89–97.

Abstract: Articulated Head and Neck Patient Model for Adaptive Radiotherapy

Hendrik Teske[1,2], Kathrin Bartelheimer[1,2], Jan Meis[1,2], Eva M. Stoiber[1,2], Rolf Bendl[1,3], Kristina Giske[1,2]

[1]Division of Medical Physics in Radiation Oncology, DKFZ Heidelberg
[2]National Center for Radiation Research in Oncology (NCRO),
Heidelberg Institute for Radiation Oncology (HIRO), Heidelberg
[3]Faculty of Computer Science, Heilbronn University
h.teske@dkfz.de

State of the art radiotherapy enables for precise shaping of dose distributions to maintain tumor control while sparing organs at risk. Online adaptive radiotherapy improves that by taking into account inter-fractional changes of the anatomy throughout the treatment course. Especially variations in the posture of head and neck cancer patients cause large deformations in the anatomy, potentially leading to considerable deviations from the planned dose distributions. Adapting the treatment plan to compensate for such changes requires an accurate assessment of anatomical deformations. Commonly used models do not distinguish between bony tissue and soft tissue and thus result in unrealistic deformations of the bones. We propose an articulated patient model for the head and neck region, which inherently preserves the rigidity of the bones while allowing for modelling arbitrary postures of the patient. An articulated skeleton model is assembled from the segmentations of the bones in the planning CT. For an exemplary head and neck cancer patient, 40 individual bones were connected by 45 joints. All the joints were modelled as ball and socket joints, granting rotational mobility around the three body axes. Propagation of motion within the skeletal model is achieved by using an inverse kinematics approach [1]. On a consumer PC, different postures are generated interactively at a rate of ∼25 per second. To investigate the advantages and limitations, this model was used to sample images of arbitrary postures of the patient. In addition to the skeletal model, a chainmail-based model was coupled to account for soft tissue deformation. Generation of realistic complex postures was achieved by using only up to 8 user-defined supporting vectors. The segmentations of the bones were generated manually. The resulting sampled images suggest that our model is able to accurately assess different inter-fractional postures of the patient. In combination with its time-efficient computation, it can further be used in the image registration context.

References

1. Sherman MA, Seth A, Delp SL. Simbody: multibody dynamics for biomedical research. Procedia IUTAM. 2011;2:241–61.

Shallow Fully-Connected Neural Networks for Ischemic Stroke-Lesion Segmentation in MRI

Christian Lucas[12], Oskar Maier[12], Mattias P. Heinrich[1]

[1]Institute of Medical Informatics, University of Luebeck
[2]Graduate School for Computing in Medicine and Life Sciences, University of Luebeck
lucas@imi.uni-luebeck.de

Abstract. Automatic image segmentation of stroke lesions could be of great importance for aiding the treatment decision. Convolutional neural networks obtain high accuracy for this task at the cost of prohibitive computational demand for time-sensitive clinical scenarios. In this work, we study the use of classical fully-connected neural networks (FC-NN) based on hand-crafted features, which achieve much shorter runtimes. We show that recent advances in optimization and regularization of deep learning can be successfully transferred to FC-NNs to improve the training process and achieve comparable accuracy to random decision forests.

1 Introduction

Human brain tissue requires a steady flow of oxygenated blood. Blockage in the event of an ischemic stroke can lead to the gradual death of brain tissue. Less affected tissue surrounding the stroke core (penumbra) may recover through therapy. The optimal choice of treatment options (e.g. mechanical recanalization) is of critical importance for patient outcomes and can be guided by imaging techniques such as perfusion CT and e.g. a learned multivariate prediction model (Kemmling et al. [1]). Multispectral MR imaging further enables the long-term investigation of stroke evolution and monitoring.

Automated segmentation on image data helps assessing prevalence and extents of a stroke. Several supervised machine learning algorithms have been proposed for a voxel- or region-wise classification of brain lesions, including random decision forests (RDF) and neural networks (NN). However, none of the existing methods reach expert performance as evident from the results of the Ischemic Stroke Lesion Segmentation (ISLES) workshop 2015 [2].

Since their recent breakthrough, deep convolutional neural networks (DCNN) have increased the accuracy of supervised classification and recognition in many fields of image analysis. They achieve this by jointly learning appropriate features and decision boundaries, making them an excellent choice for further investigation in the context of brain lesion segmentation. Kamnitsas et al. [3] obtained the highest segmentation accuracy for the Sub-acute Ischemic Stroke Lesion Segmentation task (SISS) of ISLES 2015 using a deep multi-scale 3D convolutional network. The complexity of a large number of multi-channel 3D convolutional kernels leads to excessive computational demand during both training (one day) and testing, making this approach less applicable for real-time assessment in clinical practice (where high-performance GPU hardware is non-standard). Note that the other CNN submission of Dutil et al. [2] takes about 6 hours for training with only average performance in the final SISS challenge tests.

Conventional machine learning algorithms such as RDF are based on hand-crafted image features and highly efficient in non-linear classification. This enables their use in time-sensitive scenarios, however, at the cost of lower accuracy. In this work we study whether classical shallow fully-connected (FC) neural networks can be employed to reduce the gap in segmentation accuracy between DCNN and RDF while using conventional hand-crafted image features. We believe there is much scope in further improvements for FC networks when integrating recent advances from the field of DCNN such as batch normalization (BN) suggested by Ioffe and Szegedy [4]. We aim to directly compare the FC classifier part (decision learning) of a deep network with the RDF classifier on the exact same input. We further want to demonstrate that a shallow network can be employed under practical time constraints.

1.1 Related work

An efficient method for stroke lesion segmentation, the RDF of Maier et al. [5], achieves a classification time of only 70 seconds for testing one case of the SISS 2015 dataset. Their approach extracts 151 features of various scales (4×intensity, 12×smoothed intensity, 132×local histogram, 3×distance to center) from the given MR modalities FLAIR, DWI, T1, and T2. The training of 200 trees with unlimited depth has proven to be a good heuristic for reaching a constant level of generalization. We reimplemented the algorithm and could replicate the average DICE coefficent of 0.58 for the training set.

The most recent applications of a non-convolutional network for voxel-wise stroke outcome prediction include a study on rats by Huang et al. [6]. They used one hidden layer with seven neurons and 50 epochs of a resilient backpropagation (BP) on cerebral blood flow and apparent diffusion coefficient data with T2-weighted images serving as ground truth. The size of infarction is not given by an expert's delineation but a clustering technique on T2 data. Their findings support the use of diffusion and perfusion data and the incorporation of spatial information, leading to an area under ROC of 0.89 for temporary and 0.95 for permanent occlusions. Unfortunately, they do not provide a comparison with other classification approaches.

Bagher-Ebadian et al. [7] performed a human study with 12 subjects on four modalities (DWI, T1, T2, PDWI). They optimized the number of neurons (one to six neurons in the second of two hidden layers) and epochs (up to 50) for reaching their final results. More than half of the samples are drawn from lesion voxels. The method was able to predict a 3-month stroke outcome with an area under ROC of 0.89. The dataset used in [7] was designed to exclude cerebral hemorrhage, prior strokes or other neurological disorders, which can have a strong influence on the algorithm's performance. Furthermore, the labeling based on T2 images still requires experts segmentation applied to the prediction map in order to interpret the result in terms of lesion prevalence.

Due to the curse of dimensionality, learning a conventional NN that generalizes well while increasing its degrees of freedom is difficult as it tends to over-fit complex functions and particular training cases. As a consequence, simpler architecture are in general favored in current work as well as for the two FC layers at the end of many DCNNs. We thus focus on shallow FC networks, since the parametrization of deeper FC architectures has seen limited success in the past.

2   Materials and methods

Our network has been trained on the 28 multi-spectral patient scans (FLAIR, DWI, T1, and T2) of the SISS challenge 2015 from the ISLES workshop [2], which can be downloaded at virtualskeleton.ch. They have been co-registered, skull-stripped and resampled to an isotropic scaling of 1 mm. All cases contain sub-acute ischemic strokes of different types and sizes (about 2.5% stroke prevalence in brain voxels on average) as well as other neural disorders, like non-stroke white matter lesions or haemorrhages, and imaging artifacts (e.g. parabolic lines). The manual segmentation of a single expert rater was provided for the training data.

Preprocessing of the data included MR bias correction as well as intensity standardization. We extracted the exact same 151 features as Maier et al. for the SISS. Since nearly normally distributed single-peak distributions can be observed in all the intensity-based image features, we apply a PCA first (based on the covariance/statistics of the training data) to whiten the input data for the NN. Besides orthogonalization of the principle components, the data has to be centered before the PCA.

2.1   Neural network learning

A k-hidden layer neural network is trained for the features of the input data that minimizes the cross-entropy loss with respect to a ground truth binary masks through BP and stochastic gradient descent using MatConvNet. The weight decay is set to 0.001 and the momentum of 0.9 is also fixed. During test, the two class output (background/target) is transformed to probability-like values by a softmax layer and the resulting maps are thresholded at $p = 0.5$ to obtain binary segmentations.

We use a sequence of varying learning rates over a fixed number of 60 epochs. In the beginning, it increases from 0.1 to 0.2 to learn as fast as possible while the error on the validation set is still converging. In order to keep amplitudes at such high learning rate fairly small, batch normalization is used and with each epoch the learning rate is further decreased to eventually one fourth of the maximum, which helps the learning to converge to a plateau of lower error. Batch normalization is applied after each hidden layer in our model, which has been shown to prevent over-fitting and leads to faster convergence than dropout (Fig. 2). Furthermore, rectifying linear units are applied due to fast convergence.

Fig. 1. Full pipeline including our final FC-NN with three hidden layers and softmax (SM). After batch normalization (BN) a rectifying linear unit (ReLu) is applied.

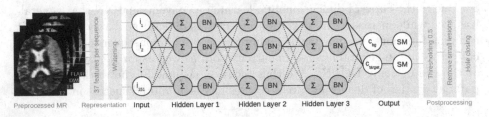

Topological and spatial regularization is hard to include for purely voxel-based classification (as opposed to the use of large receptive fields in DCNNs). Therefore, a post-processing is applied to remove very small lesions, which are supposedly non-stroke false positives. Furthermore, morphological hole closing is applied to correct missed areas of ambiguous gray values in the less visible penumbra and gives smoother closed shapes as it is prefered by human raters.

2.2 Experiments

One million samples in total have been drawn stratified across lesion and background classes (keeping the prevalence ratio), as done before by Maier et al. in [5]. We evaluated the use of k-hidden layers with $k = 1, 2, 3, 4$, each time with and without feature reduction (decreasing number of neurons per layer) to limit the degrees of freedom. A cross-validation on the training data was computed for both the NN and the implementation of Maier's RDF. The batch size was set to 4096, since using a 1D feature space (as opposed to 3D in DCNN) enables us to process more samples at once. Matrix computations of the network in MatLab as well as training and testing of the comparitive RDF in Python (scikit-learn) were processed in parallel on a standard Intel i7 CPU. For time comparison, the training in Matlab was also run on a NVidia GeForce 960 GTX using the same batch size.

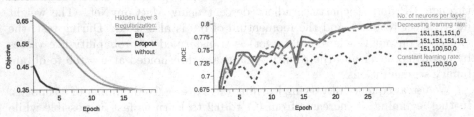

Fig. 2. Left: Objective function reaching a value of 0.35 for different regularization of the third hidden layer. (Here, BN reduces number of epochs by a factor of 3 and improves generalization compared to dropout) Right: DICE on the validation set during a training run with 3 or 4 hidden layers and constant or decreasing number of neurons.

Table 1. Mean average / standard deviation of all 36 challenge test cases for each evaluation measure. (Results from virtualskeleton.ch for selected methods)

Method	ASSD	Hausdorff D.	Precision	Recall	DICE
CNN Kamn.	07.87 / 12.63	39.61 / 30.68	0.68 / 0.33	0.60 / 0.27	0.59 / 0.31
RDF Maier	17.36 / 20.29	53.90 / 30.15	0.46 / 0.37	0.57 / 0.34	0.42 / 0.33
FC-NN (ours)	15.10 / 14.63	71.68 / 25.52	0.45 / 0.36	0.57 / 0.29	0.39 / 0.30
CNN Dutil	18.74 / 20.64	55.99 / 35.09	0.39 / 0.38	0.53 / 0.33	0.35 / 0.31

3 Results

The lowest computation times were reached with a three hidden layer network (Fig. 1) trained for 60 epochs. Due to the regularizing effect of batch normalization the use of (as many as) 151 neurons in each layer was possible and yielded the best accuracy compared to more narrow architectures, which only slightly reduced training and testing times. A similar finding was made with respect to the number of layers, where a deeper network of four layers did not further increase the DICE scores (Fig. 2). Adding more epochs increased validation measures during training on samples, but not on the overall cross-validation.

Batch normalization speeds up learning significantly (See excmplary effect for last hidden layer in Fig. 2). It allows us to use higher learning rates than with dropout or no regularization layers and the training converges more quickly. Decreasing the initial high learning rate gradually, enables the algorithm to explore the local minimum even quicker. The testing time for a feed-forward run in our shallow network is fast (30 seconds on CPU). Training our model for 8.3 minutes using MatConvNet on a GPU, we were able to compete with training time of 8.7 minutes for RDF in scikit-learn on CPU, reaching DICE values close to those of the RDF (Fig. 3, Tab. 1), while reducing test times half compared to 70 seconds for RDF and over an order of magnitude compared to DCNNs. The Hausdorff Distance indicates some strong outliers that also limited the performance of our FC-NN with respect to the other measures. Compared to all results uploaded to virtualskeleton.ch, our approach ranks in middle.

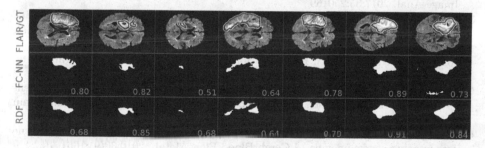

Fig. 3. The first 7 cases of the SISS training: FLAIR with ground truth, segmentation of our NN and of the RDF. The numbers show the DICE achieved with both classifiers.

4   Discussion

We have demonstrated that with recently developed techniques stemming from the deep learning field even shallow neural networks are able to compete with the efficient supervised learning of RDF when allowing the same time for training for each method. Using batch normalization is strongly recommended as it eases the tuning for an appropriate learning rate. Gradually decreasing the learning rate is a good heuristic to increase the possibility of finding a better optimum when the initial learning rate has reached the stage of an oscillating plateau.

So far we have only considered simple post-processing steps, but spatial regularization, such as Conditional Random Fields (CRF) as used by Kamnitsas et al. [3], is expected to yield further improvements to the complex task of stroke segmentation.

Without receptive fields like in DCNN, our neural network is strongly relying on the manually designed features. For comparability, we used the same set that had been optimized for the training of the RDF implementation in [5]. However, with the given feature set it seems not possible to yield better results even by increasing computational efforts (epochs, degrees of freedom). Hence, a careful selection of the given and new features may improve the process of learning the correct relation between target/background and sampled imaging values.

Furthermore, the huge class imbalance causes the log entropy loss function to assign too low penalty when a small lesion is completely missed. Incorporating a precision- and recall-related objective is expected to better guide the optimization process towards the actual target of stroke lesion segmentation.

References

1. Kemmling A, Flottmann F, Forkert ND, et al. Multivariate dynamic prediction of ischemic infarction and tissue salvage as a function of time and degree of recanalization. J Cereb Blood Flow Metab. 2015;35(9):1397–405.
2. Maier O, Menze BH, von der Gablentz J, et al. ISLES 2017: a public evaluation benchmark for ischemic stroke lesion segmentation from multispectral MRI. Med Image Anal. 2017;35:250–69.
3. Kamnitsas K, Ledig C, Newcombe VF, et al. Efficient multi-scale 3D CNN with fully connected CRF for Accurate Brain Lesion Segmentation. Med Image Anal. 2017;36:61–78.
4. Ioffe S, Szegedy C. Batch normalization: accelerating deep network training by reducing internal covariate shift. Proc Int Conf Mach Learn. 2015;37:448–56.
5. Maier O, Wilms M, Handels H; Springer. Image features for brain lesion segmentation using random forests. Brainlesion Glioma Mult Scler Stroke Trauma Brain Injuries. 2016;9556:119–30.
6. Huang S, Shen Q, Duong TQ. Artificial neural network prediction of ischemic tissue fate in acute stroke imaging. J Cereb Blood Flow Metab. 2010;30(9):1661–70.
7. Bagher-Ebadian H, Jafari-Khouzani K, Mitsias PD, et al. Predicting final extent of ischemic infarction using artificial Neural network analysis of multi-parametric MRI in patients with stroke. PLoS ONE. 2011;6(8).

Abstract: 4D Template Library Generation for Real-Time Tracking on 2D Cine MRI

Luis Paredes[1], Paul Mercea[2,3], Hendrik Teske[2,3], Rolf Bendl[2,3,4],
Kristina Giske[2,3], Ignacio Espinoza[1]

[1]Instituto de Física, Pontificia Universidad Catolica de Chile, Santiago, Chile
[2]Division of Medical Physics in Radiation Oncology, DKFZ Heidelberg
[3]National Center for Radiation Research in Oncology (NCRO), Heidelberg Institute for Radiation Oncology (HIRO)
[4]Faculty of Computer Science, Heilbronn University
lfparedes@uc.cl

In radiotherapy, fast image-based tracking of tumor motion during radiation is conventionally achieved with template matching approaches on x-ray based projection scans with limited soft-tissue contrast. Emerging MR guided radiotherapy (MRgRT) devices allow for ionization-free imaging during treatment with superior soft tissue contrast. Currently, real-time imaging with MR is only possible for single slice acquisition (2D cine MRI). In this type of acquisition, breathing-induced tumor motion may change the appearance of the target in the scanned plane. This out-of-plane target motion may affect the accuracy of tracking algorithms based on template matching. In this work, an advanced 4D multiple template library approach was developed in order to enable 3D target localization on 2D cine MRI. The image data used in this work consists of: i) training data of 84.7 seconds of parallel sequential cine MRI (4.5Hz, 11 slices, 256x256px size, 1.56 mm pixel spacing, 4.5 mm slice thickness, 35 repetitions) capturing the target throughout its motion and ii) tracking data of 200 single slices of cine MRI simulating the real-time data provided by an MRgRT device. A retrospective self-navigated phase-based 4D sorting algorithm was developed for 4DMRI reconstruction of the training data from which the phase dependent multiple templates were extracted. These templates were incorporated in a real time multiple-template matching based tracking algorithm which was executed on the tracking data. For evaluation purposes, an automatic target contouring algorithm was developed and manually generated reference data was used. The 4D self-navigated reconstruction algorithm was able to generate 4DMRIs (256x256x31px, isotropic voxel size) from the training data for up to 10 phases of the respiratory cycle. The tracking results reproduced quasi-elliptic 3D target trajectories comparable (mean error 0.76 ± 0.76 mm and max error 3.8 mm in through-plane direction) to the ones captured with a device-side 4DMRI sequence (acquisition time > 450 seconds). In comparison to the reference data, the mean tracking error in coronal orientation was 0.62 ± 0.91 mm in superior-inferior and 0.45 ± 0.80 mm in left-right direction. Out-of-plane motion effects in cine MRI can lead to reduced precision of dose administration in beam tracking. With our approach, accurate estimation of the 4D trajectory of the target volume is realized and out-of-plane motion can be assessed.

Spline-Based Multimodal Image Registration of 3D PLI Data of the Human Brain

Sharib Ali[1], Karl Rohr[1], David Gräßel[2], Philipp Schlömer[2], Katrin Amunts[2],
Roland Eils[1], Markus Axer[2], Stefan Wörz[1]

[1]Dept. of Bioinformatics and Functional Genomics,
Biomedical Computer Vision Group, BIOQUANT, IPMB,
University of Heidelberg and DKFZ, Germany
[2]Institute of Neuroscience and Medicine, Research Centre Jülich, Jülich, Germany
s.ali@dkfz-heidelberg.de

Abstract. Registration of high-resolution 3D polarized light images (PLI) to reference blockface images is necessary for the analysis of brain fiber structures. We present an automatic approach for the registration of high-resolution 3D PLI data of histological sections of a human brain that integrates automatic segmentation, rigid registration, and spline-based elastic registration. We have applied the approach to images of the temporal lobe of the human brain and assessed its accuracy and robustness.

1   Introduction

3D polarized light imaging (3D PLI) has the ability to reveal structural connectivity properties of the brain at microscopic level. This technique is applied to unstained histological brain sections [1] of optimal thickness between 100 m and 70 m. 3D PLI provides good fiber and non-fiber contrast for entire human brain sections besides local 3D fiber orientation vectors that are essential for understanding the 3D fiber architecture. However, due to the tissue sectioning and mounting process, the 3D spatial coherence between 2D sections is lost. In addition, significant local tissue deformations are caused by the sectioning process. Thus, registration of 3D PLI images is required.

In this work, we use histological sections of the human brain with 70 m thickness. Blockface (BF) images (Fig. 1, top-left) are acquired by imaging sections with a CCD camera before cutting. This yields a stack of reference BF images. Afterwards, the sections are mounted and imaged using a large area polarimeter (LAP). The acquired 3D PLI data includes (Fig. 1): Light reflectance image, transmittance image representing light extinction, retardation image showing the tissue birefringence, and directional and inclination images representing in-plane angle and out-of-plane angle respectively (i.e., local 3D fiber orientation). For the registration of 3D PLI images only little work can be found. In [2] a relatively small region of a human brain with a coarser resolution of 100 m was registered using a fluid model. Such thicker sections are less prone to sectioning artifacts. In this paper, we present an automatic approach for the registration of 3D PLI images to the reference BF images. This includes identification of brain tissue area and cropping of the region-of-interest (ROI) in the 3D PLI images using a segmentation algorithm, a rigid registration for handling very large translations and rotations, and subsequent non-linear registration to address local deformations. For non-linear registration, we use Gaussian elastic body splines (GEBS) [3] which are analytic solutions of the Navier equation and thus represent a more realistic physical deformation model compared to a fluid model in [2]. Due to the different image acquisition process (Fig. 1), the reference BF images and the 3D PLI images are multi-modal images (i.e., have significantly different intensity values). To deal with the multi-modal data, we use a local analytic measure for mutual information (MI) as similarity measure. For registration, we used the transmittance 3D PLI images and applied the computed displacement vector field to all modalities of the 3D PLI data. We applied our approach to 30 consecutive sections of 3D PLI data and registered them to the reference BF images. For a quantitative evaluation, we used three sections with manually determined ground truth.

2   Materials and methods

Our approach first performs a coarse registration of 3D PLI images to the reference BF using center-of-mass (COM) alignment and rigid registration, and then refines the result using elastic registration. Preprocessing includes segmentation of 3D PLI data.

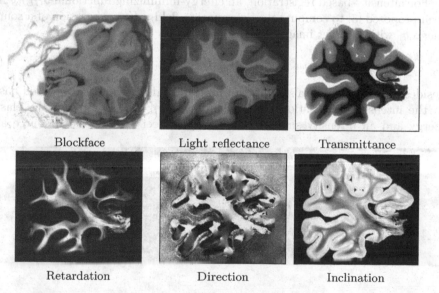

Blockface   Light reflectance   Transmittance

Retardation   Direction   Inclination

Fig. 1. Section of temporal lobe of human brain: Blockface image (top-left) and different modalities of high-resolution 3D PLI data.

2.1   Preprocessing

For registration of 3D PLI data with BF images, the brain tissue needs to be separated from artefacts like tags, borders, and small islands (isolated parts of brain caused by sectioning process, see Fig. 2, left). We use a two-step approach for localization and segmentation of the brain tissue within the 3D PLI data: 1) linear and non-linear noise reduction as well as multi-level Otsu thresholding [4], and 2) Huang thresholding [5] (Fig. 2, right).

2.2   Coarse alignment

We first calculate the COM of the segmented BF and 3D PLI images, and perform an initial alignment by matching the COMs. Subsequently, we perform rigid registration using the scheme in [6] which minimizes the mean squared intensity error. In order to initialize the rotation and to cope with a possible flip of the brain in the 3D PLI data (in case a brain section has been put upside-down on the glass plate), we apply rigid registration with 36 different rotation angles (for both the original and the flipped images).

2.3   Elastic registration

In order to compensate local deformations caused by the sectioning process, after rigid registration we use elastic registration based on Gaussian elastic body splines (GEBS). GEBS are based on the Navier equation of elasticity.

For intensity-based registration, an energy-minimizing functional J_{GEBS} has been proposed [3] to compute the deformation field $\mathbf{u}$ for registration of a source image g_1 with a target image g_2

$$J_{\text{GEBS}}(\mathbf{u}) = J_{\text{Data},I}(g_1, g_2, \mathbf{u}^I) + \lambda_I J_I(\mathbf{u}, \mathbf{u}^I) + \lambda_E J_{\text{Elastic}}(\mathbf{u}) \qquad (1)$$

Besides $\mathbf{u}$, (1) comprises a second deformation field $\mathbf{u}^I$ which is computed based on the intensity information. J_{Elastic} and $J_{\text{Data},I}$ in (1) represent the elastic energy and an intensity similarity measure between the deformed source and

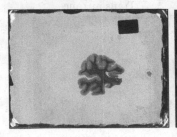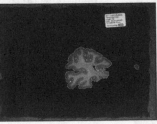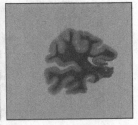

Fig. 2. Segmentation example: Original 3D PLI transmittance image with a tag, border structure, and a small island (left), ROI identification using segmentation in the light reflectance image (center), and final segmented transmittance image (right).

Table 1. Quantitative evaluation of registration steps.

Registration steps	TRE in pixels (mean±stdDev) for 3D PLI section			Mean
	#1	#2	#3	
COM alignment	573.91±225.00	529.92±224.00	517.40±210.00	540.41±220.00
Rigid registration	11.98±6.53	6.85±4.77	8.16±5.04	9.00±5.44
Elastic: MI	6.71±5.31	3.74±3.01	4.04±2.53	4.83±3.62

target images, respectively. J_I is the quadratic regularizer of the deformation field and $\{\lambda_I, \lambda_E\}$ are scalar weights. In our case, we use a local analytic measure for mutual information (MI) as similarity measure [7]

$$J_{\text{Data},I}\big(g_1, g_2, \mathbf{u}^I\big) = -\int \log_2\big(\epsilon + |\sin\theta|\big)d\mathbf{x} \tag{2}$$

with $\theta = \arccos\frac{\nabla g_1(\mathbf{x}+\mathbf{u}^I)\cdot\nabla g_2(\mathbf{x})}{\|\nabla g_1(\mathbf{x}+\mathbf{u}^I)\|\|\nabla g_2(\mathbf{x})\|}$ defined in a small neighborhood of $\mathbf{x}$ and a constant $\epsilon > 0$. Note that previously in [7] this measure was applied only to medical images such as MRI and CT. In order to handle large deformations, a multi-resolution scheme with four scales is used for the minimization of (1).

3 Results

For a quantitative evaluation, we have used three histological sections of a human brain with about 70 manually determined correspondences by an expert (serves as ground truth) in each of the 3D PLI and reference BF images. The size of each image is 1311×1103 pixels for both BF and 3D PLI images with an isotropic resolution of 64 m. Additionally, 30 histological sections have been used for visual quantification of our registration approach.

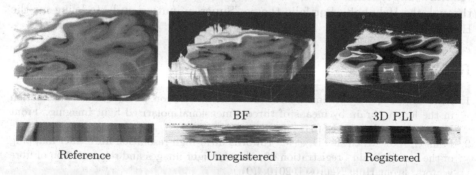

BF   3D PLI

Reference   Unregistered   Registered

Fig. 3. Registration of 30 sections of the temporal lobe of a human brain. First row: Top view with green line representing the cut-through for visualization (left), 3D stack of the reference BF images (center) and 3D stack of registered 3D PLI transmittance images to BF (right). Second row: yz slice shows the alignment of the 30 sections.

3.1   Quantitative result

Tab. 1 shows the target registration errors (TRE) for COM, rigid, and elastic registration. The large TRE values for COM show that the 3D PLI images are largely misaligned. Rigid registration robustly aligns the sections resulting in a mean TRE of 9.00 pixels (improvement by a factor of 60 compared to COM). Elastic registration further reduces the TRE by nearly a factor of two in each section and yields a mean TRE of only 4.83 pixels.

3.2   Visual assessment

We have also applied our approach to 30 consecutive sections of 3D PLI data of the temporal lobe of a human brain. Fig. 3 shows that the registered images are visually coherent to the reference BF 3D volume. It can also be observed that in the unregistered case, 3D PLI data have very large shifts. Using our approach all 30 image sections are well aligned to the reference BF images.

4   Discussion and conclusions

We have introduced an approach for registration of high-resolution 3D PLI images of histological sections of the human brain to undistorted reference BF images. Main steps include automatic segmentation, rigid registration, and elastic registration. We have performed a quantitative evaluation and found that elastic registration yields a significant improvement compared to rigid registration as well as alignment based on the center-of-mass. A qualitative assessment was also performed on a larger number of 3D PLI images. The visual coherence between the registered sections showed the effectiveness of our approach. In future work, we will investigate other local similarity measures for elastic registration.

Acknowledgement. This work was supported by the Helmholtz Association through the Helmholtz Portfolio theme "Supercomputing and Modeling for the Human Brain".

References

1. Axer M, Gräßel D, Kleiner M, et al. High-Resolution fiber tract reconstruction in the human brain by means of three-dimensional polarized light imaging. Front Neuroinformatics. 2011;5(34).
2. Palm C, Axer M, Gräßel D, et al. Towards ultra-high resolution fibre tract mapping of the human brain - registration of polarised light images and reorientation of fibre vectors. Front Hum Neurosci. 2010;4(9).
3. Wörz S, Rohr K. Spline-Based hybrid image registration using landmark and intensity information based on matrix-valued non-radial basis functions. Int J Computer Vis. 2014;106(1):76–92.
4. Otsu N. A threshold selection method from grey level histograms. IEEE Trans Syst Man Cybern. 1979;9(1):62–6.

5. Huang LK, Wang MJJ. Image thresholding by minimizing the measures of fuzziness. Pattern Recognit. 1995;28(1):41–51.
6. Thévenaz P, Ruttimann UE, Unser M. A pyramid approach to subpixel registration based on intensity. IEEE Trans Image Process. 1998;7(1):27–41.
7. Biesdorf A, Wörz S, Kaiser HJ, et al. Hybrid spline-based multimodal registration using local measures for joint entropy and mutual information. Proc MICCAI. 2009; p. 607–15.

Abstract: 3D-Rekonstruktion der Schilddrüse des Menschen mit 2D-Ultraschall-Daten im Rahmen von Routineuntersuchungen

Bastian Thiering[1], James Nagarajah[2], Hans-Gerd Lipinski[1]

[1]Biomedical Imaging Group, FH Dortmund
[2]Klinik für Nuklearmedizin, Universität Duisburg-Essen
thiering@biomedical-imaging.de

Für die Diagnostik von Schilddrüsen(SD)-Erkrankungen werden üblicherweise 2D-Ultraschall(US)-Scanner verwendet. SD Anomalien erfordern jedoch auch Kenntnisse über räumliche Verteilungen von Gewebestrukturen. Spezielle 3D-US-Scanner sind kompliziert in der Handhabung und teuer in der Anschaffung. Daher wurde ein SD Rekonstruktionsverfahren für 2D-Scandaten entwickelt. Eine SD-US-Untersuchung beginnt mit dem Ansetzen des Schallkopfes im Bereich des Brustbeins mit anschließendem Hinführen zum Zungenbein. Danach wird der Schallkopf wieder zurück zum Brustbein bewegt. Während dieses Vorgangs werden bis zu 500 zweidimensionale Bilder senkrecht zur Scanrichtung erzeugt. Bei einer konstanten Schallkopf-Geschwindigkeit ist eine lineare Zuordnung von Messzeit und korrespondierender Bildebene möglich (3D-Bildstapel-Erzeugung). Im Routinebetrieb auftretende kleine Abweichungen von einer konstanten Geschwindigkeit haben kaum einen Einfluss auf die Güte des Bilddatenstapels. Die Bilddaten werden in einem Bildanalyseprozess aufbereitet. Verwendet werden Standard Bibliotheksfunktionen von ITK und VTK. Nach einer Bildvorverarbeitung und einem Segmentationsteil (Abfolge diverser ITK Standardfilter, die sich für die Segmentation der SD-Daten als besonders geeignet herausgestellt haben), erfolgt eine räumiche SD-Rekonstruktion (Marching-Cube Methode). Um die Durchführbarkeit des Verfahrens zu überprüfen, wurden sowohl je eine US-Aufnahme als auch ein Computertomogramm (CT) der SD von 6 ausgewählten gesunden Patienten erzeugt. Sowohl die US- als auch CT-Bilddaten wurden mit den gleichen Algorithmen segmentiert und danach visualisiert. Anhand der 3D-Daten wurde das SD-Volumen in Abhängigkeit von der verwendeten Modalität bestimmt und mit konventionellen SD Volumenbestimmungsmethoden verglichen. Der Vergleich der Volumenwerte (US vs. CT) eines Patienten zeigten Abweichungen von maximal 10%. Die SD-US-Volumenwerte wiesen im Vergleich zu den mit konventionellen SD-Volumenbestimmungsmethoden gewonnenen Werten geringere Abweichungen auf als die mit dem CT gewonnenen Volumendaten. Ein visueller Vergleich der dargestellten SD-Rekonstruktionen von CT und US ergab, dass die mit den US-Daten generierten SD wesentlich detaillierter dargestellt werden können als mit CT-Bilddaten. Daher eignen sich routinemäßig gewonnene 2D-US-Bild-daten durchaus auch für eine räumliche Rekonstruktion der SD.

Systematic Analysis of Jurkat T-Cell Deformation in Fluorescence Microscopy Data

Sven-Thomas Antoni[1], Omar M. F. Ismail[1], Daniel Schetelig[2],
Björn-Philipp Diercks[3], René Werner[2], Insa M. A. Wolf[3], Andreas H. Guse[3],
Alexander Schlaefer[1]

[1]Institute of Medical Technology, Hamburg University of Technology
[2]Department of Computational Neuroscience,
University Medical Center Hamburg-Eppendorf
[3]Department of Biochemistry and Molecular Cell Biology,
University Medical Center Hamburg-Eppendorf
antoni@tuhh.de

Abstract. In the adaptive immune system, Calcium (Ca^{2+}) is acting as a fundamental on-switch. Fluorescence microscopy is used to study the underlying mechanisms. However, living cells introduce motion and for the analysis of (sub-)cellular Ca^{2+} activity a precise motion analysis is necessary. We present an image based workflow to detect and analyze cell motion. We evaluate our approach on Jurkat T-cells using cell motion as observed from actual time series of cell images. Results indicate, that our method is able to detect deformation with an error of $0.2222 \pm 0.086 \mu m$ which is in the range of the image resolution, showing that accurate cell deformation detection is possible and feasible.

1 Introduction

Calcium (Ca^{2+}) is essential for T-cell activation, the fundamental on-switch for the adaptive immune system. Fluorescence microscopy (FM) can be used to study the underlying mechanisms of the initial, short-lived, localized Ca^{2+} signals and their formation and propagation [1]. The spatial and temporal resolution of image sequences necessary for dynamic Ca^{2+} signal analysis results in large data sets, requiring automated segmentation and processing to identify the actual signal [2, 3]. Although the initial Calcium signals are evoked in milliseconds after stimulation, we are further interested in the Ca2+ signal propagation. When analyzing time series of cell image data, signal distribution over time and space is of interest. Jurkat T-cells are known to move and change their shape. Hence, while tracking subcellular Ca^{2+} dynamics in living Jurkat T-cells over time, cell deformation needs to be considered and detection and compensation of cell deformation could improve the detail of Ca^{2+} signal analysis. Cell motion and deformation has been analyzed by various means [4, 5] but only for very specific applications, i.e., co-localization of nuclear structures, a compensation has been performed [6]. We propose to identify landmarks on the cell's perimeter and to estimate the local deformation based on these landmarks. We evaluate our approach using deformations obtained from actual cell motion. The results indicate that accurate cell deformation detection is possible and feasible. As our method does not distinguish between motion and deformation we use both concepts synonymously for the sake of this work.

2 Methods and material

2.1 Deformation detection

Our deformation detection approach is based on three main steps. First, we use an entropy based information criterion to select potential landmarks on the cell's perimeter. Second, we identify landmark correspondence in subsequent image frames. Third, we apply landmark based thin-plate-spline (TPS) registration to compute the deformation.

Landmark detection. Due to noise in the signal, the contour's shape changes slightly between frames, not accounting for any deformation. Hence, instead of using the whole contour for deformation detection, we only use a limited number of specific landmarks. Before selecting the landmarks (2.1), we need to detect potentially interesting landmarks. Let C_i be the set of points on the perimeter of the cell in image I_i, then, for all points $q \in C_i$ on the perimeter we select the 21×21 neighborhood R_q centered around q. Using the Shannon entropy $E(R_q)$ of the gray values in R_q, we estimate the information criterion

$$I_q = 1 - \frac{E(R_q)}{\max_{\hat{q}} E(R_q)} \tag{1}$$

Out of all perimeter points q, we select the $n \gg 1$ with the highest I_q value. They form the elements of the landmark candidate set $L_i^{\text{cand.}}$.

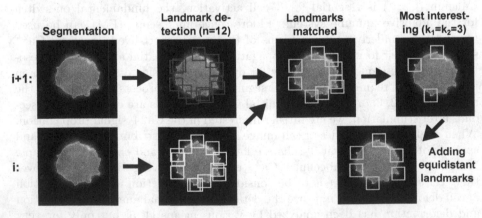

Fig. 1. The landmark workflow. First, landmarks are selected on the segmented surface of two consecutive frames. In a second step, the landmarks are matched and in the last step the landmarks for future computations are selected.

Landmark selection and correspondence establishing. In order to obtain a proper representation of the cell surface, we select landmarks on each of two subsequent images I_i and I_{i+1}. Connected landmarks in both images should mark similar structures, hence, we introduce a correspondence score and choose $k \leq n, k > 0$ corresponding landmarks. The correspondence score $m_i^{a,b}$ between two landmarks $a \in L_i^{\text{cand.}}$ and $b \in L_{i+1}^{\text{cand.}}$ is defined by the euclidean distance between the landmarks and the normalized sum-of-squared differences (SSD) between R_a and R_b, i.e.

$$m_i^{a,b} = \|a - b\|_2 + \text{nSSD}(R_a, R_b) \tag{2}$$

We say a and b are connected, if $m_i^{a,b} = \min_{\hat{a}} m_i^{\hat{a},b}$. We sort the n connected landmarks by their correspondence score and choose the $k_1 \leq k$ landmarks with the highest score. These k_1 connected landmarks are assumed to represent very similar structures. In order to obtain a proper representation of the surface we select another $k_2 = k - k_1$ corresponding landmarks equidistantly between the already selected k_1 landmarks. The result is a set $M_i = \{L_i, L_{i+1}\}$ with $L_j \subset L_j^{\text{cand}}, |L_j| = k, j = i, i+1$ of k corresponding landmarks. An example for landmark selection is shown in Fig. 1.

Determining cell deformation. We use TPS landmark-based registration to compute the deformation of the cell's shape and save the deformation grid $\omega \colon \mathbb{R}^2 \mapsto \mathbb{R}^2$. The landmarks used for registration are those that have been selected in the previous steps. See [7] for details on the registration.

2.2 Evaluation

To evaluate our approach, we need realistic shapes with known ground truth. A manual matching of landmarks is not typically done, i.e., there is no established protocol available. Moreover, this would be virtually impossible for a larger set of data. To evaluate our method on realistic data with fully known ground truth, we follow a three step approach. First, we sample sets of subsequent image frames I_i, I_{i+1} representing actual cell motion and establish a deformation ω_i between corresponding landmarks M_i on the cell shapes. Note that we cannot prove this registrations to be true. Second, we apply a random deformation ω_1 obtained in the first step to a random image frame. Hence, we get a deformed version of that frame for which we know the deformation, and we can store the two images and the deformation. Third, we apply our deformation detection method to a set of cell shapes for which we now know the true deformation and get the deformation ω_2. This allows estimating the error of our method. We express this error by means of the RMSE of the euclidean distance between the original landmarks displaced by ω_1 and by ω_2.

2.3 Material

We are working with preprocessed fluorescence microscopic image series consisting of $i = 4000$ frames I_i acquired at 38.5 frames per second per series. See [3] for

Table 1. Statistics of the RMSE of the analysis for each cell. All values in μm.

Cell	1	2	3	4	5	6	7	8
$\bar{e}$	0.2540	0.2628	0.2292	0.2708	0.2313	0.2255	0.2245	0.2452
$\sigma(e)$	0.0597	0.1091	0.0400	0.1018	0.0340	0.0369	0.0303	0.0589
RMSE	0.2608	0.2842	0.2326	0.2889	0.2337	0.2284	0.2265	0.2521
Cell	9	10	11	12	13	14	15	16
$\bar{e}$	0.3253	0.2560	0.2218	0.2305	0.2623	0.2379	0.2132	0.3096
$\sigma(e)$	0.1017	0.0372	0.0265	0.0338	0.0722	0.0596	0.0254	0.1078
RMSE	0.3405	0.2586	0.2234	0.2329	0.2719	0.2451	0.2147	0.3275

details on the preprocessing and [1] for details on the bleach correction. In total, 16 series are analyzed. Dimensions of the digital images range from 118×193 to 160×190 pixels and the resolution is 0.1537μm per pixel.

3 Results

We sampled approximately 64000 sets of subsequent image frames. For each of 16 available Jurkat T-cells we simulated 50 instances. For creating the database of deformations we used parameters $n = 100$ and $k_1 = 10$, $k_2 = 10$, $r = 1.537\mu$m (10 pixel). The same parameters were used for the evaluation. The TPS landmark based registration was performed without regularization. We separate our results on a per cell basis. Over all experiments, we observed a mean error of $\bar{e} = 0.2222 \pm 0.086\mu$m. See Tab. 1 for an overview on the statistics of our result. Also see Fig. 2 for examples of different deformations and the corresponding results.

4 Discussion

Overall, we analyzed 64000 frames for deformations. Our results show, that at least for the analyzed cells severe deformation are observable. Over all frames, our method reliably detects the deformation with a mean error below 0.23μm which is in the order of the image resolution. Our workflow shows good results for cells of all shapes, compare Fig. 2. Even for strong deformations this error stays below 0.3μm which is less than 2 pixel, compare Fig. 2(c). Note that while the depicted deformations may not seem strong, they only represent deformations between two subsequent frames. I.e., on a whole dataset approximately 4000 deformations of that range result in a very noticeable difference between frame 1 and 4000. Hence the need for compensation in order to track the signal propagation. Due to the application of the deformation, the simulated cells may be smoother than the original cells. However, the effect on the boundary and hence on the landmarks and their detection should be negligible, which is also illustrated in Fig. 2, row 2, where the original and deformed contours are shown. For our analysis we used deformations that were obtained from the cells using our method. The results of the evaluation indicate, that these deformations could reflect the actual deformation but, by design, can not prove this. As with every landmark based approach, the overall quality is heavily dependent on the proper choice of the landmarks. Currently, our correspondence score is not a metric and the impact of a more sophisticated score should be investigated. Especially the deformation of Fig. 2(c) seems stronger than what we would have expected to occur in the about 26ms between two consecutive frames. While the deformation is still reliably detected, the cause of the strong deformation is not entirely clear. We assume this is due to using unregularized registration. Hence,

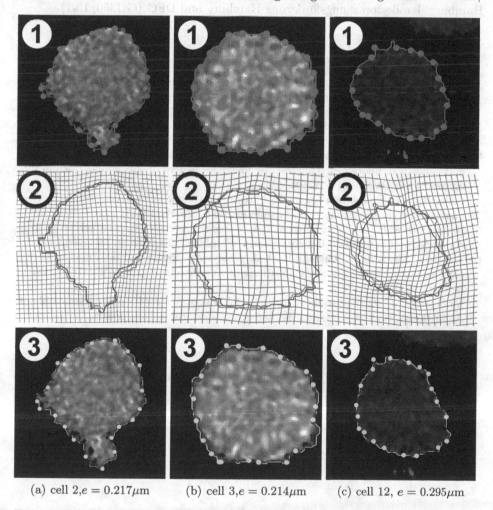

   (a) cell 2,$e = 0.217\mu$m   (b) cell 3,$e = 0.214\mu$m   (c) cell 12, $e = 0.295\mu$m

Fig. 2. Three examples of differently deformed cells. Depicted are the original cell (1) with contour and landmarks in red, the applied deformation (2) with original (red) and deformed contour (blue) and the deformed cell (3) with deformed contour and landmarks in blue and by our method calculated contour and landmarks in green. Note the strong deformation of (b) and (c).

In future experiments, different concepts to formalize the transformation caused by the deformation should be investigated. Overall, we showed that our method reliably detects cell deformations with errors in the range of the image resolution. Robust and precise motion compensation for cell signal processing seems feasible. For future work, the deformation of primary T-cells should be further analyzed and the compensation should be included in the general workflow to allow for a more precise calcium signal propagation analysis.

Acknowledgement. Partially funded by Forschungszentrum Medizintechnik Hamburg, Landesforschungsförderung Hamburg and DFG (GU360/15-1).

References

1. Wolf IMA, Diercks BP, Gattkowski E, et al. Frontrunners of T cell activation: Initial, localized Ca2+ signals mediated by NAADP and the type 1 ryanodine receptor. Sci Signal. 2015;8(398):ra102.
2. Antoni ST, Dabrowski A, Schetelig D, et al. Segmentation of T-cells in fluorescence microscopy. Proc EMBC. 2015.
3. Schetelig D, Wolf IM, Diercks BP, et al. A modular dramework for post-processing and analysis of fluorescence microscopy image sequences of subcellular calcium dynamics. Proc BVM. 2015; p. 401–406.
4. Soll DR, Voss E, Johnson O, et al. Three-dimensional reconstruction and motion analysis of living, crawling cells. Scanning. 2000 7;22(4):249–257.
5. Rosenbluth MJ, Lam WA, Fletcher DA. Force microscopy of nonadherent cells: a comparison of leukemia cell deformability. Biophys J. 2006;90(8):2994–3003.
6. Mattes J, Nawroth J, Boukamp P, et al. Analyzing motion and deformation of the cell nucleus for studying co-localizations of nuclear structures. Proc IEEE ISBI. 2006; p. 1044–1047.
7. Modersitzki J. Fair: Flexible Algorithms for Image Registration (Fundamentals of Algorithms). Society for Industrial and Applied Mathematics; 2009.

Comparison of Default Patient Surface Model Estimation Methods

Xia Zhong[1], Norbert Strobel[2], Markus Kowarschik[2], Rebecca Fahrig[2], Andreas Maier[1,3]

[1]Pattern Recognition Lab, Friedrich-Alexander-Universität Erlangen-Nürnberg
[2]Siemens Healthcare GmbH, Forchheim, Germany
[3]Erlangen Graduate School in Advanced Optical Technologies (SAOT)
xia.zhong@fau.de

Abstract. A patient model is useful for many clinical applications such as patient positioning, device placement, or dose estimation in case of X-ray imaging. A default or a-priori patient model can be estimated using learning based methods trained over a large database. Different methods can be used to estimate such a default model given a restricted number of the input parameters. We investigated different learning based estimation strategies using patient gender, height, and weight as the input to estimate a default patient surface model. We implemented linear regression, an active shape model, kernel principal component analysis and a deep neural network method. These methods are trained on a database containing about 2000 surface meshes. Using linear regression, we obtained a mean vertex error of 20.8 ± 14.7 mm for men and 17.8 ± 11.6 mm for women, respectively. While the active shape model and kernel PCA method performed better than linear regression, the results also revealed that the deep neural network outperformed all other methods with a mean vertex error of 15.6 ± 9.5 mm for male and 14.5 ± 9.3 mm for female models.

1 Introduction

Many medical applications even in the field of X-ray imaging using C-arm angiography systems, can benefit from the use of a default patient model. Such a model can be generated using only a limited set of patient parameters (or measurements). Although these default patient models cannot be expected to fit perfectly to the patient, their accuracy is much better than what can be achieved with a stylized model. In fact, if additional sensor data is available, a default patient model can be used as initialization for further model refinement. When a learning-based method is used to estimate a priori patient models, a large database is needed for the training process. The accuracy of the estimation approach depends not only on quality and the quantity of the available data but also on different estimation methods. In this paper, we evaluate different statistical estimation approaches and propose a deep neural network based approach. These methods are implemented and evaluated on a database comprising surface models and associated patient meta data such as gender, height, and weight, to highlight the performance of different approaches. This paper is structured as follows. First, we introduce the related work in the field of shape representation learning and shape estimation. Second, we provide descriptions of the implemented methods. Afterwards, we evaluate on all of the different methods and compare the results. We wrap up by discussing the proposed deep neural network approach for our particular application.

1.1 Related work

One can put our approach into prior context in two ways. Seen from one direction, our approach is related to methods which learn the shape representation in a low dimensional space. In general, this is a difficult problem as changes in pose between models need to be accounted for as well as differences in body shape. The most widely used solution for this task is the shape completion and animation for people (SCAPE) method [1]. This approach assumes that shape and pose are uncorrelated and solves the two problems separately at first and jointly afterwards. Hasler et al. [2] encodes in the shape representation further information, e.g., height and joint angle and trains a combined representation of shape and pose simultaneously. Based on the SCAPE method, Pishchulin et al. [3] proposed an improved method by incorporating mesh sampling into the training loop. The second set of methods revolves around patient shape generation base on different input parameters. Seo et al. [4] introduced a framework to generate a surface model using different input parameters. Rather than using parameters, Wuhrer et al. [5] uses anthropological measurements e.g., arm length, waist circumference as an input to both initialize and refine the surface model estimate.

2   Materials and methods

In this paper, we implemented and evaluated different methods for default patient model estimation using patient gender, height, and weight as input. The approaches can be summarized in three steps: data transform, regression, and shape reconstruction. During the data transform step, we map the input data

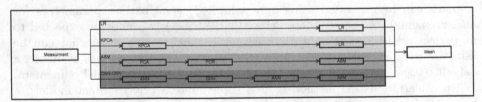

Fig. 1. Pipeline of evaluated methods, from top: linear regression (LR), kernel PCA (KPCA), active shape model (ASM) comprising principle component analysis (PCA) and principle component regression (PCR), and finally deep neural network (DNN) made up of a convolutional neural network (CNN) and an artificial neural network (ANN).

into a different space for the successive regression step. The mapping function can be linear, e.g., principal component analysis (PCA), or non-linear. In this case, a kernel function or artificial neural network (ANN) may be applied. The regression step maps the transformed data to the patient model itself or its low dimensional representation. The reconstruction step, in turn, maps the representation of the patient model to its original space. In this paper, we evaluated four different methods for patient model estimation. An overview of our approaches is shown in Fig. 1. All these methods are learning based methods, and a database is used for training. The data comprised male and female surface mesh data and corresponding measurements. We can summarize the estimation method using the equation

$$\hat{x} = \mathcal{F}(X, g) \tag{1}$$

where $\hat{x}$ denotes the estimated patient model, g is the measurement of the patient, and X refers to the collection of surface meshes stored in the database. The function $\mathcal{F}$ is the regression function that needs to be found. It depends on the database contents.

2.1   Linear regression

Linear regression (LR) is the most straightforward method for solving the regression problem. Let $G = [g_1, \cdots, g_k, \cdots, g_N] \in \mathbb{R}^{K \times N}$ denote the measurement matrix combining every measurement g_i for surface mesh x_i. Similarly the surface mesh matrix is defined as $X = [x_1, \cdots, x_k, \cdots, x_N] \in \mathbb{R}^{M \times N}$. The variable N refers to the number of meshes, M denotes the number of single mesh dimensions, e.g., the number of vertices, and K is the dimension of the measurements. The LR introduces a regression matrix $A \in \mathbb{R}^{M \times K}$ where

$$AG = X \tag{2}$$

This problem can be solved simply by using singular value decomposition (SVD) as $A = XG^+$. Then the estimation patient model $\hat{x}$ with given g is

$$\hat{x} = Ag \tag{3}$$

2.2   Kernel principal component analysis (PCA)

The kernel PCA method tries to improve the result of linear regression by introducing feature mapping using a kernel. In this case, the input measurements are mapped to a feature space using kernel PCA. The feature space is mapped to meshes using linear regression as introduced in the previous subsection. We use Gaussian and linear kernels for the kernel PCA. The reason for feature mapping is that the measurements, e.g., height and weight, may not be linearly related to the mesh vertex positions. Take the weight, for example. An integral is needed to relate it to the vertex positions. Using a linear or Gaussian kernel function Φ the estimation can be fomulated as

$$\hat{x} = A\Phi(g) \tag{4}$$

2.3 Active shape model

The motivation to use an active shape model (ASM) is to learn a joint subspace between shape and measurement. To this end, we assume that shape and measurements are correlated and that they can be described in the same subspace. By using the method proposed in [6], the measurement vector g and the shape x can be described as

$$x = \bar{x} + Q_sc \tag{5}$$
$$g = \bar{g} + Q_mc \tag{6}$$

where c is the low dimensional representation of both shape and measurement, and $\bar{x}$ and $\bar{g}$ denote the average shape and measurement. The matrix Q_s and Q_m are the corresponding modes of variation of shape, and measurement respectively. Except the low dimensional representation c, all other parameters are derived from the database by solving a matrix decomposition problem [7]. The estimation equation of the method is

$$\hat{x} = \bar{x} + Q_sQ_m^+(g - \bar{g}) \tag{7}$$

2.4 Deep neural network

The default model estimation problem can also be approached using a deep neural network (DNN) approach. The advantage of using a DNN is that we can learn a potentially non-linear mapping between measurements and shape. We propose a different neural network topology here than the general regression neural networks [8] as we try to estimate a high-dimensional output (mesh model) using a low-dimensional input (height, weight). Instead of regressing to the mesh model directly, we estimate a low dimensional representation of the mesh model. The low dimensional representations we used here is the ASM parameter c trained as described above. Other low dimensional representations e.g. bottleneck features

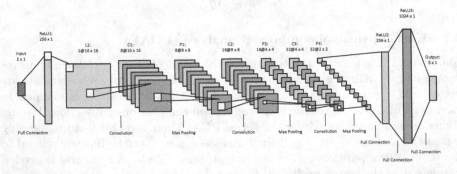

Fig. 2. An illustration of the proposed regression network topology. Input parameters are height and weight. Two DNNs were set up, one for meshes associated with women, another one for meshes representing men.

Fig. 3. The mean vertex error for male and female models using (from left to right): LR, ASM, kernel PCA with linear kernel (KPCA-LK), kernel PCA with Gauss kernel (KPCA-GK), and DNN.

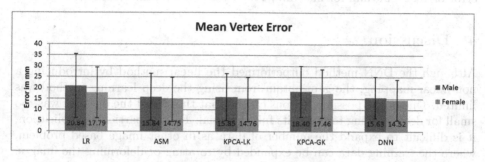

can also be used. We applied patch normalization to all the layers for robust training.

An illustration of the network architecture is shown in Fig. 2. This network takes height and weight as input and uses an ANN to expand the input vector. The output of the ANN is then converted to an image and we use a convolution neural network (CNN) layout (alternating convolution and max pooling layer) in the following layers. The result of the CNN is being flatted into the ANN layout and to the output layer. The combination of CNN followed by ANN is well established as a robust method for multi-label classification [9] of images. The proposed network also benefits from this structure and the evaluation showed that this architecture works well for our regression problem.

Estimating a surface model using a DNN can be fomulated as

$$\hat{x} = \bar{x} + Q_s \mathcal{F}^{\text{DNN}}(g) \tag{8}$$

In Eq. 8, the symbol $\mathcal{F}^{\text{DNN}}$ represents a trained network mapping function.

3   Evaluation and results

For evaluation, we used a database to comprising surface meshes and corresponding meta data (measurement data) such as height and weight. In all, there were 865 male data sets and 1063 female data sets. In the evaluation, we randomly picked ten percent of the data as the test set. The remaining 90% were used for training. The error measure is the mean vertex error distance in mm between the estimated surface mesh and the original surface mesh associated with the corresponding height and weight. Female and male surface meshes were treated separately. The results of the different methods are shown in Fig. 3.

From Fig. 3 we learn that linear regression had the largest mean vertex error with 20.8 ± 14.7 mm for male and 17.8 ± 11.6 mm for the female surface model. Kernel PCA with Gaussian kernel improved the result for male and female model to 18.4 ± 11.7 mm and 17.5 ± 11.1 mm, respectively. The active shape model and kernel PCA with linear kernel lead to almost identical results with 15.8 ± 10.8 mm for male and 14.7 ± 10.1 mm for female models. The deep neural network outperformed all the methods, albeit sightly, with a mean vertex error of 15.6 ± 9.5 mm for male and 14.5 ± 9.3 mm for female models.

4   Discussion

Although the DNN method outperformed the linear method by introducing a non-linear mapping, the gain obtain from using the deep learning method was limited. One of the possible reasons can be that the size of the data set was too small for deep learning to reveal its full potential. For our particular application, it is difficult to expand the number of data as in other image based problem, where the training data can be expanded by rotating or deforming the images. In our case, we could deform surface meshes, but the corresponding changes in heigh and weigh would be unknown.

Acknowledgement. We gratefully acknowledge the support of Siemens Healthineers, Forchheim, Germany. We also thank Siemens Corporate Technology for providing the avatar database. Note that the concepts and information presented in this paper are based on research, and they are not commercially available.

References

1. Anguelov D, Srinivasan P, Koller D, et al. SCAPE: Shape completion and animation of people. ACM Trans Graph. 2005 Jul;24(3):408–16.
2. Hasler N, Stoll C, Sunkel M, et al. A statistical model of human pose and body shape. Comput Graph Forum. 2009;28(2):337–46.
3. Pishchulin L, Wuhrer S, Helten T, et al. Building statistical shape spaces for 3D human modeling. CoRR. 2015.
4. Seo H, Magnenat-Thalmann N. An automatic modeling of human bodies from sizing parameters. In: Proc Symp Interact 3D Graph; 2003. p. 19–26.
5. Wuhrer S, Shu C. Estimating 3D human shapes from measurements. Mach Vis Appl. 2013;24(6):1133–47.
6. Edwards GJ, Lanitis A, Taylor CJ, et al. Statistical models of face images improving specificity. Image Vis Comput. 1998;16(3):203 – 11.
7. Cootes TF, Taylor CJ, Cooper DH, et al. Active shape models : their training and application. Comput Vis Image Underst. 1995 Jan;61(1):38–59.
8. Specht DF. A general regression neural network. IEEE Trans Neural Netw. 1991 Nov;2(6):568–76.
9. Krizhevsky A, Sutskever I, Hinton GE. ImageNet classification with deep convolutional neural networks. In: Pereira F, Burges CJC, Bottou L, et al., editors. Adv Neural Inf Process Syst; 2012. p. 1097–105.

Robotergestützte Ultraschallbildgebung zur Lagekontrolle von Zielgewebe während der Strahlentherapie

Bewegungskompensation und Einbindung in ein medizinisches Bildverarbeitungsprogramm

Peter Karl Seitz, Rolf Bendl

Medizinische Informatik, Hochschule Heilbronn
peter.seitz@hs-heilbronn.de

Kurzfassung. Eine Strahlentherapie von Tumorpatienten erfolgt in der Regel fraktioniert über mehrere Wochen. Die Qualität der Therapie hängt entscheidend davon ab, ob sichergestellt werden kann, dass in jeder Fraktion die Strahlung, wie ursprünglich geplant, appliziert wird. Durch Lagerungsungenauigkeiten des Patienten, Organbewegungen, Deformationen, Gewichtsabnahme etc. kann es zu relevanten Veränderungen kommen. Die Bestrahlung erfolgt dann nicht mehr nach dem ursprünglich optimierten Plan. Adaptive Therapieansätze versuchen die Bewegung der Zielstrukturen abzuschätzen und durch geeignete Maßnahmen zu kompensieren. Diese Arbeit verfolgt das Ziel, Organbewegungen während der Therapie mit Hilfe von Ultraschall (US)-Bildgebung zu detektieren. Um sicherzustellen, dass trotz leichter Bewegungen des Patienten der Schallkopf korrekt positioniert bleibt und den Kontakt zur Patientenoberfläche nicht verliert, wird ein Leichtbauroboter eingesetzt. Der Roboter verfügt über eine Sensorik, um Bewegungen der Patientenoberfläche zu erkennen und durch eine Nachführung des Schallkopfes zu kompensieren. Damit können Atembewegungen berücksichtigt werden und der Roboter kann in Gefahrensituationen ausweichen. Die Roboterapplikation wurde in das MITK eingebettet. Der Schallkopf kann während der Therapie über einen Joystick neu positioniert werden. Erste Tests an Probanden zeigen, dass die Ultraschallbilder zur Lagekontrolle eingesetzt werden können.

1 Einleitung

Die Planung und Simulation in der Strahlentherapie hat das Ziel, die Konfiguration zu ermitteln, bei der das Zielvolumen mit einer ausreichenden Dosis bestrahlt wird, damit die Tumorzellen zerstört werden. Gleichzeitig soll das umgebende gesunde Gewebe so gering wie möglich belastet werden. Unsicherheiten über die Tumorausdehnung, die Lage und Orientierung des Tumors aufgrund von Organbewegungen und Positionierungsungenauigkeiten versucht man konventionell durch Sicherheitsabstände zu verringern. D.h. das Zielvolumen wird durch verschiedene standardisierte Sicherheitszonen vergrößert. Dabei steigt zwangsläufig die Belastung des gesunden Gewebes. Konzepte der adaptiven Strahlentherapie versuchen Lagerungs- und Positionierungsunsicherheiten durch Bildgebung während der Therapie zu reduzieren und damit die Notwendigkeit für Sicherheitsabstände zu minimieren. Etabliert ist z.B. eine Bildgebung mit dem Therapiestrahl, die aber nur einen sehr begrenzten Weichteilkontrast ermöglicht. Ein weiterer Nachteil dieses Ansatzes ist die zusätzliche Dosis, die für die Bildgebung benötigt wird. Alternativ versucht man Linearbeschleuniger und MR-Geräte zu integrieren. Diese Geräte werden voraussichtlich sehr teuer und zu groß für konventionelle Bunker sein. In unserem Ansatz realisieren wir eine Bildgebung mit Ultraschall. Der Einsatz von Ultraschall zur Lagekontrolle wurde bereits 2002 untersucht [1]. Der Schallkopf wurde mit einer starren Halterung am Patienten positioniert. Die starre Positionierung hat den Nachteil, dass bei Bewegungen des Patienten (Atmung) die Ankoppelung des Schallkopfes nicht mehr gewährleistet ist, außerdem schränken die fixe Schallkopfhalterung die möglichen Einstrahlrichtungen erheblich ein. Der Einsatz von Robotern zur Akquisition von Ultraschallbildern wurde bereits in anderen Arbeiten untersucht [2, 3, 4]. Ipsen et al. [5] untersuchten in einer Phantomstudie in der Strahlentherapie die dosimetrischen Konsequenzen einer Bewegungskompensation mit Hilfe eines Multi-Leaf-Kollimators auf Basis von Ultraschallbildern.

In dieser Arbeit untersuchen wir folgende Fragestellungen: Kann die Robotersteuerung die Veränderung des Anpressdrucks des Schallkopfes durch Atembewegungen oder kleinere Patientenbewegungen messen und kompensieren, so dass der Anpressdruck ausreichend konstant gehalten werden kann, um eine kontinuierliche US-Bildgebung zu ermöglichen? Kann der Roboter in Notsituationen ohne Gefährdung für den Patienten/Probanden aus dessen direkter Umgebung entfernt werden?

2   Material und Methoden

In unserem Ansatz erweitern wir die bisherigen Konzepte. Wir verwenden einen siebenachsigen KUKA Leichtbauroboter lbr iwa 7 800, der über eine eingebaute Kraftsensorik Bewegungen der Patientenoberfläche detektieren kann und als Halterung für den Ultraschall-Kopf dient. Detektierte Bewegungen sollen durch Nachführung des Schallkopfes kompensiert werden, um die korrekte Ankoppelung des Schallkopfes an der Patientenoberfläche sicherzustellen. Gleichzeitig kann eine Gefährdung des Patienten durch einen autonom arbeitenden Roboter auch bei außergewöhnlichen Patientenbewegungen minimiert werden. Falls der Roboter oder der Schallkopf bei einer Therapie mit multiplen Einstrahlrichtungen von einem Strahl erfasst würde, soll er unter Beibehaltung der Pose des US-Kopfs umkonfiguriert werden. Die Koppelung des US-Systems mit einer MITK Workbench über das OpenIGT-Link Protokoll [6] soll in Zukunft eine automatisierte Auswertung der US-Bilder ermöglichen. Die Implementierung der Robotersteuerung erfolgt mit Hilfe der KUKA Sunrise Umgebung. KUKA stellt Java Klassen zur Verfügung, mit der unterschiedliche Sensoren ausgelesen und die Roboterpose im kartesischen Achsraum modifiziert werden kann.

2.1   Bewegungskompensation

Über die KUKA-Impedanzklasse lässt sich eine Steuerungskomponente erstellen. Diese kann einen einwirkenden Kraftvektor auf das Werkzeug bestimmen. Die gemessene Kraft wird danach entsprechend in eine Ansteuerung der Achsmotoren umgesetzt, so dass das Werkzeug auf die Kraft reagieren kann. Die Nachgiebigkeit des Roboters wurde hierzu in Schallrichtung (Werkzeugkoordinatensystem) festgelegt. Um einen vorgegebenen Anpressdruck zu gewährleisten, wird eine zusätzliche Kraft in Schallrichtung definiert. Diese Kraft sorgt dafür, dass der Roboter (Schallkopf) selbstständig einer bewegenden Oberfläche folgen kann.

2.2   Sicherheitskonzept

Die Fähigkeit des Roboters, autonom einer zurückweichenden Oberfläche zu folgen, birgt die Gefahr, dass bei abrupten Lageveränderungen des Probanden/ Patienten eine Bewegungsfolge initiiert oder abgebrochen wird, die denjenigen einklemmen könnte. Eine klassische Stopp-Reaktion des Roboters würde hier die Situation verschärfen. Deshalb überprüft eine zusätzliche Steuerungskomponente kontinuierlich und richtungsunabhängig die Kraft, die auf den Roboter ausgeübt wird und bricht die Bewegungskompensation ab, wenn diese Kraft 20N übersteigt. Die Steuerung bewegt den Schallkopf dabei orthogonal um 10 cm von der Oberfläche weg, die zuvor verfolgt werden sollte. Währenddessen ist der Roboter in allen Achsen nachgiebig und hält anschließend, weiter nachgiebig, die aktuelle Position. Der Roboter kann so während und nach der Ausweichbewegung vom Probanden leicht weggeschoben werden.

2.3   Positionierung des Schallkopfes

Im Prinzip erlaubt der Roboter im KUKA-eigenen Handführmodus, dass der Ultraschallkopf manuell an einer bestimmten Oberfläche ausgerichtet wird. Um nachträglich kleinere Korrekturen zu ermöglichen, können dem Roboter im Smart Servo Modus zyklisch neue Positionen bzw. Posen übermittelt werden. Mit Hilfe eines Joysticks als Eingabegerät kann sowohl die Orientierung als auch die Position des Schallkopfes nachträglich verändert werden. Die Achsenbewegungen des Joysticks werden dabei auf die Achswinkel des Werkzeugkoordinatensystems (Ultraschallkopfspitze) abgebildet.

2.4   Einbindung in ein med. Bildverarbeitungsprogramm

Ein MITK (Medical Imaging Interaction Toolkit [7]) Plugin übernimmt über OpenIGTLink die Kommunikation mit der Robotersteuerung. Damit wird die Grundlage geschaffen, die Positionsdaten des Roboters mit aufgenommenen Ultraschallbildern zu kombinieren und die Lage der Bilder im Raum und der darin erkennbaren Strukturen detektieren zu können. Das Plugin zeigt die aktuellen Achsstellungen inklusive der Einstellbereiche. Die Position kann wie in Posititionierung des Schallkopfes beschrieben über das Plugin modifiziert werden. Generelles Konzept ist, dem Roboter nur Befehle zu schicken, z.B. ein String mit dem

Kommandonamen und weiteren Parameter. Die Bewegungsplanung wird durch die Robotersteuerung übernommen. OpenIGTLink wurde hierzu erweitert.

2.5 Probandentests

Das generelle Anwendungskonzept wurde mit 2 Probanden evaluiert. Ziel hierbei war eine Plausibilitätskontrolle. In der Evaluation wurde untersucht, inwieweit das Setup die zuvor definierten Randbedingen erfüllt und die Robotersteuerung in der Lage ist, bei unterschiedlichen Atmungsintensitäten der Probandenoberfläche zu folgen. Als leicht zu detektierende Zielstruktur wurde die Gallenblase ausgewählt (Abb. 2.5). Der Schallkopf bzw. der Roboter wurden im Handführmodus an eine geeignete Stelle auf dem Abdomen der Probanden aufgesetzt. Über MITK und den Joystick wurde der Schallkopf so ausgerichtet, dass in einer sagittalen Schnittführung die Gallenblase sichtbar war. Anschließend erfolgte die US-Akquisition sowohl bei flacher Atmung, als auch beim tiefen Ein- und Ausatmen, jeweils mit unterschiedlichen Atemfrequenzen. Abschließend wurde getestet, wie die Robotersteuerung auf Ausnahmesituationen reagiert, in dem der Proband stärkere willkürliche Bewegungen mit Positionsveränderungen um die 10 cm in beliebige Richtungen ausführte.

3 Ergebnisse

Der Roboter lässt sich von Hand positionieren. Dabei werden die Achsstellung an das erstellte MITK Plugin übermittelt. Dadurch lässt sich eine gut Ausgangsstellung sowohl für das Ultraschall als auch für den Roboter finden. Nach der Positionierung des Ultraschallkopfes reagiert der Roboter nachgiebig und führt autonom die Kompensationsbewegung durch. Während der Kompensation lässt sich der Ultaschallkopf im erstellten MITK Plugin über einen handelsüblichen Joystick neu ausrichten. Dabei wird der Ultraschallkopf stufenfrei in allen Achsen gedreht und bewegt. Die Umorientierung mit Joystick kann nahtlos aktiviert und

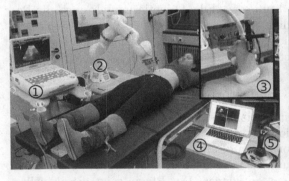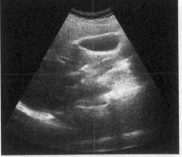

Abb. 1. Genereller Versuchsaufbau: 1 Ultraschall, 2 Roboter, 3 Halterung Ultraschall mit Rigid Body, 4 Steuerungscomputer mit MITK, 5 Joystick (links) und mit Roboter erstelltes Ergebnisbild (rechts).

deaktiviert werden. Durch Koppelung des Ultraschallgeräts mit dem Applikationsrechner können die US-Bilder über einen Frame-Grabber in MITK dargestellt werden. Das wichtigste Ergebnis ist somit die Gesamtintegration der verschiedenen Systeme in einem Programm und das Konzept, wie der Roboter gesteuert wird. Im Probandenexperiment konnte gezeigt werden, dass damit eine kontinuierliche US-Akquisition möglich ist. Damit ist das Konzept prinzipiell zum Tracking anatomischer Strukturen geeignet. Durch das entwickelte Sicherheitskonzept wurde das Einquetsch- und Verletzungsrisiko des Patienten minimiert.

3.1   Bewegungskompensation und Orientierung des Ultraschallkopfes

Es wurde gezeigt, dass die Bewegungskompensation über die Impedanzklasse von KUKA realisiert werden kann. Der Anpressdruck und die zulässige Maximalkraft lassen sich hierbei einstellen. Bei der Kompensation wich die vorgegebene Kraft um maximal 4 N ab. Zusätzlich ist es während der Atemkompensation möglich, die Orientierung zu verändern oder Ausweichbewegungen zu starten. Weiter kann der Roboterarm während der Kompensation seine Achsen umkonfigurieren.

3.2   Integration in das MITK

Der Roboter wurde erfolgreich in das MITK als Plugin integriert. Damit ist es möglich, sowohl das Ultraschallbild, als auch die Robotersteuerung in einem Programm zu vereinen. Über die Achsanzeige lässt sich der Roboter sicher positionieren und zeigt an, ob dieser sich am Rande einer erlaubten Achsstellung befindet. Weiteres Ergebnis hierbei ist die Art der Kommunikation.

3.3   Probandenexperiment

Abschließendes Ergebnis ist das Probandenexperiment. Es hat gezeigt, dass der Ansatz richtig ist und funktioniert. Visuell konnte anhand des Ultraschallbildes nachempfunden werden, wie sich das Zielgewebe bewegt. Das erzeugte Ultraschallbild war stabil und die Anpressung an den Probanden war konstant. Sowohl feinere als auch gröbere Bewegungen konnten kompensiert werden. Bei zu starken Bewegungen über 20 N brach der Roboter, wie vorgegeben, die Kompensation ab und wich dem Probanden aus.

4   Diskussion

In dieser Arbeit wurde gezeigt, dass ein KUKA Leichtbauroboter lbr iiwa über OpenIGTLink, mit dem MITK verbunden werden kann und eine Steuerung über ein MITK Plugin und selbst definierten OpenIGTLink Nachrichtenklassen erfolgen kann. Es lassen sich hierbei auch weit mehr als nur einfache Positionsbefehle realisieren. Über die erstellte Kommandostruktur kann die von Haus aus mitgelieferte KUKA Roboter API vollständig genutzt werden. Die Zuordnung von Aufgaben zwischen Robotersteuerung und MITK war richtig.

Als Ergebnis kann ein am Roboter befestigter Schallkopf, unter Auswertung der Kräfte, die auf den Roboter wirken, den Schallkopf der Probandenoberfläche nachführen, wenn sich deren Position durch Atembewegungen oder kleinere Patientenbewegungen verändert. Akquirierte US-Bilder werden ebenfalls in MITK angezeigt und können künftig dazu genutzt werden, die räumliche Bewegung von anatomischen Strukturen zu erfassen und während einer Strahlentherapie Korrekturanweisungen an die Bestrahlungseinrichtung zu geben, wie in [5] in einer Phantomstudie vorgeschlagen wurde. Die Achsstellung des Roboters kann über das MITK-Plugin, während der Kompensation, umkonfiguriert werden, ohne dass die Pose des Schallkopfes verändert wird. Damit kann der Roboter während einer Strahlentherapie mit multiplen Einstrahlrichtungen ggf. aus dem aktuellen Strahlenfeld entfernt werden, ohne dass die Bildgebung beeinträchtigt wird. Sicherheitsmechanismen minimieren das Risiko, dass der Roboter den Patienten einklemmen und verletzen kann. Damit ein automatisches Nachführen oder Ausweichen des Roboters möglich ist, müssen die Achsstellung zu Beginn so konfiguriert werden, dass entsprechende Bewegungen möglich sind. Zur verlässlichen Positionsdetektion sich bewegender anatomischer Strukturen soll der Schallkopf zukünftig über ein Navigationssystem mit dem Planungs-CT verbunden werden, da auf diesem die initiale Positionierung und die Einstrahlrichtungen festgelegt wurden.

Literaturverzeichnis

1. Falco T, Shenouda G, Kaufmann C, et al. Ultrasound imaging for external-beam prostate treatment setup and dosimetric verification. Med Dosim. 2002;27(4):271–3.
2. Priester AM, Natarajan S, Culjat MO. Robotic ultrasound systems in medicine. IEEE Trans Ultrason Ferroelectr Freq Control. 2013;60(3):507–23.
3. Salcudean SE, Bell G, Bachmann S, et al. In: Taylor C, Colchester A, editors. Robot-Assisted Diagnostic Ultrasound – Design and Feasibility Experiments. Berlin, Heidelberg: Springer Berlin Heidelberg; 1999. p. 1062–71.
4. Graumann C, Fuerst B, Hennersperger C, et al. Robotic ultrasound trajectory planning for volume of interest coverage. IEEE Conf Rob Autom. 2016; p. 736–41.
5. Ipsen S, Bruder R, O Brien R, et al. Online 4D ultrasound guidance for real-time motion compensation by MLC tracking. Med Phys. 2016;43(10):5695–704.
6. Tauscher S, Tokuda J, Schreiber G, et al. OpenIGTLink interface for state control and visualisation of a robot for image-guided therapy systems. Int J Comput Assist Radiol Surg. 2015;10(3):285–92.
7. Klemm M, Kirchner T, Gröhl J, et al. MITK-OpenIGTLink for combining open-source toolkits in real-time computer-assisted interventions. Int J Comput Assist Radiol Surg. 2016; p. 1–11.

Vergleich von Verfahren zur automatischen Detektion der Position und Orientierung des Herzens in 4D-Cine-MRT-Bilddaten

Marja Fleitmann[1], Ole Käferlein[1], Matthias Wilms[1], Dennis Säring[2], Heinz Handels[1], Jan Ehrhardt[1]

[1]Institut für Medizinische Informatik, Universität zu Lübeck
[2]Fachhochschule Wedel
wilms@imi.uni-luebeck.de

Kurzfassung. Räumlich-zeitliche 4D-Cine-MRT-Bilddaten werden in der klinischen Praxis zur Untersuchung der Herzbewegung eingesetzt. Um eine automatisierte Verarbeitung dieser Daten durch Segmentierungs- oder Registrierungsverfahren zu gewährleisten, ist als erster Schritt üblicherweise die initiale Bestimmung von Position und Orientierung des Herzens notwendig. Hierfür wurden bisher sowohl einfache grauwertbasierte Verfahren als auch lernbasierte Verfahren vorgeschlagen. Da bisher Vergleiche zwischen Verfahren aus diesen beiden Kategorien fehlen, erfolgt in diesem Beitrag ein quantitativer Vergleich zwischen einem klassisches Verfahren basierend auf der Untersuchung von zeitlichen Grauwertvarianzen und einer lernbasierten Hough Forest-Methode zur Detektion von multiplen Landmarken. Die Ergebnisse unserer Evaluation anhand von 10 4D-Cine-MRT-Bilddaten zeigen bezüglich der Initialisierungsgenauigkeit keine signifikanten Unterschiede zwischen beiden Verfahren.

1 Einleitung

Räumlich-zeitliche 4D-Cine-MRT-Bilddaten eignen sich durch den hohen Weichteilkontrast und die hohe zeitliche Auflösung optimal für die Untersuchung des sich bewegenden Herzens. Um aus den Bilddaten jedoch quantitative Informationen über die Herzbewegung, wie Volumina und weitere Funktionsparameter ableiten zu können, ist zumeist eine Segmentierung des Herzens notwendig [1], die im klinischen Alltag vollautomatisch erfolgen sollte.

Cine-MRT-Bilddaten sind in der Praxis oftmals durch Rauschen, Atemartefakte und teilweise homogene Strukturübergänge gekennzeichnet, weshalb sich u.a. besonders Segmentierungsverfahren als genau und robust erwiesen haben, die Vorwissen durch ein statistischen Formmodell nutzen [2] oder die Schätzung von Segmentierung und Bewegung koppeln [3]. Ausgangspunkt all dieser Verfahren ist eine Initialisierung, bei der der zu segmentierende Bereich als ROI bereits vereinfacht abgegrenzt bzw. ein Template initial platziert wird. Die Genauigkeit der Initialisierung wirkt sich dabei in der Regel direkt auf die Qualität der Segmentierung aus.

Klassische Methoden zur Lokalisation der Herzregion in kardialen Cine-MRT-Bilddaten stützen sich auf die Annahme, dass das Herz der sich über die Zeit am stärksten verändernde Bereich in den Bildern einer Herzsequenz ist. In [4, 5] werden daher voxelweise zeitliche Grauwertvarianzen berechnet, die mit geeigneter Nachverarbeitung zur Definition einer achsenparallelen quaderförmigen ROI genutzt werden. Klarer Nachteil der Verfahren ist die ohne Erweiterung fehlende Möglichkeit zur Schätzung der Orientierung des Herzens, welche für die genaue Initialisierung eines Templates notwendig ist. Diese Möglichkeit bieten aktuelle lernbasierte Verfahren zur automatischen Lokalisierung von multiplen Landmarken in Bildern, aus denen die Skalierung und Pose von Strukturen abgeleitet werden kann. Viele dieser Verfahren basieren auf Random Forests und definieren das Lokalisierungsproblem als Klassifikations- und/oder Regressionsaufgabe [6]. Diese Forest-basierten Verfahren wurden zuletzt schon erfolgreich zur Landmarkendetektion in kardialen Cine-MRT-Bilddaten eingesetzt [7] und versprechen eine schnelle Verarbeitung und genaue Ergebnisse. Allerdings fehlt bisher ein Vergleich zwischen klassischen und neueren Forest-basierten Methoden.

In diesem Beitrag präsentieren wir deshalb einen quantitativen Vergleich zur Bestimmung von Position und Orientierung des Herzens in Cine-MRT-Bilddaten zwischen: (1) Einer klassischen Methode zur Detektion der Herzposition, welche wir um eine einfache Möglichkeit zur Orientierungsschätzung mittels Templatematching erweitern und (2) einer adaptierten Version der im Bereich Computer Vision zur ROI-/Landmarkendetektion sehr erfolgreichen Hough Forests [8].

2   Material und Methoden

Gegeben ist ein in Kurzachse aufgenommener 4D-Cine-MRT-Datensatz bestehend aus N_j 3D Bildern $I_j : \Omega_P \to \mathbb{R}$ ($\Omega_P \subset \mathbb{R}^3$) mit $j \in \{1, \ldots, N_j\}$, die den Herzzyklus abbilden. Weiterhin gegeben ist ein Template des Herzens $T : \Omega_A \to \{0, 1, 2, 3\}$ ($\Omega_A \subset \mathbb{R}^3$) im Atlasraum Ω_A mit Labeln für Hintergrund, Myokard, linker und rechter Ventrikel. Ziel ist es dieses Template mittels einer Ähnlichkeitstransformation (7-DOF) $\varphi : \Omega_A \to \Omega_P$ optimal in einer Referenzphase I_R auszurichten.

2.1   Bewegungsdetektion und Template-Matching

Zunächst wird ein zweistufiger Ansatz zur Detektion der räumlichen Lage des Herzens in 4D-Cine-MRT-Daten betrachtet. Im ersten Schritt wird mittels klassischer Bewegungsdetektion für das Herz eine Region-of-interest (ROI) bestimmt. Um die gesuchte Transformation φ des Templates zu bestimmen, wird anschließend ein Template-Matching innerhalb der detektierten ROI durchgeführt.

ROI-Bestimmung mittels Bewegungsdetektion. Für die ROI-Bestimmung wird das von Cocosco et al. [4] vorgestellte Verfahren verwendet. Hierbei wird zunächst für jeden Bildvoxel die Standardabweichung der Grauwerte über die N_j

Herzphasen hinweg berechnet, wobei angenommen wird, dass hohe Grauwertvariationen die Bewegung des Herzen repräsenticren. Anschließend wird eine Maximumsintensitätsprojektion entlang der z-Achse des geglätteten Variationsbildes berechnet, und mittels Otsu-Schwellwert und morphologischer Nachverarbeitung eine Segmentierung erzeugt. Die entstandene ROI ist zweidimensional, allerdings robust und in zylindrischer Form für alle Schichten des 3D Bildes gültig.

Template-Matching. In dem durch die ROI eingeschränkten Bereich, kann anschließend deutlich schneller und robuster als für das gesamte Bild, ein Template-Matching durchgeführt werden. Zunächst werden die Labels des Template-Bildes durch typische Grauwerte für Myokard und Ventrikel ersetzt und an das Histogramms des Eingabebildes angepasst. Das Template-Matching erfolgt der Laufzeit halber schichtweise im 2D-Format, für jede der zentralen Schichten des Cine-MRT (Enddiastole) und dazu passenden Schichten im Template. Als Optimierungskriterium dient die normalisierte Kreuzkorrelation. Um Ausrichtung und Größe des Herzens zu bestimmen wird in diesem Prozess nur ein diskreter Satz von Rotationswinkeln und Skalierungsfaktoren getestet. Das 2D-Template-Matching generiert für die betrachteten Schichten des MR Bildes jeweils eine 2D-Transformation der zugehörigen Herzkonturen in der Template-Schicht. Mittels Least-Squares-Approximation wird dann die 3D-Transformation $\varphi : \Omega_A \to \Omega_P$ des Template-Bildes aus den transformierten Schichtbildern bestimmt.

2.2 Hough Forests

Hough Forests (HF) [8] sind ein lernbasiertes Verfahren zur Lokalisierung von u.a. Landmarken in Bildern. Die Lokalisierung wird hierbei im Random Forest-Framework als kombiniertes Regressions- und Klassifikationsproblem definiert.

Trainingsphase. Für das Training werden Bilder der gewählten Referenzphase von N_P Patienten P mit zugehöriger Herzsegmentierung und einer Landmarkenposition $l_P \in \Omega_P$ benötigt, wobei die Landmarken in allen Bildern an anatomisch korrespondierenden Punkten liegen.

Jedes Bild wird durch ein Gitter mit uniformen Gitterpunktabstand Δg gerastert. Jeder Gitterpunkt definiert das Zentrum $p_i \in \Omega_P$ eines kubischen Patches i mit Kantenlänge k, aus dem ein Merkmalsvektor $f_i \in \mathbb{R}^{N_f}$ extrahiert wird. Hierfür werden zufällig N_f Paare von Bildpunkten im Patch bestimmt, deren Intensitätsdifferenzen $f_i \in \mathbb{R}^{N_f}$ bilden. Zudem wird der Verschiebungsvektor $d_i = l_P - p_i$ zwischen Patchzentrum und Landmarkenposition und die durch die Segmentierung bestimmte Klassenzugehörigkeit (Herzregion: nein/ja) $c_i \in \{0, 1\}$ von p_i gespeichert. Ziel ist es mittels eines Random Forests eine Funktion zu lernen, die Merkmalvektoren der Herzregion auf Verschiebungsvektoren abbildet.

Hierzu wird anhand der Trainingspatches ein Forest bestehend aus N_b binären Bäumen gelernt. Jeder Baum trainiert indem rekursiv von der Wurzel bis zu den Blattknoten die Trainingsmenge geteilt wird, bis ein Abbruchkriterium erreicht ist (maximale Tiefe d; minimale Patchanzahl im Knoten N_m). Die optimale binäre Teilung der Trainingsdaten A in L und R an einem inneren Knoten erfolgt anhand einer zufälligen Dimension des Merkmalsvektors. Der benötigte Schwellwert wird zufällig entweder hinsichtlich Klassifikation oder Regression optimiert. Die Klassifikation wird mittels Informationsgewinn optimiert. Für die Regression wird die Varianz der Verschiebungsvektoren der Vordergrundpatches minimiert

$$V(L,R) = \sum_{i \in L} c_i \|\overline{d}_L - d_i\|_2^2 + \sum_{i \in R} c_i \|\overline{d}_R - d_i\|_2^2 \tag{1}$$

$\overline{d}_L$ und $\overline{d}_R$ bezeichnen jeweils die mittlere Verschiebung in L und R. Jeder Blattknoten speichert dann eine Liste von Verschiebungsvektoren der Vordergrundpatches und die Vordergrundklassenwahrscheinlichkeit.

Testphase. In der Testphase werden die Patches/Merkmalsvektoren des Testbildes in den trainierten Forest eingebracht. Landet ein Patch mit Position $p \in \Omega_P$ in einem Blattknoten, wird für jeden im Knoten vorhandenen Verschiebungsvektor d die mögliche Landmarkenposition $\tilde{l} = p + d$ berechnet und für diese in der Hough Map gewichtet mit der Vordergrundwahrscheinlichkeit abgestimmt. Die Größe der Hough Map entspricht der Bildgröße und wird von allen Bäumen des Forests befüllt. Ihr Maximum ist die geschätzte Landmarkenposition.

Mehrere Landmarken können lokalisiert werden, indem alle Landmarken gemeinsam in einem Vektor der Länge $3N_l$ kodiert und geschätzt werden. Die gesuchte Transformation $\varphi : \Omega_A \rightarrow \Omega_P$ wird dann anhand dieser Landmarken ermittelt.

2.3   Experimente

Zur Evaluation der beiden Verfahren werden 10 4D-Cine-MRT-Bilddaten (Kurzachse, 30 Phasen) von Patienten mit akutem Myokardinfarkt verwendet. Jedes 3D-Bild besteht aus $256 - 320 \times 256 - 320 \times 8 - 15$ Voxeln mit Spacing $1.4 - 1.5$ mm $\times$ $1.4 - 1.5$ mm $\times 10$ mm. Manuelle Segmentierungen der Herzregion (linker und rechter Ventrikel) liegen für alle Phasen vor. Zur Vorverarbeitung werden Bias- und Intensitätskorrektur durchgeführt und alle Bilder auf eine einheitliche Schichtauflösung von 1.5 mm $\times$ 1.5 mm gesampled (Pipeline wie in [3]). Für die HF-Methode wird zur Intensitätsdifferenzberechnung zwischen Schichten durch registrierungsbasierte Interpolation die Schichtdicke auf 1.5 mm verringert.

Als Referenzphase wird die enddiastolische (ED) Phase gewählt. Die Segmentierung der Herzregion eines registrierungsbasiert ähnlich zu [9] aus der ED-Phase aller 10 Datensätze erstellten mittleren Herzatlas dient als Template. Im Atlas werden zudem manuell in der Herzregion $N_l = 5$ Landmarken definiert, die dann registrierungsbasiert in die ED-Phasen der einzelnen Patienten übertragen werden und dort als Referenzpositionen dienen.

Zum Vergleich wird mit beiden Methoden für alle 10 Datensätze in der ED-Phase die Ähnlichkeitstransformation zwischen Template und Patient bestimmt.

Tabelle 1. Mittelwerte und Standardabweichungen für Dice-Koeffizient und mittlere Oberflächendistanz $\bar{d}_O$ zwischen dem transformierten Template und der Expertensegmentierung jedes Patienten für die getesteten Verfahren. Für die HF wird zusätzlich der mittlere Landmarkenfehler $\bar{d}_L$ angegeben.

	Dice	$\bar{d}_O$ [mm]	$\bar{d}_L$ [mm]
Bewegungsdetektion+Matching	0.80 ± 0.15	4.70 ± 5.17	–
Hough Forests	0.86 ± 0.06	3.42 ± 1.79	4.66 ± 2.05
Hough Forests (nur Regression)	0.86 ± 0.06	3.37 ± 1.48	6.11 ± 4.12

Zum Training der HF wird Leave-One-Out-Kreuzvalidierung eingesetzt. Zudem werden für die HF zwei Konfigurationen getestet: (1) Standard HF (2) HF ohne Klassifikationsknoten (votingbasierte Regression). Der quantitative Vergleich erfolgt anhand des Dice-Koeff. und des mittleren Oberflächenabstandes $\bar{d}_O$ zwischen transformiertem Template und Referenzsegmentierung. Für die HF-Konfigurationen wird zudem der mittlere Landmarkenfehler $\bar{d}_L$ ermittelt.

Die Parameter der HF-Methode wurden gewählt als: $\Delta g = 7.5$ mm; $k = 16.5$ mm; $N_f = 500$; $N_b = 50$ Trees; max. Tiefe $d = 17$; $N_m = 10$ Patches.

3 Ergebnisse

Tab. 1 fasst die quantitativen Ergebnisse der Experimente zusammen. Bezogen auf die in Tab. 1 aufgeführten Mittelwerte für Dice-Koeff. und mittlere Oberflächendistanz, lassen sich mittels gepaartem t-Test keine signifikanten Unterschiede ($p > 0.05$) zwischen der klassischen Bewegungsdetektionsmethode und den beiden HF-Konfigurationen feststellen. Die Ähnlichkeit der Ergebnisse ist in den Beispielen in Abb. 1 zu sehen, die die generell gute Annäherung an die Herzregion zeigen. Auch zwischen den getesteten HF-Konfigurationen lässt sich für keines der 3 Maße ein signifikanter Unterschied feststellen. Generell ist hervorzuheben, dass die hier erzielten Landmarkenfehler im Bereich der Werte liegen, die auch andere aktuelle Forest-basierte Verfahren [7] erzielen. Die klassische Methode benötigt ca. 1 Minute für die Detektion, wohingegen die Detektion mittels HF ≈ 7 Minuten dauert (beides auf Xeon Quad-core @ 2.67GHz).

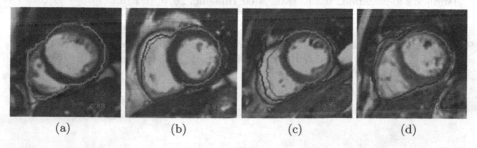

(a)   (b)   (c)   (d)

Abb. 1. Beispielkonturen des transformierten Templates für beide Methoden (blau: HF; rot: Bewegungsdetektion) für 4 verschiedene Patienten. Die Dice-Koeffizienten sind farbig im Bild markiert.

4 Diskussion

Die automatisierte Bestimmung von Position und Orientierung des Herzens in 4D-Cine-MRT-Bilddaten ist im klinischen Alltag ein wichtiger Vorverarbeitungsschritt zur automatisierten Bestimmung von Funktionsparametern des Herzens. In diesem Beitrag wurden zwei Verfahren zur initialen Posenbestimmung des Herzens in diesen Daten verglichen: Eine klassischen Methode, die auf der Untersuchung zeitlicher Grauwertvarianzen basiert, und eine Hough Forest-Methode zur Detektion von multiplen Landmarken. Die Evaluation hat gezeigt, dass beide Verfahren vergleichbare Ergebnisse liefern, die HF aber bei der Detektion wesentlich langsamer sind. Hierbei ist allerdings anzumerken, dass bei einer optimierten Implementierung Laufzeiten für die HF von unter 20 Sekunden zu erwarten sind [7].

Danksagung. Diese Arbeit wurde durch die DFG gefördert (EH 224/6-1).

Literaturverzeichnis

1. Säring D, Ehrhardt J, Stork A, et al. Computer-assisted analysis of 4D cardiac MR image sequences after myocardial infarction. Methods Inf Med. 2006;45(4):377–83.
2. Peng P, Lekadir K, Gooya A, et al. A review of heart chamber segmentation for structural and functional analysis using cardiac magnetic resonance imaging. Magn Reson Mater Phy. 2016;29(2):155–95.
3. Ehrhardt J, Kepp T, Schmidt-Richberg A, et al. Joint multi-object registration and segmentation of left and right cardiac ventricles in 4D cine MRI. Proc SPIE Med Imaging. 2014; p. 90340M.
4. Cocosco CA, Netsch T, Sénégas J, et al.; Elsevier. Automatic cardiac region-of-interest computation in cine 3D structural MRI. Proc CARS. 2004;1268:1126–31.
5. Hoffmann R, Bertelshofer F, Siegl C, et al. Automated heart localization in cardiac cine MR data. Proc BVM. 2016; p. 116–21.
6. Criminisi A, Robertson D, Konukoglu E, et al. Regression forests for efficient anatomy detection and localization in computed tomography scans. Med Image Anal. 2013;17(8):1293–303.
7. Oktay O, Bai W, Guerrero R, et al. Stratified decision forests for accurate anatomical landmark localization. IEEE Trans Med Imaging. 2016; p. n/a.
8. Gall J, Yao A, Razavi N, et al. Hough forests for object detection, tracking, and action recognition. IEEE Trans Pattern Anal Mach Intell. 2011;33(11):2188–202.
9. Ehrhardt J, Werner R, Schmidt-Richberg A, et al. Statistical modeling of 4D respiratory lung motion using diffeomorphic image registration. IEEE Trans Med Imaging. 2011;30(2):251–65.

Evaluation of Multi-Channel Image Registration in Microscopy

Sascha E.A. Muenzing[1], Andreas S. Thum[2], Katja Bühler[3], Dorit Merhof[1]

[1]Institute of Imaging and Computer Vision, RWTH Aachen University, Germany
[2]Department of Biology, University of Konstanz, Germany
[3]VRVis Research Center, Vienna, Austria
sascha.muenzing@rwth-aachen.de

Abstract. Drosophila melanogaster, commonly known as fruit fly, is an important genetic model organism for fundamental neuroscience research. The central nervous system of the larva consists of about 12,000 neurons. For efficient information retrieval and automated data mining, each patterns needs to be mapped onto a common reference space. Accurate image registration plays a key role here. We investigate standard and multi-channel image registration approaches. Our evaluation shows that multi-channel registration is beneficial in cases where the staining quality is partially compromised and can be complemented by the information contained in an additional reference channel.

1   Introduction

How is behavior output organized in a brain based on external sensory inputs, internal motivational states or even knowledge gained through prior experience?

Understanding is the most essential issue in the field of neuroscience. For centuries, researchers in the functional brain sciences have been mapping properties of behavior to areas of the brain. Yet, the step from simple maps to a generally accepted model has proven exceedingly difficult. Among the extremely reduced model organisms (e.g. C. elegans or Aplysia) that only on a constricted level allow for meaningful comparisons with humans, and more complex vertebrate systems (e.g. mouse, zebra fish) that have numerical, ethical and technical constraints, the classical genetic model organism Drosophila has acquired an important intermediate position. Even Drosophila larvae, simple foraging animals of about half a centimeter in size, were recently shown to provide relatively fast imaging of the entire nervous system with light and electron microscopes and reconstruction of complete circuits [1]. Fig. 1 shows a typical light microscopy image stack of an immunohistochemically stained sample of the central nervous system (CNS) of the Drosophila larva. The neuropil might be described in laymen terms as connective tissue in which the neurons and nerve tracts are embedded. The neuropil staining gives an overall picture of the brain anatomy, whereas the staining of the second reference channel especially highlights the nerve tracts. The relevant new information is present in the staining of specific neurons. There are three stages in the development of the larva – each stage is defined by the molting of the larva – before the metamorphosis into the adult stage where the larva develops into a fly. We aim to establish a comprehensive 4D reconstruction of the about 12,000 neurons of the larval CNS. In each image sample specific neurons are marked based on their genetic information. In order to efficiently compare specific neurons and corresponding information from functional, developmental, and behavioral studies (e.g. [2]), the neuronal expression pattern needs to be mapped onto a common reference space. Accurate image coregistration is therefore a prerequisite for reliable information retrieval and automated data mining (e.g. [3]). In this work we therefore investigate single and multi-channel registration approaches including both reference channel images of the CNS of the Drosophila larva in its third developmental stage.

2   Materials and methods

In previous work we constructed a standard template image of the CNS of the Drosophila larva in its third developmental stage, for both reference channels (Fig. 4). A standard template image is a shape and intensity averaged image representation, also called standard brain template. The construction of the template images was based on deformable registration of the neuropil channel because it is the most common reference staining and it depicts larger compact anatomical regions with fine structures of nerve tracts embedded. The staining of the tracts channel highlights nerve tracts in particular (Fig. 1).

2.1   Image data

For our experiments we used 20 images of various quality taken from a large image database [4] established at the Janelia Farm Research Campus, Howard Hughes Medical Institute, Ashburn, USA. Immunolabeled larval nervous systems were imaged on a Zeiss 510 confocal microscope using a 40× oil immersion objective (numerical aperture 1.3). Images of each nervous system were assembled

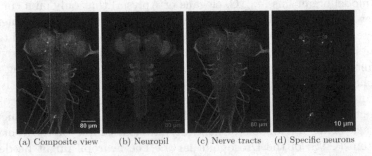

(a) Composite view   (b) Neuropil   (c) Nerve tracts   (d) Specific neurons

Fig. 1. Exemplary multi-channel image of the larval CNS. The pictures show maximum intensity projections perpendicular to the scanning plane: (a) Composite view of all three channels, (b,c) the two reference channels (Neuropil, Tracts), and (d) the expression pattern channel highlighting specific neurons.

from a 2×3 array of tiled stacks, with each stack scanned as an 8 bit image with
a resolution of 512×512 and a Z-step interval of 2 μm. The acquired images have
a size of about 980×1,430×100 voxels with in plane resolution of about 0.5 μm
and slice thickness of mostly 2 μm. We refer to Li et al. [4] for information
on the larval dissection and the employed immunohistochemistry as well as for
anatomical information about Drosophila.

2.2   Image registration approaches

The registration problem can be formulated as an optimization problem in which
the cost function $\mathcal{C}$ is minimized w.r.t. the transformation $\mathbf{T} : \Omega_F \subset \mathbb{R}^d \to \Omega_M \subset \mathbb{R}^d$, such that $\mathbf{T}(\mathbf{x}) = \mathbf{x} + \mathbf{u}(\mathbf{x})$ spatially aligns the moving image $I_M(\mathbf{T}(\mathbf{x}))$ to
the fixed image $I_F(\mathbf{x})$

$$\hat{\mu} = \arg\min_{\mu} \mathcal{C}(\mathbf{T}_\mu; I_F, I_M) \tag{1}$$

where the subscript μ indicates that the transform has been parametrized. The
vector μ contains the values of the "transformation parameters". For an affine
transformation $\mathbf{T}_\mu$ the vector μ has a length of 12. In case of parametrization
with a B-Spline grid [5], the parameters μ are formed by the corresponding B-
spline coefficients which number depends on the B-Spline control point spacing
and the image size. Standard (single-channel) image registration involves one
fixed image and one moving image, using one similarity metric to define the
fit. In multi-channel image registration, multiple fixed and moving images are
involved and therefore a combined similarity metric is needed. In this case the
registration cost function can be defined as:

$$\mathcal{C}(\mathbf{T}; I_F, I_M) = \frac{1}{\sum_{i=1}^{N} \omega_i} \sum_{i=1}^{N} \omega_i \mathcal{C}_i(\mathbf{T}; I_F^i, I_M^i) \tag{2}$$

with ω_i the weights and $\mathcal{C}_i$ the sub-metric for each channel. This way one can
simultaneously register different image channels possibly using a different similarity metric for each channel. We employ the Elastix registration toolbox [6]
version 4.8 for our experiments. In the following the employed registration setup
is described which consists of a global registration followed by a deformable registration, for both the single-channel and the multi-channel registration approach.

Single-channel registration The global registration consists of an affine transformation with a multi-resolution scheme of four levels. In the final level the full
image resolution is used and at each coarser level the image resolution is halved.
The adaptive stochastic gradient descent optimizer [7] is used along with the
normalized correlation coefficient as similarity metric. At each resolution level
1,000 iterations of random coordinate sampling of 6,000 intensity values are conducted. The deformable registration consists of a B-Spline transformation with
a control point spacing of 12×12×12 μm³ at the original image resolution and
doubled at each coarser resolution level. An image mask for the fixed image is

used that is generated by thresholding off the background of the template image (Fig. 4). Within the image mask covering the CNS, 2,000 intensity values are sampled at a randomly located region of $20{\times}20{\times}20\,\mu m^3$ in the full resolution level and doubled at each coarser level up to maximal $80{\times}80{\times}80\,\mu m^3$. The multi-resolution scheme, optimizer and similarity metric are identical to the global registration.

Multi-channel registration The parameters for the global and deformable image registration are identical to the single-channel registration setup, however, in both registration steps the cost function according to Eq. (2) is used with $i = 1 \ldots 2$ to register both reference image channels simultaneously. An alternative weighting method is evaluated using relative weights r_i for the i-th metric. The weight ω_i is computed in each iteration based on the gradient $\mathbf{g}_i = \frac{\partial \mathcal{C}_i}{\partial \mu}$ of the sub-metric

$$\omega_i = r_i \frac{|\mathbf{g}_0|}{|\mathbf{g}_i|} \tag{3}$$

with $|\mathbf{g}_0|$ the magnitude of the gradient of the first sub-metric. In the following we refer to the standard weighting in Eq. 2 by absolute weighting and to the weighting scheme in Eq. (3) by relative weighting. The weights are set to $\omega_i = 0.5$ and $r_i = 0.5$, respectively, for comparison of both weighting schemes on our image data with two reference channels to be registered.

3   Evaluation & results

We assess the image registration accuracy based on a gold standard of manually annotated landmarks. An expert in neurobiology defined 30 anatomical landmarks at distinct positions that are clearly visible in the neuropil and tracts staining and which underlie little anatomical variation. The position of the landmarks are visualized by the yellow circles in Fig. 4. The intra-rater annotation accuracy over all landmarks per scan is on average $2.0{\pm}0.3\,\mu m$ with a maximum deviation of $6.3{\pm}2.7\,\mu m$, assessed on four images annotated twice. The template image and each of the 20 images used in our experiments was annotated with up to 30 landmarks, only in two cases not all 30 landmarks could be reliably found because of partially insufficient image quality. Tab. 1 lists the registration accuracy of the single-channel and the two multi-channel registration approaches using one or both of the reference image channels, respectively. Although there is a slight improvement of the multi-channel registration approaches over the "NP" registration, the differences are not statistically significant based on the two-sided paired Student's t-test.

4   Discussion

In general, the neuropil channel appears better suited for multi-resolution image registration because it contains coarse compact as well as fine detailed structures.

However, there are cases of images where the neuropil staining is of inconsistent quality, i.e. it is partially weak, or the staining is overall weak, i.e. fine structures and the border between larger compartments are hardly visible (Fig. 4). In such cases, the inclusion of the tracts channel into the image registration can yield improved registration accuracy (Fig. 4 (c,g) and corresponding results of the registration number 3 in Tab. 1. Fig. 4 (d,h) depicts a case where the staining of the nerve tracts appears abnormal, registration number 4 in Tab. 1. Although the registration accuracy decreases in that case in the multi-channel registration approaches compared to the single-channel neuropil registration, the accuracy remains relatively good compared to the single-channel tracts registration. Overall, both multi-channel registration approaches appear robust and improved registration accuracy slightly on this challenging image data.

References

1. Ohyama T, Schneider-Mizell CM, Fetter RD, et al. A multilevel multimodal circuit enhances action selection in Drosophila. Nature. 2015;520(7549):633–9.
2. Rohwedder A, Wenz N, Stehle B, et al. Four individually identified paired dopamine neurons signal reward in larval Drosophila. Curr Biol. 2016;26(5):661–9.
3. Ganglberger F, Schulze F, Tirian L, et al. Structure-based neuron retrieval across Drosophila brains. Neuroinformatics. 2014;12(3):423–34.
4. Li HH, Kroll J, Lennox S, et al. A GAL4 driver resource for developmental and behavioral studies on the larval CNS of Drosophila. Cell Rep. 2014;8(3):897–908.
5. Rueckert D, Sonoda LI, Hayes C, et al. Nonrigid registration using free-form deformations: application to breast MR images. IEEE Trans Med Imaging. 1999;18(8):712–21.

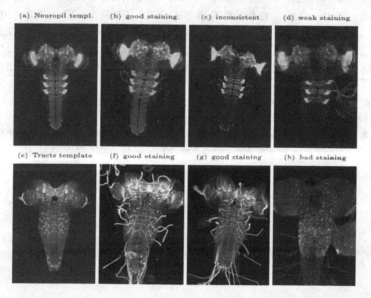

Fig. 2. Maximum intensity Z-projections of the template images (a,e) and different confocal microscopy images of the larval CNS with varying image quality.

Table 1. Evaluation of the accuracy of single and dual-channel registration approaches. NP: neuropil, TC: tracts. NP+TC: 50/50 weighted combination, abs: absolute weight, rel: relative weight, max: maximum landmark registration error.

	Landmark registration error [μm]											
	NP			TC			NP+TC abs			NP+TC rel		
#	mean	sd	max	mean	sd	max	mean	sd	max	mean	sd	max
1	7.7	(7.1)	26	13.1	(15.8)	52	7.4	(7.4)	26	7.3	(7.2)	26
2	4.2	(3.7)	14	5.5	(4.2)	16	4.3	(3.7)	14	4.2	(3.8)	14
3	7.1	(6.7)	23	5.5	(5.2)	25	4.9	(5.0)	21	4.9	(4.9)	21
4	6.8	(6.4)	21	29.0	(13.2)	53	9.8	(10.4)	38	9.3	(8.8)	35
5	7.8	(6.3)	31	8.3	(6.6)	29	7.8	(6.4)	31	7.6	(6.5)	31
6	5.0	(4.2)	16	6.2	(5.3)	21	4.9	(4.1)	17	4.9	(4.0)	16
7	6.3	(6.5)	27	5.9	(5.2)	22	6.3	(6.8)	27	6.5	(7.0)	26
8	5.2	(5.2)	24	6.7	(6.5)	29	5.0	(5.3)	22	5.1	(5.5)	24
9	4.2	(3.6)	19	5.4	(4.5)	18	4.2	(3.7)	18	4.1	(3.8)	18
10	10.0	(12.2)	46	10.1	(9.5)	31	7.6	(9.2)	33	7.3	(8.4)	31
11	4.9	(3.1)	14	11.2	(12.0)	45	4.7	(2.7)	12	4.5	(2.7)	11
12	4.5	(5.1)	25	8.4	(11.3)	43	4.3	(4.8)	23	4.4	(5.0)	25
13	4.6	(4.4)	25	6.5	(6.6)	32	4.4	(4.1)	22	4.2	(4.0)	22
14	3.5	(2.6)	10	5.4	(5.2)	25	3.6	(2.5)	11	3.3	(2.4)	10
15	4.2	(2.9)	14	4.4	(3.3)	14	3.9	(2.9)	14	3.9	(2.9)	14
16	4.6	(3.2)	14	5.1	(3.1)	15	4.5	(3.2)	15	4.5	(3.2)	15
17	5.4	(6.8)	29	6.6	(6.6)	27	5.4	(6.4)	28	5.1	(6.2)	27
18	6.4	(5.4)	20	42.6	(23.7)	95	6.8	(5.5)	20	6.3	(5.6)	21
19	6.5	(7.2)	27	13.4	(11.8)	43	6.5	(7.3)	28	6.4	(7.6)	29
20	4.3	(2.8)	12	4.6	(2.5)	10	4.0	(2.8)	11	4.0	(2.7)	11
Avg	5.66	(5.3)	21.9	10.20	(8.1)	32.2	5.51	(5.2)	21.5	5.39	(5.1)	21.3

6. Klein S, Staring M, Murphy K, et al. Elastix: a toolbox for intensity-based medical image registration. IEEE Trans Med Imaging. 2010;29(1):196–205.
7. Klein S, Pluim JPW, Staring M, et al. Adaptive stochastic gradient descent optimisation for image registration. Int J Computer Vis. 2009;81(3):227–39.

Abstract: Medical Research Data Management Using MITK and XNAT
Connecting Medical Image Software and Data Management Systems in a Research Context

Caspar Jonas Goch, Jasmin Metzger, Marco Nolden

Division for Medical and Biological Informatics, DKFZ Heidelberg
c.goch@dkfz.de

Image and data processing plays an increasingly important role in medical research. Improvements in acquisition techniques and collaborations across traditionally separate research fields, such as fusing genomics and radiological information in decision making, lead to an ever increasing, in number as well as in size, amount of data. Managing and sharing this amount of data remains an important area of study. One well-known solution to this problem is the extensible neuroimaging archive toolkit (XNAT) [1], which provides a storage and management solution for large amounts of disparate data. However the processing of data remains largely separate and requires a lot of manual interaction.

We present a free and open source solution for managing such research data integrated with powerful tools for image processing. Our solution is based on the Medical Imaging Interaction Toolkit (MITK) [2] and offers the option to manage data in an XNAT from within an MITK application.

We will present an easy and intuitive workflow, downloading data from the server, segmenting the data and uploading the results back to the server, without leaving the application. This enables faster, more convenient interaction and improves the acceptance of research data management solutions, such as XNAT. This in turn improves traceability of data and processing done on data, as well as open the door to remote, or cloud based processing using the XNAT pipeline framework.

Our goal are workflows resulting in open software and open data publications, particularily in light of the concern which has been raised regarding the reproducability of research results in recent years [3, 4].

References

1. Marcus DS, Olsen TR, Ramaratnam M, et al. The extensible neuroimaging archive toolkit. Neuroinformatics. 2007;5(1):11–33.
2. Nolden M, Zelzer S, Seitel A, et al. The medical imaging interaction toolkit: challenges and advances. Int J Comput Assist Radiol Surg. 2013;8(4):607–20.
3. Nosek BA, Alter G, Banks GC, et al. Promoting an open research culture. Sci. 2015;348(6242):1422–5.
4. Baker M. 1,500 scientists lift the lid on reproducibility. Nat. 2016;533(7604):452–4.

Fully Automated Multi-Modal Anatomic Atlas Generation Using 3D-Slicer

Julia Rackerseder[1], Antonio Miguel Luque González[1], Charlotte Düwel[2],
Nassir Navab[1,3], Benjamin Frisch[1]

[1]Computer Aided Medical Procedures, Technische Universität München, Germany
[2]Urologische Klinik und Poliklinik, Technische Universität München, Germany
[3]Johns Hopkins University, Baltimore, MD, USA
julia.rackerseder@tum.de

Abstract. Atlases of the human body have many applications, including for instance the analysis of information from patient cohorts to evaluate the distribution of tumours and metastases. We present a 3D Slicer module that simplifies the task of generating a multi-modal atlas from anatomical and functional data. It provides for a simpler evaluation of existing image and verbose patient data by integrating a database that is automatically generated from text files and accompanies the visualization of the atlas volume. The computation of the atlas is a two step process. First, anatomical data is pairwise registered to a reference dataset with an affine initialization and a B-Spline based deformable approach. Second, the computed transformations are applied to anatomical as well as the corresponding functional data to generate both atlases. The module is validated with a publicly available soft tissue sarcoma dataset from The Cancer Imaging Archive. We show that functional data in the atlas volume correlates with the findings from the patient database.

1 Introduction

Atlases of the human body have, although they might be challenging to create, a plethora of applications. A possible use case is the study of anatomic principles, such as creating a detailed model of the human heart from multi-slice computed tomography (CT) [1]. They can also serve as a basis for registering unseen subjects to a previously studied cohort of imaging volumes, allowing for a comparison of the patient's anatomy with the atlas and helping with the segmentation of structures within a certain area [2] for breast density assessment. Yet another field of application would be the better understanding of the distribution of tumors and metastases in certain cancer types in order to predict outcome and progress of the condition in patients, as done by Hegemann et al. [3].

Atlas generation is mostly based on anatomical imaging modalities such as CT and magnetic resonance imaging (MRI) that offer excellent image quality and resolution. Functional imaging modalities, in particular from nuclear medicine, are limited by their spatial resolution and lack of anatomical information. However, nuclear imaging is nowadays mostly coupled to CT or MRI, situating the functional information in its anatomic environment. Besides allowing for an improved interpretation of this information [4], it allows generating atlases of functional information based on the registered anatomical information.

The objective of this work is to present a simple, fully automated method to compute a multi-modal anatomical and functional atlas with the integrated creation and visualization of a MySQL database. We further allow for the display of text-based information, that can be included in the database, alongside structural and functional data.

State-of-the-art atlas generation tools such as AtlasWerks [5] are, although powerful in terms of algorithmic flexibility, limited to mono-modal atlas generation. They are hard to use for non-trained users because they are command-line based or restricted to special use cases, like the alignment of specific organs [6]. As an alternative to these methods, we present an easy to use framework that allows for the effortless computation of combined anatomical and functional atlas volumes and integrates text-based patient information into an automatically generated database.

2   Materials and methods

This work uses 3D Slicer [7], an open-source tool intended to analyze and visualize medical imaging data. It includes ITK (Insight Segmentation and Registration Toolkit, https://itk.org), an open-source library with a large variety of algorithms for the segmentation and registration of 2D and 3D medical images.

We introduce a module that automatically builds a patient database from text files and incorporates it with a computed anatomical atlas with additional information from a second modality, such as functional data obtained from pre-aligned multi-modal 3D patient data.

2.1   Database creation

Patient data that is intended for further examination in studies by physicians or lab staff is often stored in spread sheets or tab/comma separated files. While this may be simple to use, it renders data less accessible for evaluation or statistical analysis. Our module provides a script that reads information from such a file to automatically build a MySQL database while choosing all needed parameters and the database schema in an automated manner.

2.2   Registration pipeline

The module requires as inputs both the text file and medical image data from multiple patients, consisting of information from an anatomical imaging modality such as CT or MRI along with pre-aligned (functional) data such as from positron emission tomography (PET) or single photon emission computed tomography (SPECT). It is also possible to use manually labelled and segmented data instead of functional images. The registration pipeline starts with an affine registration of every single volume to a predefined reference volume in a pairwise fashion according to a given batch file. This brings all patient images into a common reference frame and thus allows for an accurate and fast atlas creation. Each registration is initialized with the center of mass of the two respective volumes. The user is advised to choose the template patient carefully, since it might have an influence on the quality of the resulting atlas. Then, a deformable registration can be performed. We chose to use a free-form deformation model based on B-splines [8], since it is suitable for several modalities including CT and MRI. The implementation is based on 3D Slicer's "Expert Automated Registration" module. For both registration steps, Mattes mutual information is used as a cost function in order to allow for more variability in the input data, such as different scanning protocols. The maximum number of iterations can be limited for both the affine and deformable registrations, such as to terminate the process in the case that no global minimum in the cost function can be found. Further, a multi-resolution optimization scheme is employed to avoid local minima. Each level is initialized with the result of the predecessor registration of the downsampled image and a coarser grid.

2.3   Atlas computation

For the atlas generation, the final transformation estimates of the affine and B-Spline registrations are applied to the anatomic volumes of the respective patient. The same transformations are also applied to the corresponding functional volumes. Thus both modalities are registered to the reference patient, without requiring a less accurate alignment of the functional images themselves. The anatomical atlas is created by averaging over all registered image information at each voxel. For the functional atlas preparation, the data usually needs to be normalized before computing the mean across all patients, to make the data comparable. The functional atlas is inherently aligned to the anatomical atlas due to the intra-patient pre-alignment from the multi-modal imaging device and the application of the same transformation to both patient image sets.

2.4   Visualization

After finishing the database and atlas computations, both can be visualized alongside within the 3D Slicer module and are available for further evaluation.

3   Results

We validate the presented method by building a multi-modal atlas from a soft tissue sarcoma dataset publicly available at The Cancer Imaging Archive [9, 10]. We used FDG-PET/CT images from 24 patients with histologically confirmed soft-tissue sarcoma (STS) of the lower extremities. For all patients in this retrospective study, personal and clinical data such as gender, age, histopathological type and tumor grade are available in a spread sheet. Our module's script used the sheet to create a database file that stores all information and included it into a local MySQL server that is connected to 3D Slicer. The simple database schema can be seen in Fig. 1a).

The registration pipeline was parametrized with a maximum number of 50 and 20 iterations for the affine and deformable registration, respectively. The sampling ratio was set to 0.075, which means that only 7.5% of the image information is used to estimate the transformation, making it significantly faster while preserving enough image information for a good registration result. We use a 4 level multi-resolution approach.

The PET data is normalized using the standardized uptake value (SUV), which is calculated for each voxel from the PET DICOM dataset. The SUV is a ratio of measured radioactivity at a certain voxel c and the complete injected dose d set in relation to patient weight w, elapsed time t between the injection and the acquisition of the image and half-life of the used nuclide $t_{0.5}$. It is calculated in the following way

$$SUV = c \cdot \frac{1000 \cdot w}{d \cdot e^{\frac{-0.693 \cdot t}{t_{0.5}}}}$$

The PET atlas is comprised of the average over all SUV values at each voxel. Results for the combined multi-modal atlas are shown in Fig. 2. The combined PET/CT atlas is shown in all three planes, with CT being visualized in greyscale and PET overlayed in a commonly used color map. The intensities range from dark blue (low radioactivity uptake) over red (high) to yellow (maximum uptake). In the example case, an accumulation of high SUV can be observed in the left upper thigh, which correlates with the evaluation of the counts of the "Site of primary STS" in the database, which are shown in Fig. 1b). The table

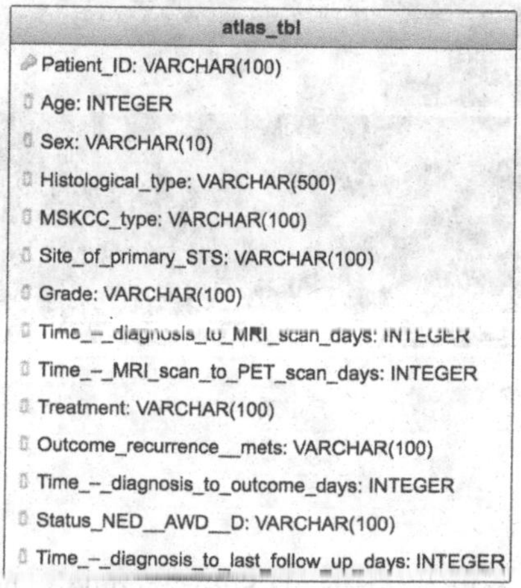

atlas_tbl
Patient_ID: VARCHAR(100)
Age: INTEGER
Sex: VARCHAR(10)
Histological_type: VARCHAR(500)
MSKCC_type: VARCHAR(100)
Site_of_primary_STS: VARCHAR(100)
Grade: VARCHAR(100)
Time_-_diagnosis_to_MRI_scan_days: INTEGER
Time_-_MRI_scan_to_PET_scan_days: INTEGER
Treatment: VARCHAR(100)
Outcome_recurrence__mets: VARCHAR(100)
Time_-_diagnosis_to_outcome_days: INTEGER
Status_NED__AWD__D: VARCHAR(100)
Time_-_diagnosis_to_last_follow_up_days: INTEGER

(a)

Site of primary STS	count
left thigh	10
right thigh	4
right calf	3
right quadricep	2
left poplietal fossa	1
left calf	1
right buttock	1
left adductur	1
right knee	1

(b)

Fig. 1. (a) Database schema automatically generated from the publicly available soft tissue sarcoma dataset. (b) Distribution of sites of primary STS as noted in the patient information database.

shows that almost 42% of the patients in this cohort suffer from sarcoma in the left thigh, whereas only 17% and 13% have cancer in the right thigh or calf, respectively. Only a small subgroup or single patients have confirmed STS in other regions of the leg. These findings are reflected in the multi-modal atlas, where mean SUV inside the volume of interest is almost 30 times higher than outside (4.7 vs. 0.16).

4   Discussion

This work introduces a fully automated 3D Slicer plugin to generate a multi-modal 3D atlas comprised of anatomical and functional data as well as a fully integrated MySQL database for a straightforward use in clinical studies. We show that the B-Spline based registration method is suitable for the creation of a PET/CT atlas and expect it to also be applicable for other imaging modalities such as PET/MRI [6]. The correlation of findings from our sample study, showing that the most probable region of high SUV coincides with the clinical findings, demonstrates that the tool allows for a fast and simple reading of functional data and interlinkage with the information gained from the incorporated database. This ease of generating and comparing information is a distinctive feature when compared with other tools, where such inter-modal analysis is hard to facilitate.

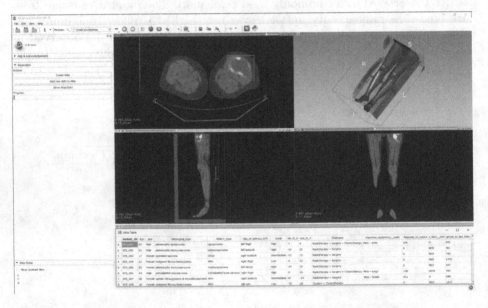

Fig. 2. Screenshot of atlas and patient database in our 3D Slicer module. The atlas volume can be viewed in all three image planes, as well as volumetric rendering. CT data is shown in greyscale, PET images are overlayed in a heatmap coloring scheme. Volume of interest is outlined in red in all three planes.

The presented 3D Slicer module can be enhanced by including further registration algorithms, diverse cost functions and several options for the final fusion of all images. An extensive set of features for the statistical analysis of the highlighted areas in the atlas and the automated computation of graphs and charts will support users of this tool. The tool will be made available to our clinical partners to support the analysis of data that has not yet been evaluated, thereby providing a final validation of its applicability to clinical studies.

References

1. Hoogendoorn C, Duchateau N, Sánchez-Quintana Dea. A high-resolution atlas and statistical model of the human heart from multislice CT. IEEE Trans Med Imaging. 2013;32(1):28–44.
2. Ortiz CG, Martel A. Automatic atlas-based segmentation of the breast in MRI for 3D breast volume computation. Med Phys. 2012;39(10):5835–48.
3. Hegemann NS, Wenter V, Spath Sea. Distribution of prostate nodes: a PET/CT-derived anatomic atlas of prostate cancer patients before and after surgical treatment. Radiat Oncol. 2016;11(1):1.
4. Evans AC, Marrett S, Torrescorzo Jea. MRI-PET correlation in three dimensions using a volume-of-interest (VOI) atlas. J Cereb Blood Flow Metab. 1991;11(1 suppl):A69–A78.
5. Institute S; 2016. AtlasWerks: An open-source (BSD license) software package for medical image atlas generation. Scientific Computing and Imaging Institute (SCI), Download from: http://www.sci.utah.edu/software/atlaswerks.html.
6. Peressutti D, Sinclair M, et al WB. A framework for combining a motion atlas with non-motion information to learn clinically useful biomarkers: application to cardiac resynchronisation therapy response prediction. Med Image Anal. 2017;35:669–84. Available from: http://www.sciencedirect.com/science/article/pii/S1361841516301815.
7. Fedorov A, Beichel R, Kalpathy-Cramer Jea. 3D slicer as an image computing platform for the Quantitative imaging network. J Magn Reson Imaging. 2012;30(9):1323–41.
8. Rueckert D, Sonoda LI, Hayes Cea. Nonrigid registration using free-form deformations: application to breast MR images. IEEE Trans Med Imaging. 1999;18(8):712–21.
9. Clark K, Vendt B, Smith Kea. The cancer imaging archive (TCIA): maintaining and operating a public information repository. J Digit Imaging. 2013;26(6):1045–57.
10. Freeman C, Skamene S, El Naqa Iea. A radiomics model from joint FDG-PET and MRI texture features for the prediction of lung metastases in soft-tissue sarcomas of the extremities. Phys Med Biol. 2015;60(14):5471.

Automatic Classification and Pathological Staging of Confocal Laser Endomicroscopic Images of the Vocal Cords

Kim Vo[1], Christian Jaremenko[1], Christopher Bohr[2], Helmut Neumann[3], Andreas Maier[1]

[1]Pattern Recognition Lab, Department of Computer Science, FAU Erlangen-Nürnberg, Germany
[2]Department of Otorhinolaryngology - Head and Neck Surgery, University Hospital Erlangen
[3]Department of Medicine 1, University Hospital Mainz
kim_vo@web.de

Abstract. Confocal laser endomicroscopy is a novel imaging technique which provides real-time in vivo examination and histological analysis of tissue during an ongoing endoscopy. We present an automatic classification system that is able to differentiate between healthy and cancerous tissue of the vocal cords. Textural as well as CNN features are encoded using Fisher vectors and vector of locally aggregated descriptors while the classification is performed using random forests and support vector machines. Two experiments are investigated following a leave-one-sequence-out cross-validation and a fixed training and test set approach. Classification rates reach up to 87.6 % and 81.5 %, respectively.

1   Introduction

Head and neck cancer is a collective term that comprises cancers of the upper aerodigestive tract including laryngeal cancer. Over 90% of laryngeal cancers are squamous cell carcinomas whereof half involve the vocal cords. To date, the standard of care for the diagnosis of laryngeal cancer is white light examination followed by biopsies and histopathology of suspicious lesions to confirm malignancy. These treatments are time consuming and resections may lead to permanent voice disorders. Moreover the accuracy of the diagnosis is highly dependent on the experience of the surgeon, the pathologist and the quality of biopsy. Recently a novel optical imaging method called confocal laser endomicroscopy (CLE) has been proposed, allowing subsurface analysis of the epithelium in real time and thus enables optical histology during ongoing endoscopy. In order to acquire high-contrast visualization of the surface epithelium, contrast agents such as fluorescein is administered intravenously to stain the cellular architecture and extracellular matrix. Thus, gained images allow the comparison between healthy epithelium and malignant lesions.

CLE has been successfully applied in gastroenterology and was recently introduced in the context of head and neck cancer. To assist the decisions of the surgeon during an ongoing endoscopy, several approaches for the automatic detection and classification of healthy and cancerous tissue exist. For example Dittberner et al. [1] propose an automated image analysis algorithm for the classification of head and neck cancer using distance map histograms. Another approach, introduced by Jaremenko et al. [2], uses various textural features for the automatic classification of CLE images of the oral cavity.

This paper presents a bag of words (BoW) approach, based on the framework of [2], to differentiate between images of healthy and cancerous tissue using vector of locally aggregated descriptors (VLAD) and Fisher vectors (FV), and additional textural features are evaluated [3].

2   Materials and methods

In this study, 45 video sequences from 5 patients were obtained using a probe-based CLE (pCLE) system from Cellvizio (UHD GastroFlex, Mauna Kea Technologies, Paris, France). These sequences are separated into single images leading to a database consisting of 1767 physiological images and 2675 images containing carcinoma. The images were labeled by an expert of the University Hospital Erlangen, Germany. While images of healthy epithelium show flat and relatively uniform scale-like cells with alternating bright and dark bands, images of carcinoma show a completely disorganized cell structure with fluorescein leakage as visualized in Fig. 1.

2.1   Features

Following the pre-processing step proposed by Jaremenko et al. [2], features are extracted from small rectangular patches with an edge length of 105 pixels and 50 % overlap. From each of the image patches, Histogram of Oriented Gradients (HoG) [4], Gray level co-occurrence matrices (GLCM) [5], Local binary patterns (LBP) [6], Local derivative patterns (LDP) [7] and CNN features are extracted as local descriptors. In [2] the average and standard deviation of each feature over all patches is used to describe each image, whereas here the concatenation of all patch descriptors depicts each image.

2.2   Convolutional neural network model design and training

For the extraction of the CNN features, a CNN architecture based on the LeNet-5 network [8] is used. LeNet-5 consists of a convolutional layer followed by a

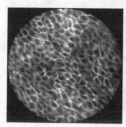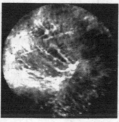

Fig. 1.   Examples of pCLE images of healthy (left) and cancerous (right) squamous epithelium.

max-pool layer, another convolutional layer followed by a max-pool layer and two consecutive fully connected layers. Additionally a fully connected layer is added and the sigmoid activations are replaced by Rectified Linear Unit (ReLU) activations. The network is trained on a training set consisting of 154440 image patches (2790 images) and 2 classes. The weights are updated by stochastic gradient descent, accompanied by momentum term of 0.9 and the learning rate is set to 0.0005 for all epochs.

Data augmentation is used to align the distribution of both classes of the original training set and to increase its variance. For this purpose, the CLE images are rotated arbitrarily and additional patches are extracted. Following this procedure, the training set is increased to 374972 image patches (7211 images).

2.3   Bag of words framework

The BoW model requires the construction of a visual codebook based on k-means clustering of features extracted from training images. The codebook consists of a set of visual words (cluster centers) which is used to compute a histogram of visual word frequencies to encode a given image. FV and VLAD have shown to outperform the classical BoW model in the context of image classification. In this study, both methods are used to encode the image features proposed in chapter 2.1, followed by a classification step using support vector machines (SVM) and random forests (RF).

Fisher vector. encoding [9] uses a Gaussian mixture model (GMM) as a generative model, where the parameters of the K components can be denoted as $\lambda = \{(\omega_k, \mu_k, \Sigma_k), k = 1, 2..., K\}$, where ω_k, μ_k and Σ_k are the mixture weight, mean and covariance matrix of the k-th component learned from a training set, respectively. Given a feature vector $X = \{x_1, ..., x_T\}$ extracted from an image, the gradients of the FV with respect to the weight parameters, mean and standard deviation can be computed with following equations

$$\mathcal{G}^X_{\alpha_k} = \frac{1}{\sqrt{w_k}} \sum_{t=1}^{T} (\gamma_t(k) - w_k) \tag{1}$$

$$\mathcal{G}^X_{\mu_k} = \frac{1}{\sqrt{w_k}} \sum_{t=1}^{T} \gamma_t(k) \left(\frac{x_t - \mu_k}{\sigma_k}\right) \tag{2}$$

$$\mathcal{G}^X_{\sigma_k} = \frac{1}{\sqrt{w_k}} \sum_{t=1}^{T} \gamma_t(k) \frac{1}{\sqrt{2}} \left[\frac{(x_t - \mu_k)^2}{\sigma_k^2} - 1\right] \tag{3}$$

where $\gamma_t(k)$ is the posterior probability. By concatenating $\mathcal{G}^X_{\alpha_k}$, $\mathcal{G}^X_{\mu_k}$ and $\mathcal{G}^X_{\sigma_k}$ for all K components, the final FV of the image is obtained with size $(2 \times D + 1)K$, where D is the dimension of the local feature vectors x. Subsequently, ℓ_2-normalization and power normalization of the form $f(z) = \text{sign}(z)|z|^\alpha$ is applied to improve the performance of Fisher vectors.

VLAD. encoding [10] is a simplification of the FV encoding. A codebook $\{\mu_1, \mu_2, ..., \mu_K\}$ is generated by using k-means. The VLAD descriptor for each μ_k can be computed by accumulating the differences $x - \mu_k$, where x is the image feature having μ_k as its nearest cluster center $\mu_k = NN(x)$

$$v_k = \sum_{x_j : NN(x) = \mu_k} x_j - \mu_k \tag{4}$$

The final VLAD encoding vector is obtained by concatenating v_k over all μ_k and has the dimension $D \times K$, where D is again the dimension of the local image feature vectors x. As for FV, the VLAD descriptor is also normalized subsequently. In this study, intra-normalization is performed, where the sum over each cluster center μ_k is ℓ_2-normalized before applying the standard ℓ_2-normalization of the entire VLAD descriptor.

3 Results

To estimate the generalization performance of the BoW approach using FV and VLAD, a leave-one-sequence-out cross-validation (LOSO-CV) model is used, to evaluate the classification performance.

As the LOSO-CV model would lead to exhausting computation times in case of the CNN approach, the performance is evaluated and compared to the textural features using a fixed train and test set following a 70:30 split ratio. To avoid correlation effects, complete sequences are used as hold out test set consisting of at least two sequences of each subject, one being physiological and one being pathological. The number of visual words are empirically set to 5 for both FV and VLAD as the performance did not improve using a larger vocabulary size in preliminary experiments.

The accuracy (Acc) and average recall (Rec) for the two feature encoding methods FV and VLAD are illustrated in Tab. 1. Overall, VLAD encoding outperformed FV and reaches the best result with an accuracy of 87.6% and average recall of 86.7% using LBP and the SVM classifier.

The results of [2] using the same image database, are listed on the bottom of Tab. 1. As comparison the two best performing features of [2] were chosen. The approach reaches an accuracy above 89.1% and average recalls above 90.3% using the SVM classifier and similar results also apply for the RF classifier.

For the evaluation of the CNN features, we only consider the approach of [2] and VLAD encoding as they consistently outperformed FV. Moreover for the comparison, we focus on the features GLCM and LBP due to their superior performances. In Tab. 2, the results of CNN features and the residual features are illustrated. Using VLAD, CNN features exceed the classification results of all residual features with an accuracy of 76.1% and an average recall of 74.7% using the RF classifier. By using data augmentation, the results further improve to an accuracy of 81.5% and an average recall of 81.7%.

Using the approach of [2], CNN features using data augmentation and LBP show comparable classification results and outperform the residual features with

Table 1. Classification results using FV, VLAD*, the approach of [2]⁺ and LOSO-CV: Accuracy (Acc) and average recall (Rec).

Features	Property	SVM		RF	
		Acc	Rec	Acc	Rec
HOG	—	66.1%	63.0%	62.0%	55.3%
GLCM	QuantLvl 8	77.1%	74.1%	76.2%	72.1%
GLCM	QuantLvl 32	78.6%	75.8%	78.1%	74.2%
LBP	R5 N16	75.8%	71.0%	72.0%	65.3%
LDP	3rd order R5	83.4%	82.5%	81.5%	79.6%
HOG*	—	75.4%	73.6%	71.9%	66.4%
GLCM*	QuantLvl 8	83.4%	82.5%	84.3%	83.7%
GLCM*	QuantLvl 32	80.0%	76.5%	78.6%	74.6%
LBP*	R5 N16	87.6%	86.7%	87.5%	86.6%
LDP*	3rd order R5	82.9%	81.9%	79.6%	76.8%
GLCM⁺	QuantLvl 8	89.8%	90.5%	86.4%	88.6%
GLCM⁺	QuantLvl 32	89.6%	90.3%	86.7%	88.7%
LBP⁺	R5 N16	89.1%	91.3%	89.3%	91.6%

Table 2. Comparison of CNN features with residual features using VLAD* and the approach of [2]⁺: Accuracy (Acc) and average recall (Rec).

Features	Property	SVM		RF	
		Acc	Rec	Acc	Rec
CNN*	–	72.6%	69.5%	76.1%	74.7%
CNN*	Data augmentation	76.0%	75.7%	81.5%	81.7%
GLCM*	QuantLvl 8	61.4%	55.1%	72.0%	70.4%
LBP*	R5 N16	72.1%	68.2%	74.2%	72.2%
CNN⁺	–	77.6%	80.1%	76.5%	78.8%
CNN⁺	Data augmentation	79.9%	80.4%	81.3%	81.7%
GLCM⁺	QuantLvl 8	77.9%	81.3%	76.4%	80.1%
LBP⁺	R5 N16	79.5%	82.1%	80.5%	81.8%

average accuracies of 79.5% and 77.9% and average recalls of 82.1% and 80.4%, respectively.

4 Discussion

Despite of the very small visual vocabulary size, FV and VLAD already reach decent classification results and may have the potential to excel the algorithm proposed by [2]. However, with the current setup, the approach of [2] outperforms our proposed method in case of all features. This might be due to the fact that Jaremenko et al. incorporated additional information in terms of the mean and standard deviation of all features and patches of an image, that is neglected within the VLAD approach.

CNN features show comparable results and slightly outperform any other of the tested features but still leave room for improvements using different CNN models. As expected, using data augmentation the performance of CNN increases as a result of the larger size and increased variance of the training set. Most likely the results could be improved further with additional augmentation, but this was not the aim of this paper. Considering the small amount of subjects of the dataset, it would be beneficial to increase its variance by investigating additional patients rather than performing augmentation using rotation. As a next step, with an increased patient database it would be possible to perform a leave-one-patient-out cross-validation to avoid intra-patient correlation effects during the training of the classifier that yet may be existent within the LOSO-CV and fixed dataset approach.

The current results are promising but nonetheless, additional effort is needed, to further develop the proposed approach to be able to reliably support and improve diagnosis of vocal cord cancer during endoscopy.

References

1. Dittberner A, Rodner E, Ortmann W, et al. Automated analysis of confocal laser endomicroscopy images to detect head and neck cancer. Head Neck. 2016;38:1419–26.
2. Jaremenko C, Maier A, Steidl S, et al. Classification of confocal laser endomicroscopic omages of the oral cavity to distinguish pathological from healthy tissue. Proc BVM. 2015; p. 479–85.
3. Razavian AS, Azizpour H, Sullivan J, et al. CNN features off-the-shelf: an oustanding baseline for recognition. Proc IEEE CVPR. 2014; p. 512–9.
4. Dalal N, Triggs B. Histograms of oriented gradients for human detection. Proc IEEE CVPR. 2005;1:886–93.
5. Haralick R, Shanmugam K, Dinstein I. Textural features for image classification. IEEE Trans Syst Man Cybern. 1973;(6):610–21.
6. Pietikäinen M, Hadid A, Zhao G, et al. Computer Vision Using Local Binary Patterns. London: Springer; 2011.
7. Zhang B, Gao Y, Zhao S, et al. Local derivative pattern versus local binary pattern: face recognition with high-order local pattern descriptor. IEEE Trans Image Process. 2010;19(2):533–44.
8. LeCun Y, Bottou L, Bengio Y, et al. Gradient-based learning applied to document recognition. Proc IEEE. 1998;86(11):2278–324.
9. Sánchez J, Perronnin F, Mensink T, et al. Image classification with the fisher vector: theory and practice. Int J Comput Vis. 2013;105(3):222–45.
10. Jegou H, Perronnin F, Douze M, et al. Image classification with the fisher vector; theory and practice. IEEE Trans Pattern Anal Mach Intell. 2013;34(9):1704–16.

Abstract: Soft Tissue Modeling with the Chainmail Approach

Kathrin Bartelheimer[1,2], Hendrik Teske[1,2], Rolf Bendl[1,3], Kristina Giske[1,2]

[1]Division of Medical Physics in Radiation Oncology, DKFZ Heidelberg
[2]National Center for Radiation Research in Oncology (NCRO),
Heidelberg Institute for Radiation Oncology (HIRO)
[3]Faculty of Computer Science, Heilbronn University
k.bartelheimer@dkfz-heidelberg.de

For deformable image registration in the context of medical applications, the choice of the transformation model determines the level of detail with which the human anatomy can be described. Transformation models, which are based on physical descriptions and allow for detailed modeling, like finite element or mass-spring models, however, require high computation times. Fast models based on e.g. splines or diffusion, on the other hand, rely on interpolation between landmarks in high contrast regions of the images and lack anatomical correctness, especially in soft tissue. Therefore, we have developed a heterogeneous transformation model based on the chainmail approach [1] with the aim of improving the characteristic deformation behavior of soft tissue within short calculation times.

We adopted the enhanced version of the original chainmail algorithm [2] to cope with heterogeneous tissue in CT-images. Deformations are initialized by anatomical landmarks and propagated into the surrounding tissue by adjusting geometrical deformation limits for every voxel. These geometrical constraints represent elastic tissue properties and are assigned automatically to each voxel according to its HU-value. Furthermore, we extended the algorithm by rotational degrees of freedom to be able to model locally decaying rotations.

With an exemplary input of a set of landmarks from a kinematic head-and-neck skeleton model we used our rotation-enabled chainmail-based algorithm to deform high resolution CT-images (512x512x126) in less than 10 s. Resampling of the image was realized via CUDA API on the GPU to obtain an artificial scan of the deformed planning CT.

This is the first time that the chainmail algorithm was extended by rotational degrees of freedom, allowing to model local rotations. Together with volume conservation, to be included in a next step, our transformation model promises to achieve high accuracy in the detection of deformations while at the same time requiring short calculation times.

References

1. Gibson SFF. 3D chainmail: a fast algorithm for deforming volumetric objects. Proc Symp Interact 3D Graph. 1997; p. 149–54.
2. Schill MA, Gibson SFF, Bender HJ, et al. Biomechanical simulation of the vitreous humor in the eye using an enhanced chainmail algorithm. Proc MICCAI. 1998; p. 679–87.

Brain Parenchyma and Vessel Separation in 3D Digital Subtraction Angiography Images

Jürgen Endres[1,4], Christopher Rohkohl[2], Kevin Royalty[3], Sebastian Schafer[3], Andreas Maier[1], Arnd Dörfler[4], Markus Kowarschik[2]

[1]Pattern Recognition Lab, Friedrich-Alexander-Universität Erlangen-Nürnberg
[2]Siemens Healthcare GmbH, Advanced Therapies, Forchheim
[3]Siemens Medical Solutions USA, Inc., Hoffman Estates, IL, USA
[4]Department of Neuroradiology, Universitätsklinikum Erlangen
juergen.endres@fau.de

Abstract. In 3D digital subtraction angiography, the propagation of iodine-based contrast agent in cerebral vessels implies a delayed enhancement of soft tissue, i.e. parenchyma, which causes inconsistencies across the acquired projection images that impair the quality of the reconstructed volumes. In order to cope with this issue, we perform an estimation of contrast-enhanced parenchyma in projection images. The estimation is based on a vessel segmentation and an iterative interpolation of segmented vessel pixels. The estimated parenchyma is subsequently separated from the projection images. Thus, only contrast-enhanced vessels remain and data inconsistencies due to late-enhancing parenchyma will be reduced. The method is applied to two datasets of cerebral vasculatures. The image series are compared prior and post to parenchyma subtraction. Reconstructed volumes show minor noise in background voxels. An average increase of 37% in signal-to-noise ratio is achieved.

1 Introduction

3D digital subtraction angiography (DSA) represents an established procedure in interventional neuroradiology. In two consecutive rotational acquisitions of an angiographic C-arm scanner, both a set of mask images as well as a set of fill images are acquired. For the fill images, contrast agent is injected into the patient's vasculature during acquisition. A subtraction of the mask from the fill images reveals the contrast-enhanced vessels by cancelling out static structures which are present in both mask and fill images [1].

During the acquisition of the mask and fill runs, the imaging device is rotated around the patient's head which depicts the contrast-enhanced vessel tree from different angulations. Subsequently, these images are used for the reconstruction of a volumetric representation of the vessels, typically using the Feldkamp-Davis-Kress (FDK) algorithm [2]. In this case, the filling of the vessels with contrast agent is required to be consistent across the range of projection images.

In practice, however, the fill images usually show variations over time. As a source of noise besides the filling of arteries and veins, surrounding brain tissue, i.e. parenchyma, lately appears as contrast blush around the vessels, as illustrated in Fig. 1. While the filling of the vessels may be optimized using altered injection/acquisition protocols, the parenchyma cannot be prevented from getting contrast-enhanced.

In the following, we present a method to preprocess the log-subtracted projection data by estimating and separating contrast-enhanced parenchyma.

1.1   Related work

Improving the image quality of computed tomography (CT) or 3D DSA images denotes an important step for medical imaging applications. Noise is typically handled using filtering operations [3, 4], which are further used for structure enhancement [5]. For image artifacts, such as metal artifacts, more sophisticated techniques like segmenting and removing the metal object from projection images are used [6]. In cardiac imaging, Chen et al. [7] investigated a similar approach based on separating an object of interest from surrounding structures within a tomographic image. Subsequently, numerical projections of the remaining volume are used to generate images without the object; i.e., background projection images. These images are then subtracted from the original projection images, hence increasing the contrast of the desired object. Blondel et al. [8] proposed a method to estimate, segment, and separate contrast-enhanced coronary arteries from background for generating DSA-like image sequences from a single rotational acquisition run, with the purpose of artifact reduction for reconstructed volumes. A related approach has been recently proposed by Unberath et al. [9] for applications in material decomposition.

2   Materials and methods

2.1   Parenchyma estimation

Compared to vessels, contrast-enhanced soft tissue varies smoothly on DSA images. We hence estimate the contrast-enhanced parenchyma as a low-frequent image by applying Gaussian filtering to the subtracted input image sequence. The parameter of the filter, the standard deviation σ, has to be chosen sufficiently high to preserve a smooth image character, while on the other hand, σ is

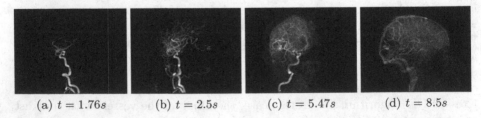

(a) $t = 1.76s$ (b) $t = 2.5s$ (c) $t = 5.47s$ (d) $t = 8.5s$

Fig. 1. In (a) and (b), contrast agent is only visible in large arteries at the base of the brain, whereas later, additional parenchyma (c) and veins (d) become visible. t denotes the time passed since the beginning of the acquisition.

required to be small enough to keep the spatial information of the parenchyma. Gaussian filtering also blurs high-contrast vessels, which results in increased intensities and hence an overestimation of surrounding parenchyma.

In order to overcome this issue, we first performed a segmentation of vessels on the subtracted image data. We computed an initial reconstruction from the original log-subtracted projection data, resulting in a volume f. Using a ray-based maximum intensity projection (MIP) and a subsequent thresholding operation on that projection data results in set of binary vessel masks v_j, where pixels with value 1 represent vessels and pixels with value 0 represent non-vessels, see Fig. 2 (b). $n_j = 1 - v_j$ represents the inverse vessel mask. As initial estimate for the parenchyma images $b_j^{(0)}$, the original images i_j, where the values of vessel pixels are set to 0, were used. The threshold was set to 500 Hounsfield Units (HU).

As a second step, the pixels which had been masked out were interpolated. For that purpose, we performed a Gaussian filtering of the initial estimate $b_j^{(0)}$ with zeroed vessel pixels. Thus, these holes received a certain intensity from neighboring pixels due to the blurring. Subsequently, the pixel values for non-vessel pixels n_j were replaced with the pixel values from the original data i_j. These steps were repeated until the change of intensity values for the vessel pixels converged or a certain predefined number k of iterations was reached, i.e.

$$b_j^{(n+1)} = \left(\left(b_j^{(n)} \right)^T v_j + (i_j)^T n_j \right) * g(\sigma) \qquad (1)$$

where b_j denotes the estimated parenchyma image for frame j, i_j the corresponding original input image, and $g(\sigma)$ the Gaussian kernel with parameter σ (standard deviation). The superscript n denotes the current iteration. For our experiments, we chose $\sigma = 20$ for an image size of 1240×960 and a fixed number of $k = 20$ iterations.

The purpose of this iterative scheme is to lower the intensities of the pixels belonging to vessels onto an intensity level of the surrounding non-vessel pixels, while keeping them at an approximately constant intensity level. The resulting rotational projection images that show the estimated brain parenchyma only are finally used to separate the vessels by subtracting the parenchyma images from the original projection images.

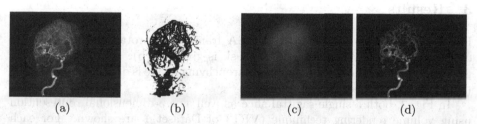

(a)   (b)   (c)   (d)

Fig. 2. Original projection frame $i_{j=164}$ (a), the corresponding vessel mask (b), estimated parenchyma (c), and resulting vessel image (d).

2.2 Data

Two rotational DSA datasets acquired using an angiographic C-arm device (Artis zee biplane, Siemens Healthcare GmbH, Forchheim, Germany) were used, for which we separated the parenchyma. Each of the two datasets consists of both a mask and a fill run, which were preprocessed and subtracted before processing. During the acquisition, contrast agent was injected such that at the beginning of the fill sequence the arterial inflow phase of contrast agent was visible.

2.3 Evaluation

For evaluation, we reconstructed the unmodified original log-subtracted projection data as well as the data where parenchyma had been estimated and removed. We used identical reconstruction parameters for both reconstructions. The resulting volumes were presented using volume rendering, and we assessed the effect of parenchyma subtraction qualitatively. Note that for the evaluation using volume rendering, we applied a scaling of the parenchyma-subtracted projection data prior to reconstruction in a way that selected voxels within vessels shared an approximately equal intensity value for the reconstructed data without and with parenchyma removal. This scaling had to be applied due to the change in projection image content, removing the parenchyma resulted in a reduced HU value in the reconstructions. With the scaling applied, an equal HU window could be selected for visualization of both volumes. The scaling factors were 1.04 and 1.02, respectively, and had been determined heuristically.

Additionally, the signal-to-noise ratio (SNR) was calculated on the reconstructed data. For that purpose, we separated each volume into vessel voxels r and background voxels s using thresholding of voxel intensities. The threshold had been determined such that a 1% vessel and 99% background voxel split was achieved for each reconstructed volume. The numbers of vessel and background voxels were given by $|r|$ and $|s|$, respectively. The SNR was then calculated as

$$\text{SNR} = \frac{\frac{1}{|r|}r^T r}{\frac{1}{|s|}s^T s} \tag{2}$$

3 Results

Fig. 2 (a) depicts an original, plane DSA frame of the rotational image series of Dataset 1. The segmented vessel mask is given in (b). After applying the parenchyma separation, the estimated parenchyma image is depicted in (c), while (d) denotes the remaining vessel image.

In Fig. 3, both a single sagittal slice as well as a 3-dimensional represention using volume rendering technique (VRT) of Dataset 1 are shown. For each representation, the images are depicted prior and post parenchyma removal as well as the calculated difference thereof.

Table 1. Signal-to-noise ratios for both datasets. The values in the 'Diff' column refer to the differences in SNR between original and parenchyma-subtracted reconstruction.

Dataset	SNR w/o parenchyma removal	SNR w/ parenchyma removal	Diff
1	312	450	+44%
2	348	453	+30%

Finally, Tab. 1 lists the calculated SNRs for the investigated datasets both for input data without and with parenchyma removed. The datasets show an average increase in SNR of 37% when parenchyma removal is applied.

Compared to the reconstruction and vessel mask generation, the interpolation was not yet optimized for performance, hence the algorithm resulted in a runtime of about 1s per projection image.

4   Discussion

While contrast-enhanced parenchyma appears as noisy blush between vessels in Fig. 3 (a), that noise could be reduced using parenchyma removal, Fig 3 (b). The difference images, Fig. 3 (c), clearly outlines that the estimated parenchyma is restricted to the surrounding of vessels, while important structures, i.e., the vessels themselves, virtually remain unaffected.

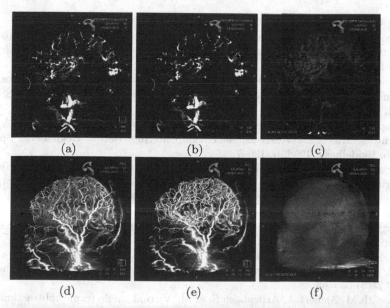

(a)   (b)   (c)

(d)   (e)   (f)

Fig. 3. Sagittal slice (first row) and VRT (second row) of reconstructed Dataset 1, both prior (first column) and post (second column) parenchyma removal and the difference thereof (third column).

In the VRT representation, Fig. 3 (d), blush causes smaller vessels in the background to be hardly visible, while for the rendering of the dataset with parenchyma being removed, Fig. 3 (e), these vessels are easier to spot.

Beneath the visual impression, which may also be improved using an adjusted HU windowing function, the presented method may further facilitate automatic image processing algorithms due to an increased signal-to-noise ratio between vessels and background as stated in Tab. 1.

We presented a basic preprocessing method for estimating and separating brain parenchyma from vessels in 3D digital subtraction angiography images. This serves the purpose of eliminating inconsitencies caused due to late-enhancing soft tissue. Applications in reconstruction and planar image sequence processing may benefit from an increased signal-to-noise ratio between vessels and background.

Disclaimer. The concept and software presented in this paper are based on research and are not commercially available. Due to regulatory reasons its future availability cannot be guaranteed.

References

1. Brody WR. Digital subtraction angiography. IEEE Trans Nucl Sci. 1982;29(3):1176–80.
2. Zeng GL. Medical Image Reconstruction. Springer; 2010.
3. Lanzolla A, Andria G, Attivissimo F, et al.; IEEE. Denoising filter to improve the quality of CT images. Instrumentation and Measurement Technology Conference, 2009 I2MTC'09 IEEE. 2009; p. 947–50.
4. Manhart M, Kowarschik M, Fieselmann A, et al. Fast dynamic reconstruction algorithm with joint bilateral filtering for perfusion C-arm CT. Proceedings NSS/MIC 2012. 2012; p. 2304–11.
5. Frangi AF, Niessen WJ, Vincken KL, et al. In: Wells WM, Colchester A, Delp S, editors. Multiscale Vessel Enhancement Filtering. Berlin, Heidelberg: Springer Berlin Heidelberg; 1998. p. 130–7.
6. Psychogios MN, Scholz B, Rohkohl C, et al. Impact of a new metal artefact reduction algorithm in the noninvasive follow-up of intracranial clips, coils, and stents with flat-panel angiographic CTA: initial results. Neuroradiology. 2013;55(7):813–8.
7. Chen M, Zheng Y, Mueller K, et al.; IEEE. Enhancement of organ of interest via background subtraction in cone beam rotational angiocardiogram. Proc IEEE Int Symp Biomed Imaging. 2012; p. 622–5.
8. Blondel C, Malandain G, Vaillant R, et al. Reconstruction of coronary arteries from a single rotational X-ray projection sequence. IEEE Trans Med Imaging. 2006;25(5):653–63.
9. Unberath M, Aichert A, Achenbach S, et al. Virtual single-frame subtraction imaging. Proc CT Meeting. 2016; p. 89–92.

Classification of DCE-MRI Data for Breast Cancer Diagnosis Combining Contrast Agent Dynamics and Texture Features

Kai Nie, Sylvia Glaßer, Uli Niemann, Gabriel Mistelbauer, Bernhard Preim

Department of Simulation and Graphics, OvG-University Magdeburg
kai@isg.cs.uni-magdeburg.de

Abstract. Classification of breast tumors via dynamic contrast-enhanced magnetic resonance imaging is an important task for tumor diagnosis. In this paper, we present an approach for automatic tumor segmentation, feature generation and classification. We apply fuzzy c-means on co-occurrence texture features to generate discriminative features for classification. High-frequency information is removed via discrete wavelet transform and computation is simplified via principal component analysis before extraction. We evaluate our approach using different classification algorithms. Our experimental results show the performances of different classifiers with respect to sensitivity and specificity.

1   Introduction

In 2012, breast cancer was estimated in 1.7 million cases and 521,900 deaths world wide [1]. Dynamic contrast-enhanced magnetic resonance imaging (DCE-MRI) can characterize more details of breast tumors than standard MRI, through the contrast agents (CA) motion over time. In comparison with conventional X-ray mammography, DCE-MRI has higher sensitivity [2]. The average relative enhancement (RE) curve of a region of interest (ROI) reflects blood vessels and tissue permeability in this region. Based on the RE curve, Degani et al. presented the three-time-point (3TP) method [3], which allows for automatic classification of the RE curves. Glaßer et al. [4] clustered spatially connected tumor regions with similar 3TP classes to identify a "most suspect region" per lesion from which CA perfusion features were derived as input for the classification of malignant and benign breast tumors.

Data mining and machine learning have gained increasing popularity for benign and malignant tumors separation. Chang et al. [5] proposed to use co-occurrence texture features combined with kinetic curves to classify breast tumor types via fuzzy clustering. Zhang et al. [6] combined discrete wavelet transform (DWT) and principal component analysis (PCA) for feature extraction and classify brain images via a neural network (NN) classifier. Zheng et al. [7] used k-means to derive features from the membership probability of cluster that were learned on a set of malignant and a set of benign tumors, respectively. This reduced set of features was used for training the support vector machines (SVM) classifier.

We use fuzzy c-means (FCM) to generate new texture features based on the co-occurence matrix, and combine with Gabor square energy and Gabor mean amplitude to improve the diagnosis in classifying breast tumors. The tumor region is segmented with the 3TP method. We employ three classifiers with the newly generated features and test their performance.

2   Material and methods

2.1   Image data

In this study, we use a collection of 282 slices of tumor images from 50 patients, which include 141 slices of benign tumors and 141 slices of malignant tumors (see Preim et al. [8]). All data sets were acquired with a (rather old) 1T scanner (Philips Medical Systems) with the following parameters: matrix $\approx 500 \times 500$ pixels, slice thickness = 3 mm, slice gap = 1.5 mm, echo time = 6 ms, number of acquisitions = 5–6 s, total acquisition time = 300–400 s. We select 25 patients of benign tumors and 25 patients of malignant tumors from our data sets randomly. Each patient provides one slice breast tumor image, which can reflect typical traits of the tumor, and these 50 slices are used to establish the training sets after features extraction. All these images have already been segmented by an expert radiologist.

2.2   Methods

Fig. 1 shows the general steps of the presented approach, which is separated into two parts: tumor region of interest (ROI) identification and tumor classification.

The temporal features of the DCE-MRI data can effectively distinguish lesions from normal tissue. Thus, we segment the data via the 3TP method. The 3TP method [3] provides an automatic classification of the tumor's perfusion characteristics based on the RE curve. The RE is calculated with $RE = (SI_c - SI)/SI \times 100$, where SI is the pre-contrast and SI_c is the post-contrast signal intensity [2]. We extract the three time points t'_1, t'_2, t'_3, where t'_1 is the first time point before contrast agent injection, t'_2 is 2 min after t'_1 and t'_3 is 4 min after t'_2. Fig. 2 shows the RE curves classification via the 3TP method. At t'_2

Fig. 1. The workflow of the presented approach.

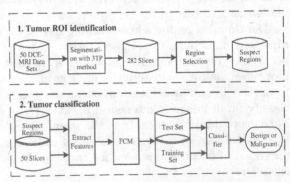

the RE curve is classified into three types: slow, normal and fast. If the result is normal or fast, the lesion areas will be identified as suspicious and be segmented. We use 3×3 median filter and bilateral filter to reduce noise. Meanwhile, the texture features have strong relationship with the size of image and the position of lesion, therefore we use rectangular ROIs to select the regions and remove the background.

We use two level discrete wavelet transform (DWT) to capture the frequency characteristics of the tumor ROIs and use principal component analysis (PCA) to reduce the number of dimensions. We remove high-frequency detail information and simplify computation via two level DWT and PCA. We extract 12 features, including contrast, correlation, energy, homogeneity, mean, standard deviation, entropy, root mean square, variance, smoothness, kurtosis, skewness, inverse difference moment, from the tumor image using the gray-level co-occurrence matrix (GLCM) method combined with Gabor square energy and Gabor mean amplitude.

In k-means clustering, each data point is assigned to exactly one cluster. We choose its extension, FCM, where the degree of cluster membership is given as probability. We employ FCM to extract malignant and benign tumor features separately, as described in [7]. We extract the features from training sets and recognize their patterns, which reflect the average distance of each feature to its cluster centroid. After this, we measure the similarity of each feature of the test sets and the detected patterns via FCM, which shows how well the features are fitted. For each feature, the clustering result reflects its effectiveness in classification. If the result is < 0.3 in both malignant and benign measurement, this feature is considered as irrelevant and is removed.

We assess the performance of the subsequent classifiers: decision tree C4.5, support vector machine with a linear kernel and radial basis function (RBF) kernel, probabilistic neural network. We use the new features sets to learn these classifiers.

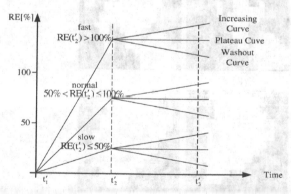

Fig. 2. The three-point method for evaluating DCE-MRI data (adapted from [3]).

3   Results

In this section, we study the performance of the 3TP segmentation methods, the impact of the ROI selection and the performance of different classifiers. Our implementation is done in Matlab 2015a on a Windows 7 platform with an Intel Core i5 CPU at 3.3GHz and 8GB memory.

Fig. 3 shows two example tumors with different traits and shapes. Fig. 3(a) depicts a benign tumor with an irregular shape and Fig. 3(d) depicts a regular malignant sample. Blue lines highlight the tumor boundaries. Fig. 3(b) shows the segmented result of a benign tumor, Fig. 3(e) shows the segmented result of a malignant tumor. Fig. 3(c) and Fig. 3(f) show the ground truth segmented by an experienced radiologist. The average 3TP segmentation accuracy is 98.2% for benign data and 98.3% for malignant data.

The proportion of the foreground pixel is calculated with $R = N_t/N_i$, where N_t is the number of foreground pixels, N_i is the number of the whole image pixels. Table. 1 shows the effect of the rate R on classification accuracy using probabilistic neural network (PNN) classifier. Thus, we set the rate R to 55%–60% for regular tumors and 50%–55% for irregular tumors, and all the lesions are set in the center of the regions to keep the classification result more stable.

The sensitivity and specificity are as follows: the sensitivity of decision tree C4.5, SVM with linear kernel, SVM with RBF kernel and PNN classifiers are 57.4%, 80.9%, 79.4% and 92.2%, the specificity are 63.1%, 97.2%, 98.6% and 95.8%, respectively.

Glaßer et al. [9, 10] combined the 3TP method with J4.8 decision tree to classify the breast tumors, and the correctly classified instances are approximately 67% based on the same data set we use in this work.

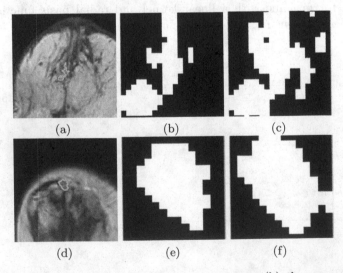

Fig. 3. Tumor segmentation result, (a) a benign tumor; (b) the segmented benign tumor; (c) the ground truth of the benign tumor; (d) a malignant tumor; (e) the segmented malignant tumor; (f) the ground truth of the malignant tumor.

Table 1. Classification accuracy of ROI selection using PNN Classifier.

Rate R		Classification accuracy (%)			
		< 50%	50%–55%	55%–60%	> 60%
Regular	Benign	87.6	90.5	93.3	94.3
tumors	Malignant	98.1	94.5	94.5	92.7
Irregular	Benign	86.1	91.7	94.4	94.4
tumors	Malignant	98.8	97.7	95.3	93.0

4   Discussion

The 3TP method takes advantage of dynamic curves, which reflect the tissue's pharmacokinetic characteristics or CA accumulation, to segment the suspected regions. Although the segmentation results can be easily obtained via the 3TP method, it is sensitive to artifacts, such as noise and tissue displacement, and time points selection.

Compared to the results of Glaßer et al. [9, 10], we achieved a higher classification accuracy by integrating texture features. The combination of pharmacokinetic features and features representing the tumor's texture enable a high accuracy even for this data with only moderate quality.

Despite the SVM having the highest accuracy in malignant tumor classification, the PNN classifier shows the best discriminative power among these three classifiers. Furthermore, the accuracy of classifying a tumor of benign is far below than the accuracy of malignant. The reason is that our data sets include numerous small tumors. These small tumors which can only be detected in DCE-MRI data, are very hard to distinguish and classify, even for a human expert, and these tumors have a substantial impact on the classification performance.

The ratio of foreground/background reflect the relationship between textural features and lesions. However, the ratio can not exceed a value cause the rectangular ROIs must include the whole lesion, and consider the diversity of data sets, the ratio should be set in a certain range. The influence of region selection on the classification result is shown in Tab. 1. Thus, we defined the size and position of ROIs before the classification, to reduced the impact of subjectiveness from manual region selection.

We presented a comprehensive workflow which includes feature extraction, feature selection and classification to separate between malignant and benign tumors in DCE-MRI data. 282 slices of tumor images, which had been confirmed as either malignant or benign, were considered in this study. We used the 3TP method to segment the tumors, which provide a high accuracy. We could not eliminate all the errors in preprocessing and registering, which have influence on the segmentation. A total of 12 features are extracted and the invalid features are automatically removed by FCM. We compared different classifiers and concluded that the PNN classifier has a good performance in both benign and malignant tumors. Although the SVM shows the highest accuracy in malignant tumor classification, its poor stability for benign tumors does not make it suitable for small tumors with similar textures.

One limitation of our approach is the low classification accuracy for very small tumors. For future work, a hybrid classifier, improved segmentation methods, and the combination of temporal informations and textural informations will be taken into consideration. Then, the connectivity and correlation of tumors can be described, and the accuracy of tumor segmentation will be improved. Moreover, the combination of various features and classifiers ensemble can overcome the disadvantage of a single classifier.

References

1. Torre LA, Bray F, Siegel RL, et al. Global cancer statistics, 2012. CA Cancer J Clin. 2015;65(2):87–108.
2. Kuhl C. The current status of breast MR imaging part I. Choice of technique, image interpretation, diagnostic accuracy, and transfer to clinical practice. Radiology. 2007;244(2):356–78.
3. Degani H, Gusis V, Weinstein D, et al. Mapping pathophysiological features of breast tumors by MRI at high spatial resolution. Nat Med. 1997;3(7):780–2.
4. Glaßer S, Preim U, Tönnies K, et al. A visual analytics approach to diagnosis of breast DCE-MRI data. Comput Graph. 2010;34(5):602–11.
5. Chang RF, Chen HH, Chang YC, et al. Quantification of breast tumor heterogeneity for ER status, HER2 status, and TN molecular subtype evaluation on DCE-MRI. Magn Reson Imaging. 2016;34(6):809–19.
6. Zhang Y, Dong Z, Wu L, et al. A hybrid method for MRI brain image classification. Expert Syst Appl. 2011;38(8):10049–53.
7. Zheng B, Yoon SW, Lam SS. Breast cancer diagnosis based on feature extraction using a hybrid of K-means and support vector machine algorithms. Expert Syst Appl. 2014;41(4, Part 1):1476–82.
8. Preim U, Glaßer S, Preim B, et al. Computer-aided diagnosis in breast DCE-MRI-quantification of the heterogeneity of breast lesions. Eur J Radiol. 2012;81(7):1532–8.
9. Glaßer S, Niemann U, Preim B, et al. Can we distinguish between benign and malignant breast tumors in DCE-MRI by studying a tumor's most suspect region only? Proc IEEE Comput Based Med Syst. 2013; p. 77–82.
10. Glaßer S, Niemann U, Preim U, et al. Classification of benign and malignant DCE-MRI breast tumors by analyzing the most suspect region. Proc BVM. 2013; p. 45–50.

Registrierung von nicht sichtbaren Laserbehandlungsarealen der Retina in Live-Aufnahmen des Fundus

Timo Kepp[1,3], Stefan Koinzer[2], Heinz Handels[3], Ralf Brinkmann[1]

[1]Medizinisches Laserzentrum Lübeck GmbH
[2]Klinik für Ophthalmologie, Universitätsklinikum Schleswig-Holstein, Campus Kiel
[3]Institut für Medizinische Informatik, Universität zu Lübeck
kepp@mll.uni-luebeck.de

Kurzfassung. Die Laserphotokoagulation ist eine wirksame thermische Therapie für zahlreiche Netzhauterkrankungen. Schonendere Behandlungsmethoden vermeiden die klassischen, starken Verödungen, indem das Gewebe kontrolliert erwärmt wird. Dadurch sind die Behandlungsareale unsichtbar, wodurch während der Behandlung nicht mehr nachvollziehbar ist, an welchen Stellen behandelt wurde. In dieser Arbeit wird ein Verfahren vorgestellt, das diese nicht sichtbaren Laserbehandlungsareale der Retina zur Orientierungshilfe in Echtzeit erkennt und darstellt. Durch die Verwendung eines featurebasierten Registrierungsansatzes werden die Behandlungsareale zu einem Mosaik zusammengefügt, auf das die Laserspots eingezeichnet werden. Dabei wird jede Position über ein Konturextraktionsverfahren ermittelt. Die Genauigkeit und Robustheit unseres Ansatzes konnte in drei Experimenten gezeigt werden.

1 Einleitung

Die Laserphotokoagulation ist seit Jahrzehnten Standardbehandlungsmethode für verschiedene Erkrankungen der Retina. Als Weiterentwicklung zu dieser bereits etablierten Behandlungsweise wurden schonendere Behandlungsmethoden vorgestellt wie die selektive Retina-Therapie (SRT) [1], die sich als gute Alternative zur konventionellen Behandlung von Makulopathien wie dem diabetischen Makulaödem herausstellt. Vorteile solcher sanften, nicht verödenden Behandlungen bestehen in verminderten Schmerzen während der Behandlung und reduzierten Nebenwirkungen, etwa dem Vermeiden von narbenbedingten Gesichtsfeldausfällen. Problematisch ist jedoch, dass die Lasereffekte, d. h. verödete Netzhautareale, während der Therapie für den behandelnden Arzt nicht sichtbar sind und nicht als Orientierungshilfe für die Gesamtbestrahlung dienen können. Hierdurch lassen sich die Dichte der Behandlung und eine unkontrollierte Mehrfachbestrahlung gleicher Stellen nur mit großer Unsicherheit kontrollieren.

In unserer Arbeit wird die Position des Lasers zu jeder Zeit in einem Live-Bild des Fundus verfolgt, wobei Bestrahlungsorte auf einer Behandlungskarte eingetragen werden. Die Besonderheit der Aufnahmen ist ein sehr großer Einblickwinkel auf den Fundus. Dieser wird über eine spezielle Funduskamera ermöglicht, die an einer Spaltlampe integriert ist. Die Behandlungskarten werden mithilfe eines Mosaicking-Ansatzes aus der Live-Aufnahme des Fundus erzeugt.

Einen ersten Mosaicking-Ansatz von Spaltlampenbildern stellte Asmuth et al. vor [2]. Hierbei wurde das Spaltbild durch eine geeignete Wahl von Farbmittelwerten und Formbeschränkungen in Einzelbildern einer Videosequenz segmentiert. Anschließend wurde die Translation zwischen den einzelnen Zeitpunkten durch Minimierung der Sum of Squared Differences (SSD) bestimmt. Durch Verwendung einer Laplace-Pyramide wurden die Einzelbilder überblendet.

In der Arbeit von Richa et al. wurde ein gleichzeitiges Tracking und Mosaicking von Spaltlampenaufnahmen unter der Verwendung eines Kontaktglases vorgestellt [3]. Sie verwendeten ein featurebasiertes Tracking in Kombination mit der SSD, das neben den drei Bildkanälen auch Belichtungsparameter berücksichtigte.

Der Mosaicking-Ansatz wird in unserer Arbeit durch ein simultanes Lasertracking erweitert. Durch eine GPU-basierte Registrierung können die Einzelbilder einer Videosequenz des Fundus in Echtzeit getrackt und zu einem Mosaik zusammengesetzt werden. Gleichzeitig wird die Position des Pilotlasers, welcher während der Behandlungssitzung mit schwacher, unschädlicher Laserstrahlung die Stelle der Behandlung markiert und somit auch die des Behandlungslasers, durch das Tracking erfasst. Anschließend werden die registrierten Behandlungsorte auf das Mosaik übertragen. Unser Ansatz wurde auf Videoaufnahmen des Fundus angewandt, um Behandlungskarten zu erzeugen, auf denen die Bestrahlungsorte automatisiert eingetragen werden.

2   Material und Methoden

Unsere Arbeit gliedert sich in mehrere Abschnitte, die im Folgenden detailliert vorgestellt werden: Bildakquisition, Vorverarbeitung, Mosaicking und Lasertracking. Eine gute Übersicht über unseren Ansatz gibt eine schematische Darstellung in Abb. 1.

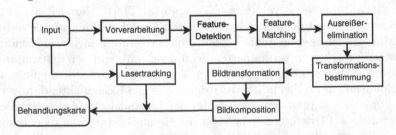

Abb. 1. Schematische Darstellung des Algorithmus.

2.1 Bildakquisition

Die Fundusvideoaufnahmen wurden mit dem Scanning Slit Ophthalmoscope (SSO) der Firma RS Medizintechnik GmbH aufgenommen, das an einer Spaltlampe (Zeiss LSL 532s) montiert wurde. Das SSO erstellt über ein Scanning-Verfahren reflexionsarme Aufnahmen mit einem großen Bildwinkel, die Papille, Makula und die zentralen Netzhautgefäße darstellen. Der Aufbau sowie eine Beispielaufnahme des SSO werden in Abb. 2 gezeigt. In dem SSO ist eine USB 3 uEye CP Kamera der Firma IDS Imaging Development Systems GmbH verbaut, mit der wir Videosequenzen des Fundus mit einer Auflösung von 1200 × 1024 Pixeln bei 15 fps aufnahmen. Üblicherweise wird bei der Lasertherapie des Fundus ein Kontaktglas auf die Kornea aufgesetzt. Daher wurden Aufnahmen sowohl mit einem Diagnosetubus als auch mit einem Kontaktglas (Volk SuperQuad 160, Mainster focal grid) erstellt.

2.2 Vorverarbeitung

Damit Störeffekte in den Bildaufnahmen, wie Reflexionen oder inhomogen beleuchtete Bildareale, spätere Verfahren nicht negativ beeinflussen, müssen diese maskiert werden. Wie in [3] vorgeschlagen, wird in einem ersten Schritt eine binäre Maske erzeugt, um Bildpixel, die zur Retina gehören, zu selektieren und gleichzeitig die Vignettierung und störende Reflexionen zu kompensieren. Ein Bildpixel gehört demnach zur Retina, wenn $R - 0.7G > 0$, wobei R bzw. G den roten bzw. grünen Bildkanal repräsentieren. Für den weiteren Verlauf wird lediglich der grüne Bildkanal verwendet. Dessen Kontrast wird in einem zweiten Vorverarbeitungsschritt verbessert. Hierzu wird CLAHE (Contrast Limited Adaptive Histogram Equalization) benutzt [4]. Durch den Einsatz von CLAHE wird außerdem die Feature-Detektion unterstützt.

2.3 Mosaicking

Beim Mosaicking werden aufeinanderfolgende Einzelbilder einer Szene miteinander registriert und anschließend zu einem Gesamtbild zusammengefügt, was ein Optimierungsproblem darstellt. In dieser Arbeit entsprechen die Einzelbilder

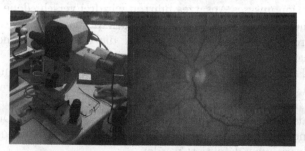

Abb. 2. Links: Scanning Slit Ophthalmoscope der Firma RS Medizintechnik GmbH. Rechts: Weißlichtaufnahme des SSO vom Fundus.

den Bildframes der Videosequenz, die vom Fundus aufgenommen werden. Zwischen jeweils zwei aufeinanderfolgenden Bildframes der Videosequenz wird eine Transformationsmatrix $\varphi_{k-1\rightarrow k}(\boldsymbol{p})$ bestimmt, die jeden Bildpixel $\boldsymbol{x}$ aus I_k auf das vorherige Einzelbild I_{k-1} $(k = 1 \ldots N)$ abbildet. Hierbei besteht das Optimierungsproblem darin, die geeigneten Parameter $\boldsymbol{p}$ zu finden. Für diese Arbeit wird eine partielle affine Registrierung mit insgesamt vier Freiheitsgraden (Rotation θ, Skalierung s, Translation t) gewählt und ist bestimmt durch

$$\varphi_{k-1\rightarrow k} = \begin{bmatrix} p_1 & -p_2 & p_3 \\ p_2 & p_1 & p_4 \end{bmatrix} \tag{1}$$

mit $p_1 = \cos(\theta)s$, $p_2 = \sin(\theta)s$, $p_3 = t_x$ und $p_4 = t_y$. Nach der Bestimmung von $\varphi_{k-1\rightarrow k}$, wird I_k transformiert und zum Mosaik hinzugefügt. Für das erste Einzelbild I_0 wird die Transformationsmatrix mit $\varphi_0 = Id$ initialisiert. Alle weiteren Transformationsmatrizen $\varphi_{k-1\rightarrow k}$ werden in jeder Iteration miteinander konkateniert. Für die Bestimmung der Transformationsmatrizen wird ein featurebasierter Registrierungsansatz gewählt. Hierbei wird SURF (Speeded Up Robust Features) verwendet. Zur Eliminierung von Ausreißern wird der RANSAC-Algorithmus (Random sample consensus) genutzt.

2.4 Lasertracking

Für die ortsrichtige Eintragung der Bestrahlungsorte auf der Behandlungskarte wird die Position des Behandlungslasers ermittelt. Durch die Verwendung einer Schwellenwertsegmentierung des Subtraktionsbilds von rotem und grünem Bildkanal $(R - G)$ kann idealerweise der Laserspot mit geeignetem Schwellenwert maskiert werden. Mithilfe des Ansatzes aus [5] wird die Kontur des Laserspots berechnet. Da sich der Durchmesser des Laserspots im Bild kaum ändert, wird über einen weiteren Schwellenwert die Kontur mit der geeigneten Länge übernommen, wodurch das Verfahren robuster gegenüber Störungen wird. Schließlich beschreibt der Schwerpunkt der ermittelten Kontur den Bestrahlungsort.

2.5 Experimente

Für die Evaluation unseres Ansatzes führten wir drei verschiedene Experimente durch, bei denen sowohl synthetische als auch probandenbezogene Bilddaten verwendet wurden. Zunächst evaluierten wir die Genauigkeit und Robustheit von Mosaicking und Lasertracking getrennt voneinander.

Im ersten Experiment erzeugten wir synthetische Videosequenzen aus Fundusaufnahmen, indem wir eine ROI entlang einer vordefinierten Trajektorie über das jeweilige Bild verschoben. Für jede Pixelposition wurde dann der Bildinhalt der ROI als Bildframe in einer Videosequenz abgespeichert. Die Trajektorie dient als Grundwahrheit. Durch sie können mögliche Registrierungsfehler des Mosaicking-Algorithmus detektiert werden.

Ähnlich wie beim Mosaicking wurde bei der Evaluation des Lasertrackings verfahren. Hier beschreibt ebenfalls eine vordefinierte Trajektorie die Bewegung eines simulierten Pilotlaserspots. Wie beim ersten Experiment repräsentiert die Trajektorie eine Grundwahrheit, wodurch die Genauigkeit des Lasertrackings evaluiert wird.

In einem letzten Versuch wurde der Ansatz auf probandenbezogene Bilddaten angewandt, die an der Klinik für Ophthalmologie am Universitätsklinikum Schleswig-Holstein in Kiel aufgenommen wurden. Leider konnte während der Studie kein Pilotlaser für die Aufnahmen benutzt werden, sodass dieser wie im zweiten Experiment simuliert wurde. Ziel des Experiments sollte die Erstellung von Behandlungskarten mit gleichzeitiger Eintragung von fiktiven Laserspots sein. Dabei war es wichtig zu überprüfen, dass der Laserspot das Mosaicking nicht stört und das Lasertracking in den probandenbezogenen Aufnahmen zuverlässig funktioniert.

Unser Ansatz wurde in C++ mithilfe der Softwarebibliothek OpenCV implementiert. Durch die Verwendung von Nvidia CUDA ist unser Ansatz echtzeitfähig.

3   Ergebnisse

Für die ersten beiden Experimente wurde jeweils der Abstand zwischen den geschätzten Trajektorien beider Algorithmen mit der jeweiligen Grundwahrheit verglichen. Sowohl das Mosaicking als auch das Lasertracking zeigten gute Ergebnisse. Ausgehend von der geschätzten Trajektorie wurde für jeden Punkt der nächstliegendste Punkt der Grundwahrheit gesucht. Für den Mosaicking-Algorithmus ergab sich eine mittlere Distanz zur Trajektorie von $3,02 \pm 2,57\,px$. Das Tracking des simulierten Laserspots lieferte eine mittlere Distanz von $0.45 \pm 0.44\,px$ zur Grundwahrheit. Die Ergebnisse des letzten Experiments sind in Abb. 3 dargestellt. Das Experiment zeigte, dass beide Algorithmen gut in Kombination funktionieren und sich nicht gegenseitig stören. In den Behandlungskarten fanden sich keine Artefakte des Laserspots. Darüber hinaus wurden Laser-

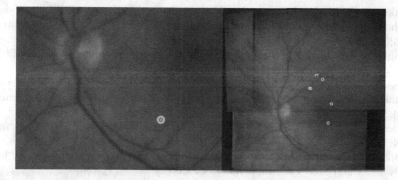

Abb. 3. Links: Die Genauigkeit des Lasertrackings wurde mithilfe von synthetischen Bilddaten ermittelt. Sobald der Algorithmus den Laserspot registriert, wird dieser markiert. Rechts: Erstellte Behandlungskarte aus probandenbezogenen Bilddaten mit simuliertem Pilotlaser. Die Markierungen zeigen hierbei simulierte Bestrahlungsspots.

spotmarkierungen auf der Behandlungskarte eingetragen, sobald ein künstliches Triggersignal betätigt wurde. Der Algorithmus läuft bei 15 − 20 fps in voller Auflösung.

4 Diskussion

In diesem Beitrag wurde ein Ansatz zur Registrierung und Dokumentation von unsichtbaren Bestrahlungsorten vorgestellt. Unser Ansatz aus kombiniertem Mosaicking und Lasertracking konnte in den Experimenten gute Ergebnisse erzielen. Beide Verfahren zeigten nur eine geringe Abweichung zur Grundwahrheit.

Ähnlich wie bei [3] konnten zum Teil größere Abweichung zur Trajektorie beim Mosaicking beobachtet werden, die bei unserem Ansatz mit fortschreitender Laufzeit größer wurde. Daher wird in zukünftigen Arbeiten die Registrierung robuster gestaltet, um die Genauigkeit zu erhöhen. Ebenso wird eine Überarbeitung der Maskierung dazu führen, dass störende Effekte die Feature-Detektion nicht negativ beeinflussen. Darüber hinaus werden Artefakte aus den erstellten Behandlungskarten durch entsprechende Korrekturmaßnahmen entfernt. Da der Lasertracker bis jetzt nur auf simulierten Bilddaten getestet werden konnte, sind Aufnahmen am Probanden mit Pilotlaser angedacht, um die Robustheit des Algorithmus weiter evaluieren zu können. Neben den Weißlichtaufnahmen sollen zukünftig Nahinfrarotlichtaufnahmen (NIR) aufgezeichnet werden. Da NIR-Licht für das menschliche Auge nicht sichtbar ist, würde die Anwendung dieser Aufnahmetechnik die Behandlung für den Patienten angenehmer gestalten.

Ziel des Projektes ist eine optimale Navigationsunterstützung, bei der die getrackten Laserspots ins Okular der Spaltlampe eingespiegelt werden, sodass ein Blick zum Monitor sich erübrigt.

Literaturverzeichnis

1. Brinkmann R, Roider J, Birngruber R. Selective retina therapy (SRT): a review on methods, techniques, preclinical and first clinical results. Bull Soc Belge Ophtalmol. 2006;(302):51–69.
2. Asmuth J, Madjarov B, Sajda P, et al. Mosaicking and enhancement of slit lamp biomicroscopic fundus images. Br J Ophthalmol. 2001;85(5):563–5.
3. Richa R, Linhares R, Comunello E, et al. Fundus image mosaicking for information augmentation in computer-assisted slit-lamp imaging. IEEE Trans Med Imaging. 2014;33(6):1304–12.
4. Zuiderveld K. Contrast limited adaptive histogram equalization. Graph Gems IV. 1994; p. 474–85.
5. Suzuki S, et al. Topological structural analysis of digitized binary images by border following. Computer Vis Graph Image Process. 1985;30(1):32–46.

Abstract: Real-Time Online Adaption for Robust Instrument Tracking and Pose Estimation

Nicola Rieke[1], David Joseph Tan[1], Federico Tombari[1], Josué Page Vizcaíno[1], Chiara Amat di San Filippo[2], Abouzar Eslami[2], Nassir Navab[1]

[1]Computer Aided Medical Procedures, Technische Universität München, Germany
[2]Carl Zeiss MEDITEC München, Germany
nicola.rieke@tum.de

In [1], we propose a novel method for instrument tracking in Retinal Microsurgery (RM) which is apt to withstand the challenges of *in-vivo* RM visual sequences. The proposed approach is a robust closed-loop framework to track and localize the instrument parts in real-time, based on a dual-random forest (RF). First, a tracker employs the pixel intensities in a RF to infer the bounding box around the tool tip. In the second step, this region of interest is forwarded to another RF, which predicts the locations of the tool joints based on HOG features. We propose to "close the loop" between the tracking and 2D pose estimation by obtaining a joint prediction for the template position: the outcome of the two separate forests is merged in a synergic way according to the confidence of their estimation. Such cooperative prediction will in turn provide pose information for the tracker, improving its robustness and accuracy. To cope with the strong illumination changes affecting the RM sequences, we adapt the offline RF model to online information while tracking, so to incorporate the appearance changes learned by the trees with real photometric distortions witnessed at test time. This offline learning - online adaption leads to a substantial capability regarding the generalization to unseen sequences. These key drivers allow our method to outperform state-of-the-art methods on two benchmark datasets.

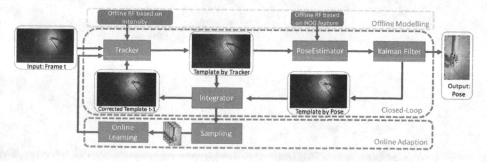

Fig. 1. Pipeline.

References

1. Rieke N, Tan DJ, Tombari F, et al. Real-time online adaption for robust instrument tracking and pose estimation. Proc MICCAI. 2016; p. 422–30.

Abstract: Wound Imaging in 3D Using Low-Cost Mobile Devices

Ekaterina Sirazitdinova, Thomas Deserno

Department of Medical Informatics, Uniklinik RWTH Aachen, Germany
ekaterina.sirazitdinova@rwth-aachen.de

The state-of-the-art method of wound assessment is manually performed by clinicians. Such procedure has limited reproducibility and accuracy, large time consumption and high costs. Novel technologies such as laser scanning microscopy, multi-photon microscopy, optical coherence tomography and hyperspectral imaging [1], as well as devices relying on the structured light sensors [2, 3] have limitations due to high costs and may lack portability and availability. The high prevalence of chronic wounds, however, requires inexpensive and portable devices for 3D imaging of skin lesions.

We present a low-cost wound assessment system and architecture for fast and accurate cutaneous wound assessment using inexpensive consumer smartphone devices [4]. We reconstruct wounds in 3D as dense models, which are generated from images taken with a built-in camera of a smartphone device. For that, we adapt the method of Ondruska et al. [5], where dense tracking is performed in each recorded frame: camera positions are estimated using a dense feature-free monocular camera tracking method. The system architecture includes imaging, processing and storage devices. It supports tracking over time by alignment of 3D models, color correction using a reference color card placed into the scene and automatic segmentation of wound regions. Using our system, we are able to detect and document quantitative characteristics of chronic wounds, including size, depth, volume, rate of healing, as well as qualitative characteristics as color, presence of necrosis and type of involved tissue.

References

1. Zhou A. A survey of optical imaging techniques for assessing wound healing. Int J Intell Control Syst. 2012;17.
2. Fuel3D. Eykona: Medical scanning solutions from fuel 3D technologies [Internet]; 2016. Accessed: 2016-03-22. Available from: https://www.fuel-3d.com/de/eykona/.
3. Bills JD, Berriman SJ, Noble DL, et al. Pilot study to evaluate a novel three-dimensional wound measurement device. Int Wound J. 2015; p. 1–6.
4. Sirazitdinova E, Deserno TM. System design for 3D wound imaging using low-cost mobile device (forthcoming 2017). Proc SPIE. 2017.
5. Ondruska P, Kohli P, Izadi S. MobileFusion: real-time volumetric surface reconstruction and dense tracking on mobile phones. IEEE Trans Vis Comput Graph. 2015;21(11):1251–8.

Interpatientenübertragung von Atemmodellen für das Virtual-Reality-Training von Punktionseingriffen

Andre Mastmeyer, Matthias Wilms, Heinz Handels

Institut für Medizinische Informatik, Universität zu Lübeck
mastmeyer@imi.uni-luebeck.de

Kurzfassung. Aktuelle VR-Trainingssimulatoren von Punktionen gehen oft von statischen 3D-Patientendaten aus oder verwenden eine unrealistisch-periodische Animation der Atembewegung. Existierende Methoden zur Modellierung der Atembewegung schätzen personalisierte Atemmodelle, die auch in VR-Trainingssimulatoren verwendet werden können. Für jeden neuen Patienten ist jedoch eine stark belastende bzw. teure 4D-Datenakquisition als Vorraussetzung der Modellbildung notwendig. Die hier entwickelte Methodik erlaubt, eine plausible Übertragung existierender Atembewegungsmodelle eines Referenzpatienten auf einen neuen statischen Patienten. Dieser kosten- und dosissparende Ansatz wird hier als Proof-of-Concept für das VR-Training im Leberbereich atmender virtueller Patienten gezeigt.

1 Einleitung

Das virtuelle Training und die Planung von minimalinvasiven chirurgischen Eingriffen mit Virtual-Reality-Simulatoren bietet Medizinern eine intuitive, visuohaptische Benutzeroberfläche für das risikolose Erlernen und die Planung von Eingriffen. Unsere Arbeitsgruppe beschäftigt sich seit Jahren mit der Simulation von Leberpunktionen [1, 2, 3].

Wichtig ist neben der optischen Darstellung der Anatomie virtueller Patientenkörper die haptische Simulation (1) der Gegenkräfte durch die manuelle Interaktion mit dem Patienten und (2) in neueren Entwicklungen die Simulation der Kräfte durch Patienteneigenbewegungen (Atmung) mit haptischen Ein- und Ausgabegeräten [3, 4, 5].

Die bisher bekannten VR-Trainingssimulatoren verwenden zumeist zeitinvariante 3D-Patientenmodelle. Eine Punktion des Spinalkanals kann hinreichend plausibel durch solche Modelle simuliert werden. Im thorakalen und oberen abdominalen Bereich sind jedoch Atem- und Herzbewegungen fortlaufend präsent. Im Zwerchfellbereich wurden Bewegungsunterschiede von bis zu 5 cm gemessen [6]. Unser Ziel ist hier, diese physiologisch-funktionalen Bewegungen realistisch in die Modellbildung aufzunehmen, um dem Benutzer eine realitätsnähere visuo-haptische VR-Punktionssimulation anzubieten. Dies bedeutet z.B. auch die Intra- und Interzyklenvariabilität (Hysterese, variable Amplitude bei Ein-/Ausatmung) zu berücksichtigen.

Von anderen Gruppen publizierte Ansätze [7, 8] modellieren nur eine sinusförmige Atembewegung ohne Hysterese und Unregelmäßigkeit. Eine akkurate Simulation der Atembewegung abhängig von Surrogatsignalen ist z.B. in der Strahlentherapie relevant. Da jedoch zur personalisierten Atemmodellbildung ein patientenspezifischer 4D-Volumendatensatz benötigt wird und dessen Aquisition mit einer hohen Strahlenbelastung bei der 4D-CT ($\geq$ 20-30 mSv (eff.)) einhergeht [9], ist unser Ansatz die Übertragung bereits existierender Atemmodelle auf neue Patienten. Zum Vergleich sei genannt: Die durchschnittliche natürliche Hintergrundstrahlung beträgt ca. 2,1 mSv (eff.) pro Jahr[1].

Andererseits ist für Trainingszwecke keine Indikation gegeben und auch aus Kostengründen eine Modellbildung aus dafür aufzunehmenden 4D-MR-Daten nicht vertretbar.

Wir zeigen hier eine Machbarkeitsuntersuchung mit ersten qualitativen Ergebnissen zur Übertragung eines existierenden Atemmodells [10] auf statische Patientendaten, bei denen nur eine 3D-CT-Thorax-Leber-Aufnahme mit maximaler Einatmung als Referenzphase notwendig ist (ca. 2-13 mSv (eff.))[2]

2 Material und Methoden

2.1 VR-Leberpunktionssimulator für Planung und Training

In [1, 2, 11, 12] wurden bereits Konzepte für einen 3D-VR-Simulator und die Patientenmodellierung für das Training verschiedener Punktionseingriffe (z.B. Leberpunktionen) vorgestellt. Die manuelle Steuerung und haptische Kraftrückkopplung übernimmt ein Geomagic Phantom Premium 1.5 HighForce. Eine Nvidia Shutterbrille und ein stereoskopisches Display sorgen für die räumlich plausible Darstellung der Simulationsszene. Dieses System verwendet zeitinvariante 3D-CT-Datensätze als Grundlage des Patientenmodells. Bei der manuellen Interaktion mit dem Modell auftretende Gewebedeformationen bzw. Kräfte werden durch ein direktes visuo-haptisches Volume-Rendering-Verfahren dargestellt.

Neue Entwicklungen von VR-Simulatoren [2] erlauben in Echtzeit für den zu visualisierenden Patienten anstatt eines statischen 3D-CT-Datensatzes einen zeitvarianten 4D-CT-Datensatz zu verwenden. Die Atembewegung kann als Keyframe-Modell oder mit einem Atemmodel, das im Folgenden beschrieben wird, visuo-haptisch dargestellt werden.

2.2 Atemmodellierung

Grundlage für die Atemmodellierung ist in der Regel ein 4D-Datensatz mindestens eines Atemzyklus und ein Surrogatsignal (z.B. mittels Spirometrie), um die Patientenatmung niedrigdimensional zu parametrisieren [10].

---

[1] Interkontinentalflug max. 0,11 mSv (eff.): https://goo.gl/8VQoKV
[2] Siemens Somatom Defintion AS: https://goo.gl/S8ZdIk

Wir verwenden ein gemessenes Spirometersignal $v(t)$ [ml] und seine zeitliche Ableitung in einem zusammengesetzten Surrogatsignal: $(v(t), v'(t))^T$. Dies ist begründet in der Forderung, verschiedene Tiefen der Atmung und die Unterscheidung zwischen Ein-/Ausatmung zu ermöglichen (Atemhysterese). Unter der Annahme der Linearität zwischen Signal und Bewegung werden für das personalisierte Atemmodell mit einer linearen multivariaten Regression die Koeffizienten $a_{1..3}^{\text{pat4D}}$ als Vektorfelder über den Positionen $\mathbf{x}$ geschätzt

$$\hat{\varphi}^{\text{pat4D}}(\mathbf{x}, t) = a_1^{\text{pat4D}}(\mathbf{x}) \cdot v(t) + a_2^{\text{pat4D}}(\mathbf{x}) \cdot v'(t) + a_3^{\text{pat4D}}(\mathbf{x}) \tag{1}$$

Somit kann zu einem Patientenzustand repräsentiert durch ein ggf. bisher ungesehenes Atemsignal und zu jedem Zeitpunkt t das zugehörige verschobene Referenzbild $I_{j_{\text{ref}}}^{\text{pat4D}} \circ \hat{\varphi}^{\text{pat4D}}(\mathbf{x}, t)$ angegeben werden. Die nun zeitvariant modellbasiert animierbaren CT-Daten $I_{j_{\text{ref}}}^{\text{pat4D}}$ können in einer neuen Variante des Simulators aus [2] dargestellt und zum Training genutzt werden.

2.3   Übertragung existierender Atemmodelle auf neue, statische Patientendaten

Mit der bisher geschilderten Methode lassen sich personalisierte Atemmodelle erstellen, deren Flexibilität genügt, um auch in der Beobachtungsphase der Modellbildung nicht gesehene Atemzustände des Patienten zu approximieren.

Allerdings ist bisher damit für jeden Patienten die dosisbelastende bzw. teure Aufnahme mindestens eines 4D-Datensatzes notwendig.

Daher wird im Folgenden die Idee verfolgt, einmal z.B. anhand eines 4D-Referenzpatienten erstellte Atemmodelle für neue statische Patientendaten pat3D nutzbar zu machen und im in Abschnitt 2.1 beschriebenen VR-Simulator zu zu animieren.

Dazu ist es notwendig, die anatomischen Variabilitäten zwischen dem Referenzpatienten mit den Bilddaten $I_{j_{\text{ref}}}^{\text{pat4D}}$ und den neuen Patientenbilddaten $I_{\text{ref}}^{\text{pat3D}}$ anhand einer möglichst ähnlichen Atemphase auszugleichen. Dies wird bspw. durch eine Hold-Breath-Aufnahme (ref) in maximalem Einatemzustand erreicht, der in einem standardisierten 4D-Aufnahmeprotokoll eine bestimmte Phase j_{ref} entspricht. Eine nichtlineare Interpatientenregistrierung $\varphi(\mathbf{x}) : \Omega_{\text{pat3D}} \to \Omega_{\text{pat4D}}$ unter Minimierung einschlägiger Bilddistanzmaße D sorgt für den notwendigen Ausgleich

$$\varphi_{j_{\text{ref}}}^{\text{pat3D}\to\text{pat4D}} = \underset{\varphi}{\text{argmin}} \left(D... \left[I_{\text{ref}}^{\text{pat3D}}, I_{j_{\text{ref}}}^{\text{pat4D}} \circ \varphi \right] + \alpha \cdot R(\varphi) \right) \tag{2}$$

wobei '...' hier einen Distanzmaßtyp und R ein gewichtetes Regularisierungsmaß repräsentiert. Das Distanzmaß kann je nach Modalität und Qualität der Bilddaten gewählt werden. Die in der nichtlinearen Interpatientenregistrierung bestimmte Transformation $\varphi_{j_{\text{ref}}}^{\text{pat3D}\to\text{pat4D}}$ kann nun zur morphologischen Übertragung der einmalig für den Referenzpatienten bestimmten Deformationen φ_j^{pat4D}

verwendet werden und die Bewegungsinformationen φ_j^{pat4D} als plausible Schätzung $\hat{\varphi}_j^{\text{pat3D}}$ übertragen ($j \in \{1, \ldots, n\}$, $\circ$: v.r.n.l.)

$$\hat{\varphi}_j^{\text{pat3D}} = \left(\varphi_{j_{\text{ref}}}^{\text{pat3D} \rightarrow \text{pat4D}} \right)^{-1} \circ \varphi_j^{\text{pat4D}} \circ \varphi_{j_{\text{ref}}}^{\text{pat3D} \rightarrow \text{pat4D}} \tag{3}$$

Der Ansatz zur Schätzung der Atembewegung für den neuen Patienten kann nun analog zum Referenzpatienten (siehe Abschnitt 2.2) angewendet werden. Mit dieser effizienten Methode kann die Atembewegung virtueller Patientenmodelle, die nur auf einem mit vergleichsweise geringer Dosis aufgenommener 3D-CT-Daten basieren plausibel realisiert werden

$$\hat{\varphi}^{\text{pat3D}}(\mathbf{x}, t) = \hat{a}_1^{\text{pat3D}}(\mathbf{x}) \cdot v(t) + \hat{a}_2^{\text{pat3D}}(\mathbf{x}) \cdot v'(t) + \hat{a}_3^{\text{pat3D}}(\mathbf{x}), \ \mathbf{x} \in \Omega_{\text{pat3D}} \tag{4}$$

Wahlweise können in irgendeiner Weise simulierte Surrogatsignale $v(t)$ zur 4D-Animation der 3D-CT-Daten verwendet werden. Einfache Alternativen sind zudem, das ggf. skalierte Surrogatsignal des Referenzpatienten oder auch ein Signal des neuen Patienten zu verwenden, das einfach nur mit der entsprechenden spirometrischen Meßvorrichtung ohne Bildakquise aufgenommen werden kann.

2.4 Evaluation

Wir verwenden in Gl. (2) die Summe der quadrierten Intensitätsunterschiede an korrespondierenden Voxel-Stellen als Distanzmaß D_{SSD} und eine diffusive nichtlineare Regularisierung R, $\alpha = 1$. Beiderseits wird die Atemlage maximaler Einatmung als Referenzphase (ref) gewählt.

Die Interpatientenübertragung realistischer variabler Atembewegungen von einem Referenzpatienten auf einen nur durch einen statischen 3D-CT-Datensatz ($512^2 \times 318$ Voxel zu 1^3 mm) repräsentierten neuen Patienten wird in einer qualitativen Machbarkeitsstudie im 4D-VR-Trainingssimulator [2] anhand der Bereiche mit plausibler Atemsimulation und der noch störenden Problemstellen gezeigt.

Die DICE-Koeffizienten der übertragenen Lebermasken werden zur Einordnung der Qualität der Interpatientenregistrierung der Referenzatemphasen (Single-Atlas-Ansatz) auf der quantitativen Seite dargelegt.

Seitens des 4D-Referenzpatienten wurde ein 4D-CT-Datensatz des Thorax und oberen Abdomens mit 14 Atemphasen ($512^2 \times 462$ Voxel zu 1^3 mm) und ein Spirometersignal $v(t)$ genutzt. Als Referenzatemphase für das Training des Atemmodells wird jeweils ebenfalls die Phase mit maximaler Einatmung herangezogen. Alle Volumenbilddaten wurden aufgrund des begrenzten Grafikkartenspeichers des verwendeten Referenzsystems (GPU: Nvidia GTX 680 mit 3 GB RAM) auf eine Größe von 256^3 Voxel reduziert.

3 Ergebnisse

Die DICE-Koeffizenten der Single-Atlas-Übertragung der Lebermasken auf den neuen statischen Patienten pat3D ergeben befriedigende Werte von 0,86±0,01 mit dem von uns hier implizit verwendeten Single-Atlas-Segmentierungs-Ansatz bei stark unterschiedlichem Scan-Bereich (Abb. 1 oben links). Die Animation der relevanten Strukturen anhand eines variablen echten Atemsignals des Zielpatienten pat3D (Abb. 1 oben rechts) ist in Abb. 1 unten exemplarisch dargestellt. Im punktionsrelevanten Leberbereich werden die Atemzustände des neuen Patienten pat3D visuell plausibel simuliert.

4 Diskussion

Die hier beschriebene Methode zur Übertragung der retrospektiv modellierten Atembewegung eines Referenzpatienten auf einen neuen Patienten erlaubt die plausible Animation realistischer Atembewegungen in einem 4D-VR-Trainings-simulator mit visuo-haptischer Interaktion. Wir erreichen in dieser Machbar-keitsuntersuchung bereits qualitativ plausible Ergebnisse für den Leberbereich. Im Hinblick auf die Punktion z.B. im unteren Lungenbereich mit Perforation des Zwerchfells müssen jedoch weitere Optimierungen vorgenommen werden, da sich am Lungenrand (Zwerchfell, Rippen) stärkere Artefakte [2] bei geringem Atemzugvolumen zeigen könnnen (Abb. 1 unten, drittes Bild). Die bisherige Annahme [10], der notwendigen dosisrelevanten bzw. teuren Akquisition eines

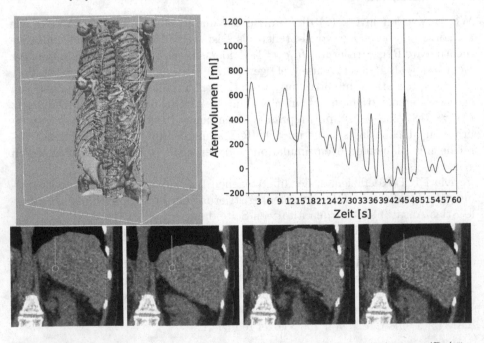

Abb. 1. Oben links: Field-of-View-Unterschied zwischen Referenzpatient pat4D (tür-kis) und Zielpatient pat3D (gelb). Unten: Coronale Ansicht der mit dem Modell von pat4D deformierten CT-Daten des Zielpatienten pat3D zu den markierten Zeitpunkten des Spirometersignals von pat3D (oben rechts).

4D-CT-Datensatzes für jeden Patienten, kann durch das vorgestellte Konzept mitigiert werden.

Zukünftige Arbeiten beschäftigen sich mit der besseren Adaption und Simulation des Atemsignals. Weitere Themen sind die Optimierung der Interpatientenregistrierung und die Konstruktion von alternativ wählbaren Referenzatemmodellen.

Literaturverzeichnis

1. Fortmeier D, Mastmeyer A, Schröder J, et al. A virtual reality system for PTCD simulation using direct visuo-haptic rendering of partially segmented image data. IEEE J Biomed Health Inform. 2016;20(1):355–66.
2. Fortmeier D, Wilms M, Mastmeyer A, et al. Direct visuo-haptic 4D volume rendering using respiratory motion models. IEEE Trans Haptics. 2015;8(4):371–83.
3. Mastmeyer A, Hecht T, Fortmeier D, et al. Ray-casting based evaluation framework for haptic force-feedback during percutaneous transhepatic catheter drainage punctures. Int J Comput Assist Radiol Surg. 2014;9:421–31.
4. Fortmeier D, Mastmeyer A, Handels H. Image-based palpation simulation with soft tissue deformations using ChainMail on the GPU. Proc BVM. 2013; p. 140–5.
5. Fortmeier D, Mastmeyer A, Handels H. GPU-based visualization of deformable volumetric soft-tissue for real-time simulation of haptic needle insertion. Proc BVM. 2012; p. 117–22.
6. Seppenwoolde Y, Shirato H, Kitamura K, et al. Precise and real-time measurement of 3D tumor motion in lung due to breathing and heartbeat, measured during radiotherapy. Int J Rad Oncololgy Biol Phys. 2002;53(4):822–34.
7. Villard PF, Vidal FP, Cenydd L, et al. Interventional radiology virtual simulator for liver biopsy. Int J Comput Assist Radiol Surg. 2014;9(2):255–67.
8. Villard PF, Boshier P, Bello F, et al. In: Takahashi H, editor. Virtual reality simulation of liver biopsy with a respiratory component. InTech; 2011. p. 315–34.
9. Matsuzaki Y, Fujii K, Kumagai M, et al. Effective and organ doses using helical 4DCT for thoracic and abdominal therapies. J Radiat Res Tokyo. 2013;54(5):962–70.
10. Wilms M, Werner R, Ehrhardt J, et al. Multivariate regression approaches for surrogate-based diffeomorphic estimation of respiratory motion in radiation therapy. Phys Med Biol. 2014;59:1147–64.
11. Mastmeyer A, Fortmeier D, Handels H. Efficient patient modeling for visuo-haptic VR simulation using a generic patient atlas. Comput Methods Programs Biomed. 2016;132:161–75.
12. Mastmeyer A, Fortmeier D, Maghsoudi E, et al. Patch-based label fusion using local confidence-measures and weak segmentations. Proc SPIE. 2013; p. 86691N-1–11.

Automatic Initialization and Failure Detection for Surgical Tool Tracking in Retinal Microsurgery

Josué Page Vizcaíno[1], Nicola Rieke[1], David Joseph Tan[1], Federico Tombari[1,4],
Abouzar Eslami[3], Nassir Navab[1,2]

[1]Computer Aided Medical Procedures, Technische Universität München, Germany
[2]Computer Aided Medical Procedures, Johns Hopkins University, Baltimore, USA
[3]Carl Zeiss MEDITEC München, Germany
[4]DISI, University of Bologna, Italy
josue.page@tum.de

Abstract. Instrument tracking is a key step for various computer-aided interventions in retinal microsurgery. One of the bottlenecks of state-of-the-art template based algorithms is the (re-)initialization during the surgery. We propose an algorithm for robustly detecting the bounding box around the tool tip together with a failure detection of the tracking algorithm. Hereby, the user input dependent algorithm is transformed into a completely automatic framework without the need of an assistant. The performance was compared to two state-of-the-art methods.

1 Introduction and related work

In Retinal Microsurgery (RM), the surgeon has to handle surgical instruments with high precision while observing them through a stereo-microscope. Recent research has aimed at introducing real-time instrument tracking algorithms within RM, which allow to simplify the surgical workflow and increases safety during surgical maneuvers. Bouget et al. [1] recently presented an overview of the latest vision-based approaches in this field, including a mutual information approach [2], a Bayesian filtering problem [3] and a gradient boosted regression tree [4]. An online learning approach was presented by Li et al. [5] and a combination of offline learning with online adaption via random forests was suggested by Rieke et al. [6]. One of the missing links for a seamless template-based tracking framework is the initial localization of the bounding box around the tool tip. The vision based detection of this region of interest in in-vivo is still challenging, mainly due to illumination changes and variable instrument appearances. In this paper, we introduce a detector which provides this region of interest around the tool tip and analyses the possibilities of a failure detection. In this way, an initialization dependent algorithms can be transformed into a fully automated system (Fig. 1). The performance of the proposed approach is quantitatively evaluated on an in-vivo RM dataset, and demonstrate comparable performance with respect to ground truth initialization when combined with the state-of-the-art in terms of robustness and generalization.

2 Materials and method

In the following sections, we elaborate how to integrate the proposed algorithm into the overall pipeline (Sec. 2.1) and present details of the detector for the template initialization (Sec. 2.2) and the failure detection (Sec. 2.3). The method is exemplarily combined with the tracking algorithm proposed by Rieke et al. [6] and tested on an in-vivo RM dataset (Sec. 2.4).

2.1 Pipeline

Our pipeline begins with requesting the location of the bounding box around the tool tip from the detector, considering the entire image information in the frame. This region of interest is passed on as an initialization for a template tracking and pose estimation, as for example by Rieke et al. [6]. The output of this algorithm defines a template, which is forwarded to a failure detection module, which evaluates the performance via a similarity measure. Depending on a threshold applied to this result, the inner loop of the tracking remains either uninterrupted or new initialization is requested to the detector. This is a closed loop approach without any user input, as depicted in Fig. 1.

2.2 Detector

The detector supplies a tracker with a template initialization by following the steps shown in Fig. 2. In the first step, the optical flow (OF) of the video sequence using the Shi-Tomasi corner detection [7] reduces the region of interest from the entire frame to locations where movement is present. Since the background and the light are not static in RM, the OF encompasses not only the tool but also some anatomic structures of the retina. Therefore, in a second step, the region is further reduced by classifying every pixel in the masked image as either tool part or background via a random forest (RF). For this, the gradient image is computed and a sliding window extracts patches on the considered locations. The gradient magnitude is hereby sampled from every patch in a grid-like fashion and used as an input to the RF. During training, the binary splitting function of the RF partitions the samples based on one dimension of the input in a way that

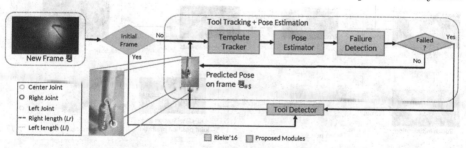

Fig. 1. Diagram of our framework (Sec. 2.1).

the information gain is maximized. The leaves of the RF store a normalized histogram with 4 bins, which represent the probability of belonging to one of the classes for a sample reaching this leaf. During prediction, the sample is navigated through the trees until it reaches a leaf. The resulting histograms with the lowest standard deviations are averaged and the class with the highest value in the average histogram is selected as the final prediction for the current window position. In the third step, this prediction is refined to the most probable solution. For this, a separate heat-map is created for every class by considering the respective candidates. A non maximal suppression is applied to these heat-maps in order to find the point with the lowest standard deviation and thereby the most probable location. As in RM the tool is inserted through a trocar into the eye, the possible orientations of the tool are limited allowing the introduction of mechanical constrains based on the predicted joint position, for example: the center joint can't be above the left or right tips, and the right tip can't be on the left of the left tip. The tool parts are described in Fig. 1. Then every prediction in the corresponding joint heat-map contributes to the position of the final tool part prediction as follows

$$C = C_0 + \frac{1}{255 \cdot N} \cdot \sum_{n=0}^{N} \sigma_n \cdot P_n \tag{1}$$

Where N is the number of points found for the current tool part, σ_n the standard deviation of current prediction, P_n the position of the current prediction, C_0 the position found through non-maximal suppression and C is the final predicted position. A crucial requirement is the robustness to different tool sizes. The detector overcomes this by using a multi-scale approach, in which the upper three-step procedure is performed on 5 different scales. In order to pick the correct scale, we introduce a score S for every scale. For every joint that couldn't be found, S is multiplied by a factor to discourage picking this scale as the final result. If all 3 points are found, the score S is computed as follows

$$S = w_1 \cdot |L_l - L_r| + w_2 \cdot (|\frac{L_l}{s} - L_a| + |\frac{L_r}{s} - L_a|) \tag{2}$$

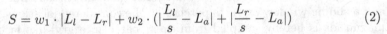

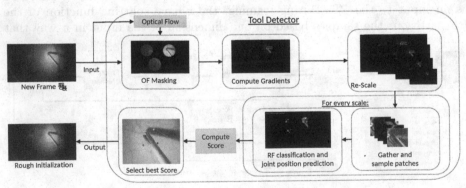

Fig. 2. Structure of detector (Sec. 2.2).

where L_l and L_r correspond to the predicted length of the left and right tool part respectively as shown in Fig. 1, L_a to the expected constant length of the tool and w_1 and w_2 to the score weighting factors. These calculation enforces a similar length of the right and left joints as that is normally the topology of the instrument. The detector then picks the scale with the lowest score. The final template for the tracker is then defined by the three points prediction of this scale via a homography.

2.3 Failure detection

We propose to consider the frame provided by the detector (Sec. 2.2) as a reference template and employing the Sum of Squared Differences (SSD) between it and the predicted template on the current frame as a performance metric. If a failure is indicated, a re-initialization by the detector is requested. Different similarity measures were investigated and SSD delivered the best results.

2.4 Analysis design

We evaluated our approach on a *in-vivo* RM sequence dataset [8], which comprises 4 sequences with 200 consecutive frames at 1920×1080 pixels of resolution each, with high illumination, blurriness and background color changes and were no tool occlusions are observed. First, we evaluate the proposed template detector regarding the accuracy when using different features for the random forest. However we expect the detector to provide a tracking algorithm a usable template initialization, rather than a precise prediction. Therefore we evaluate in the second step, if the proposed method combined with the tracking algorithm by [6] achieves similar results as the tracking algorithm with the ground truth initialization. In the third experiment, we examine the influence of the failure detection when tested on a longer sequence consisting of 350 frames, in which the instrument exits the frame. The performance was evaluated by means of a pixel threshold distance as suggested by Sznitman *et al.* [9]. The parameters $w_1 = 400$, $w_2 = 100$ and $L_a = 100$ were defined by using a grid search approach.

3 Results

In the following section, we present the results on the mentioned experiments.

3.1 Detector accuracy evaluation

The accuracy of the detector is evaluated by means of a thresholded distance which considers a prediction as correct if the distance between a prediction and the ground truth is lower than a threshold. This criteria was used on the 4 RM sequences using three different feature spaces. The experiment indicates that gradient features yield the best performance (Fig. 3). The predicted center joint positions of the 4 sequences were averaged in this graph.

Fig. 3. Comparison of features for RF classification (Sec. 3.1).

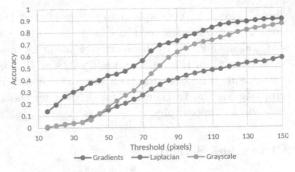

Fig. 4. Evaluation on sequence with re-initialization (Sec. 3.3).

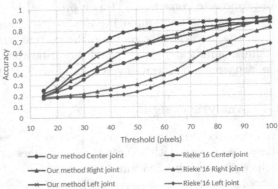

3.2 Evaluation of entire framework

A leave-one-out approach is used to evaluate the robustness of the proposed method where the RF is trained on 3 RM sequences and tested on the 4th one The performance is compared to the approaches presented by Rieke *et al.* [6, 8]. In both the state-of-the-art methods, the tracking is initialized with the ground truth, while in our method it is initialized by the detector. Fig. 3 shows very similar results between these methods, which means that the detector can be used to start the tracking when no ground truth is available.

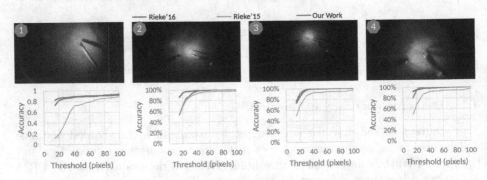

Fig. 5. Accuracy comparison regarding the center joint prediction (Sec. 3.2).

3.3 Evaluation on sequence with re-initialization

In the 4 RM sequences of the previous experiment, the tool is always visible. For evaluating the failure detection and re-initialization we tested both methods on a sequence consisting of 350 frames, in which a re-initialization is required, and trained the RF with the leave-one-out approach. As indicated in Fig. 4, our approach is able to detect failure and to re-initialize the tracker, delivering better results when compared to Rieke'16 [6], where this feature is absent. This sequence comes closer to the situation in medical practice as it's common that the instrument goes out of the field of view during RM.

4   Discussion

In this article we explore the possibility of providing an initialization and a failure detection to a template based tracking algorithm, allowing it to be independent from user interaction. The experiments show that from the investigated feature spaces the gradients deliver the best results, however it is possible that there are feature spaces providing even more reliable information. The current available data sets are limited, as the tool is usually visible and the illumination of the sequences is generally constant. A next step could be to test the proposed method on a more extensive experiment to evaluate the robustness of the algorithm regarding more complex light changes and frequent tool disappearances.

References

1. Bouget D, Allan M, Stoyanov D, et al. Vision-based and marker-less surgical tool detection and tracking: a review of the literature. Med Image Anal. 2017; p. 633–54.
2. Richa R, Balicki M, Meisner E, et al. Visual tracking of surgical tools for proximity detection in retinal surgery. Proc IPCAI. 2011; p. 55–66.
3. Sznitman R, Basu A, Richa R, et al. Unified detection and tracking in retinal microsurgery. Proc MICCAI. 2011; p. 1–8.
4. Sznitman R, Becker C, Fua P. Fast part-based classification for instrument detection in minimally invasive surgery. Proc MICCAI. 2014; p. 692–9.
5. Li Y, Chen C, Huang X, et al. Instrument tracking via online learning in retinal microsurgery. Proc MICCAI. 2014; p. 464–71.
6. Rieke N, Tan DJ, Tombari F, et al. Real-time online adaption for robust instrument tracking and pose estimation. Proc MICCAI. 2016; p. 422–30.
7. Shi J, Tomasi C. Good features to track. Proc CVPR. 1994; p. 593–600.
8. Rieke N, Tan DJ, Alsheakhali M, et al. Surgical tool tracking and pose estimation in retinal microsurgery. Proc MICCAI. 2015; p. 266–73.
9. Sznitman R, Ali K, Richa R, et al. Data-driven visual tracking in retinal microsurgery. Proc MICCAI. 2012; p. 568–75.

Automatic Viewpoint Selection for Exploration of Time-Dependent Cerebral Aneurysm Data

Monique Meuschke[1], Wito Engelke[2], Oliver Beuing[3], Bernhard Preim[1],
Kai Lawonn[4]

[1]Dept. of Computer Graphics and Simulation, OvG-University Magdeburg, Germany,
and Research Campus STIMULATE
[2] Simulation and Software Technology, German Aerospace Center, Braunschweig,
Germany
[3] Institute of Neuroradiology, University Hospital of Magdeburg, Germany, and
Research Campus STIMULATE
[4] Institute of Computational Visualistics, University of Koblenz – Landau, Germany
meuschke@isg.cs.uni-magdeburg.de

Abstract. This paper presents an automatic selection of viewpoints,
forming a camera path, to support the exploration of cerebral aneurysms.
Aneurysms bear the risk of rupture with fatal consequences for the patient. For the rupture risk evaluation, a combined investigation of morphological and hemodynamic data is necessary. However, the extensive
nature of the time-dependent data complicates the analysis. During exploration, domain experts have to manually determine appropriate views,
which can be a tedious and time-consuming process. Our method determines optimal viewpoints automatically based on input data such as
wall thickness or pressure. The viewpoint selection is modeled as an
optimization problem. Our technique is applied to five data sets and
we evaluate the results with two domain experts by conducting informal
interviews.

1 Introduction

Cerebral aneurysms are abnormal dilatations of intracranial arteries, resulting
from a pathological weakness in the vessel wall. Their rupture leads to a sub-
arachnoid hemorrhage and is associated with a high mortality and morbidity
rate. The aneurysm's initiation and outcome depends on different morphological and hemodynamic factors, whose impact on the individual rupture risk is not
yet well understood. Computational Fluid Dynamic (CFD) simulations enable
the investigation of the patient-specific internal wall mechanics and blood flow
during the cardiac cycle. Experts are interested in correlations between hemodynamic factors that are associated with an increased risk of rupture. Therefore,
hemodynamic and morphological parameters are visualized on the aneurysm
surface simultaneously [1]. The problem of analyzing aneurysm data is twofold:
first, the obtained flow data are very complex, and secondly, adjacent vessels
could lead to occlusions. Domain experts have to manually search for suspicious

352

regions by selecting views that enable an occlusion-free exploration. This can be a tedious and time-consuming process. Therefore, a camera control including an adequate viewpoint selection is crucial for an efficient analysis.

There are several methods to determine good views for polygonal [2, 3], volume data [4] and vector fields [5, 6]. They mainly based on entropy [2], which is a measure to assess the quality of a view with the aim of maximizing its information content. For polygonal meshes, the relation between visible polygons and visible area [2] or surface parameters [3] were maximized. For volume data, voxel-based entropy functions were optimized and for vector fields, the visibility as well as flow parameters of streamlines were used. The suitability of a view also depends on application-specific characteristics, e.g., familiar and preferred views in surgery. Mühler et al. [7] integrated geometric aspects with such preferences.

In this work, we present an automatic calculation of a camera path to support the exploration of simulated aneurysm data. The camera path is composed of optimal viewpoints that present the most interesting regions during the cardiac cycle based on user-selected morphological and hemodynamic parameters. With our method, we enable the detection of suspicious surface regions without a time-consuming manual search. Our collaborating domain experts confirmed that our method supports the analysis of the time-dependent data.

2   Material and methods

In this section, we describe the acquisition of simulated aneurysm data as well as our selection of appropriate viewpoints for the camera path.

2.1   Data acquisition and preprocessing

First, contrast-enhanced CT image data of the vessel morphology are acquired. Based on this, the vessel surface is reconstructed using the pipeline by Mönch et al. [8]. The 3D aneurysm surface and its parent vessel were extracted by using a threshold-based segmentation followed by a connected component analysis and Marching Cubes. The results are evaluated by medical experts to ensure anatomical plausibility. From the surface mesh, an unstructured volumetric grid is generated, on which a CFD simulation with a temporal resolution of 93 time steps is performed, using the STAR-CCM+ (CD-adapco, USA) solver.

2.2   Best viewpoint selection

This section explains our viewpoint selection. We describe the formulation of the target function, the start point sampling and the generation of the camera path.

Target function. To select viewpoints, a target function $f : V \rightarrow \mathbb{R}$ has to be formulated that covers the criteria of an optimal viewpoint $\mathbf{x} \in V$. Selected viewpoints are local maxima of the target function that consists of two parts. The first one is the size of the visible aneurysm surface area, because mostly, domain experts are interested in regions on the aneurysm. The second part is the significance of a surface area according to a user-selected parameter combination. For the first criteria, we separate the aneurysm from the parent vessel by segmenting it. This is done by an approach that determines the geodesic distance on the surface. For this, we place a start point on the aneurysm dome and compute the geodesic distance based on the heat equation [9]. Afterwards, we specify the distance that restricts the region of the aneurysm, including the ostium. For the second criteria, the user has to select two scalar parameters s_1 and s_2 that she wants to explore. Moreover, the user has to define if lower or higher values of the respective parameter should be weighted stronger. Based on the aneurysm segmentation, we implement a GPU-based approach to determine the target function's value for a specific viewpoint.

In the following, we explain how the target function $f(\mathbf{x})$ is defined for a viewpoint $\mathbf{x}$. Every fragment $p(\mathbf{x})$ in the current viewpoint $\mathbf{x}$ is assigned a value $t(p(\mathbf{x}))$. The sum of the fragment's values yields the target function $f(\mathbf{x}) = \sum_i t(p_i(\mathbf{x}))$. If the fragment p does neither belong to the segmentation nor to the front faces, we assign $t(p) = 0$. If $t(p)$ is not equal to zero, the two scalar values per fragment $s_1, s_2 \in [0, 1]$ are multiplied by 10 and truncated to the nearest integer values, yielding $s_{i1}, s_{i2} \in \{0, \ldots, 10\}$. Moreover, s_{i1} and s_{i2} are squared to stronger weight interesting values. Additionally, we divide the framebuffer in $n \times n$ subimages and assign a constant factor $B_{ij} = \binom{n-1}{i} \cdot \binom{n-1}{j}$ to each subimage (i, j) in the design of a binomial filter. We used $n = 5$. Then, B_{ij} is added to s_{i1} and s_{i2}, depending on the subimage the current fragment belongs to, which yields the updated values s'_{i1} and s'_{i2}. This leads to a stronger weighting of s_{i1} and s_{i2}, if they occur in the center of the camera view. Lower values of n result in a too strong weighting of uninteresting surface regions, while higher values lead to an excessive weighting of small areas. We set $t(p) = s'_{i1} + s'_{i2}$, which represents the scalar value for a fragment p. Finally, we determine the target function $f(\mathbf{x})$ and store the value on an image, which allows a later CPU-based access.

After we used f to find appropriate starting points. The gradient ascent method is applied to each of them. The goal is to further optimize the two camera angles and the view direction (x, y, z), which results in five Degrees Of Freedom (DOF). Each DOF is changed iteratively, $f(\mathbf{x})$ is evaluated and the gradient of $f(\mathbf{x})$ is calculated. The new viewpoint $\mathbf{x}_{new}$ is calculated by $\mathbf{x}_{new} = \mathbf{x}_{old} + s \cdot \nabla f(\mathbf{x}_{old})$, where $\mathbf{x}_{old}$ is the current viewpoint, s is the step size and $\nabla f(\mathbf{x}_{old})$ is the gradient of $f(\mathbf{x}_{old})$. The gradient ascent stops if the gradient magnitude falls below a threshold t with $t = 0.001$. Moreover, f is evaluated for different values of s, where the integer values range from 1 to 5.

Starting point selection. The camera path should indicate interesting surface regions during the cardiac cycle. Within a time step, there are mostly several positions where significant parameter correlations arise. To find these local optima, we select multiple starting points per time step. It would be possible to define an arbitrary number of points at arbitrary positions around the aneurysm. However, possibly the optimization would require many iterations to find local optima. Thus, we try to select starting points close to local optima on an approximated ellipsoid around the aneurysm. The ellipsoid's axes are the eigenvectors scaled by twice the eigenvalues of the covariance matrix of all aneurysm's vertices. The ellipsoid is sampled by using polar coordinates $\theta = 2\pi/36 \cdot i$, $i \in \{0, \ldots, 18\}$ and $\phi = 2\pi/m \cdot j$, with $m = 2 \cdot (9 - |i - 9|) + 1$, $j \in \{0, \ldots, m\}$. The scaling of the ellipsoid's eigenvalues ensures that the camera has an appropriate distance to the aneurysm, yielding the viewpoints $\mathbf{x}_i$. For each of these candidates, f is sampled. From this scalar field, we calculate the 90 % quantile and keep the remaining viewpoints as candidates for possible starting points. To further reduce their number, we cluster the candidates by using *DBSCAN*, a density-based clustering [10] that does not need a priori selection of the cluster number, because the number of optimal viewpoints is unknown. For each cluster, the averaged position is used as a starting point. However, for *DBSCAN* two thresholds must be specified, the minimum number of objects to form a valid cluster, and a maximum allowed dissimilarity between two objects of a cluster. In our case, each cluster must contain at least one candidate, and a maximum difference of 20 degrees for both angles, θ and ϕ, between a candidate and the cluster center is allowed. Smaller values lead to clusters, where the resulting starting points are very similar. With greater values the clusters are too large so that not all belonging candidates lie within the view frustum of the averaged camera position.

Camera animation. For each simulated time step, our approach calculates a set of optimal viewpoints. We order these viewpoints by their ϕ angle within a time step and connect them to a camera path. Moreover, the viewpoints are combined between adjacent time steps to generate a global camera animation during the cardiac cycle. Therefore, for each time step the viewpoint is used first that has the smallest distance of ϕ to the last viewpoint in the previous time step. We move the camera from one viewpoint in time to the next, where the camera position and view direction is interpolated from their known camera settings in each render pass. For the interpolation factor t, a cubic easing function is used with $t < .5 ? 4 \cdot t^3 : (t - 1) \cdot (2 \cdot t - 2) \cdot (2 \cdot t - 2) + 1$. With this the camera accelerates until halfway between two adjacent viewpoints and decelerates then. The resulting path enables a smooth animation between two adjacent viewpoints.

3   Results

We calculated camera animations for five data sets, where the results were evaluated with two domain experts by conducting informal interviews. The computation time per time step is between 8 and 10 s, depending on the amount of starting points. Our testing system uses an Intel Core i7 CPU with 2 GHz, 12

GB RAM and an NVidia GeForce GT 540M. The experts are one neuroradiologist with 16 years of work experience and one CFD engineer working on blood flow simulations for cerebral aneurysms with three years of work experience. They should assess if the automatic camera path supports the exploration and navigation within time-dependent data. Moreover, the experts had to manually search for suspicious surface regions depending on the selected parameters s_1 and s_2. Fig. 1 shows the optimal viewpoints for two data sets at the systolic peak. The left part shows the segmented aneurysm together with the manually selected results of our neuroradiologist. In both cases, three optimal views (1,2,3) are detected, presented in the right part of the subimages. In Fig. 1(a) and (b) the Wall Shear Stress (WSS) and wall thickness are color-coded, respectively, and the wall deformation and pressure are depicted with illustrative techniques, respectively, as introduced in [1]. Reddish, dense hatched areas indicate suspicious surface regions. The experts described the camera path as very helpful for the exploration of the time-dependent data. The automatically selected views correlated with the manual results within that time step. However, for the manual searching a series of rotations was necessary. Further, the time-dependent behavior of the data increases the manual exploration effort, because it is difficult to find critical regions during animation, since the rotation process itself needs a certain amount of time. Moreover, the experts liked that no further specification of thresholds is necessary for the calculation of the camera path. In addition, they described the animation as helpful for the navigation in 3D. However, it depends on which part of the aneurysm the users want to navigate their way around. If the users only want to navigate in a small region such as a bleb, a manual rotation was preferred. For the time-dependent navigation over the whole aneurysm surface, the automatic rotation was preferred.

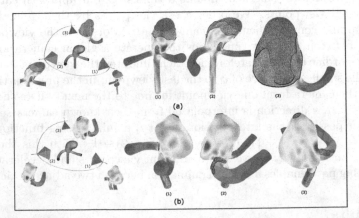

Fig. 1. Exemplary viewpoint selections for two data sets at the systolic peak. The left part shows the segmented aneurysm together with the manually selected results of our medical expert. For both, three optimal views (1,2,3) are detected, presented in the right part of the subimages. In (a) and (b), WSS and wall thickness are color-coded, respectively, and wall deformation and pressure are depicted by hatching, respectively. The camera is moving to all positions in a smooth way indicated by the purple spline.

4   Discussion

We present an automatic selection of occlusion-free views on suspicious surface regions for cerebral aneurysms based on user-selected parameters. From the viewpoints, a camera path is generated over the cardiac cycle. Our domain experts confirm the importance of camera paths to support the data exploration, because they enable the detection of suspicious regions without a time-consuming manual search. A possible application of our method is to get a quick overview of the aneurysm data, where rupture-prone areas are presented. In addition, our method could support the clinical report generation and serve as a summary of a patient's rupture risk. In the future, the camera path should be calculated in real time. Moreover, we want to integrate information about specific blood flow patterns such as vortices into the target function. Then, it would be possible to select views that present the time-dependent vortex behavior. A possible criterion in this context could be the optimization of the vortex core line visibility.

Acknowledgement. This work was funded by the BMBF (STIMULATE-OV -GU:13GW0095A). The authors thank Samuel Voss and Philipp Berg for providing us the data sets.

References

1. Meuschke M, Voss S, Beuing O, et al. Combined visualization of vessel deformation and hemodynamics in cerebral aneurysms. IEEE Trans Vis Comput Graph. 2017; p. 761–70.
2. Vázquez PP, Feixas M, Sbert M, et al. Viewpoint selection using viewpoint entropy. Proc VMV. 2001; p. 273–80.
3. Neugebauer M, Lawonn K, Beuing O, et al. AmniVis. A system for qualitative exploration of near-wall hemodynamics in cerebral aneurysms. Comput Graph Forum. 2013;32(3):251–60.
4. Bordoloi UD, Shen HW. View selection for volume rendering. Proc Conf Vis. 2005; p. 487–94.
5. Lee TY, Mishchenko O, Shen HW, et al. View point evaluation and streamline filtering for flow visualization. IEEE Pacific Vis Symposium. 2011; p. 83–90.
6. Tao J, Ma J, Wang C, et al. A unified approach to streamline selection and viewpoint selection for 3D flow visualization. IEEE Trans Vis Comput Graph 2013;19(3):393–406.
7. Mühler K, Neugebauer M, Tietjen C, et al. Viewpoint selection for intervention planning. IEEE Eurographics Symp Vis. 2007; p. 267–74.
8. Mönch T, Neugebauer M, Preim B. Optimization of vascular surface models for computational fluid dynamics and rapid prototyping. Workshop Dgit Eng. 2011; p. 16–23.
9. Crane K, Weischedel C, Wardetzky M. Geodesics in heat: a new approach to computing distance based on heat flow. ACM Trans Graph. 2013;32.
10. Ester M, Kriegel HP, Sander J, et al. A density-based algorithm for discovering clusters in large spatial databases with noise. Proc Knowl Discov Data Min. 1996; p. 226–31.

Abtract: Shape Analysis in Human Brain MRI

Martin Reuter[1,2], Christian Wachinger[3]

[1]German Center for Neurodegenerative Diseases (DZNE), Bonn, Germany
[2]Department of Radiology, Harvard Medical School, Boston, USA
[3]Department of Child and Adolescent Psychiatry, LMU, Munich, Germany
mreuter@nmr.mgh.harvard.edu

Structural magnetic resonance imaging data are frequently analyzed to reveal morphological changes of the human brain in dementia. Most contemporary imaging biomarkers are scalar values, such as the volume of a structure, and may miss the localized morphological variation of early presymptomatic disease progression. Neuroanatomical shape descriptors, however, can represent complex geometric information of individual anatomical regions and may demonstrate increased sensitivity in association studies. Yet, they remain largely unexplored. We have recently introduced *BrainPrint* [1] – an ensemble of shape descriptors computed for cortical and subcortical structures derived via longitudinal *FreeSurfer* segmentations [2]. *BrainPrint* naturally augments the contemporary region of interest-based volume and thickness analysis with shape information. Using *BrainPrint* to quantify lateral asymmetry, we demonstrated that neurodegeneration of subcortical structures in Alzheimer's disease is not symmetric across hemispheres [3]. The hippocampus shows a significant increase in asymmetry longitudinally and both hippocampus and amygdala show a significantly higher asymmetry cross-sectionally concurrent with disease severity above and beyond an aging effect. Based on longitudinal asymmetry measures we studied the progression from mild cognitive impairment to dementia, demonstrating that shape asymmetry in hippocampus, amygdala, caudate and cortex is predictive of disease onset. The same analyses based on lateral volume differences did not produce any significant results, indicating that shape asymmetries, potentially induced by morphometric changes in subnuclei, are associated with disease progression and can yield powerful imaging biomarkers for early classification and prediction of Alzheimer's disease. Because research has focused on contralateral volume differences, subcortical disease lateralization may have been overlooked thus far.

References

1. Wachinger C, Golland P, Kremen W, et al. BrainPrint: A discriminative characterization of brain morphology. Neuroimage. 2015;109:232–48.
2. Reuter M, Schmansky NJ, Rosas HD, et al. Within-Subject Template Estimation for Unbiased Longitudinal Image Analysis. NeuroImage. 2012;61(4):1402–18.
3. Wachinger C, Salat DH, Weiner M, et al. Whole-brain analysis reveals increased neuroanatomical asymmetries in dementia for hippocampus and amygdala. Brain. 2016;in press. Available from: http://dx.doi.org/10.1093/brain/aww243.

Abstract: Learning of Representative Multi-Resolution Multi-Object Statistical Shape Models from Small Training Populations

Matthias Wilms, Heinz Handels, Jan Ehrhardt

Institute of Medical Informatics, University of Lübeck
wilms@imi.uni-luebeck.de

Statistical shape models learned from a population of training shapes are frequently used as a shape prior. A key problem associated with their training is to provide a representative and large training set of (manual) segmentations. Therefore, models often suffer from the high-dimension-low-sample-size (HDLSS) problem, which limits their expressiveness and directly affects their performance.

We present a new approach for learning representative multi-resolution multi-object statistical shape models from small training populations. It is specifically designed to handle the challenges of multi-object scenarios: adequate modeling of individual objects and their relations. Our key assumption is that local shape variations have only limited effects in distant areas, which allows us to model those parts (nearly) independently. As the exact minimum distance between independent parts is unknown, a multi-resolution scheme is developed by learning models at different levels of locality. These models are subsequently fused into one compact model to eliminate redundancies. Furthermore, by introducing a distance between parts of different objects multi-object scenarios can be handled. The proposed multi-resolution multi-object modeling process can be integrated into the standard statistical shape modeling framework [1] by setting covariances of distant landmarks to zero. The resulting combined and compact representation of global and local variability allows the use of the active shape model strategy for segmentation and, hence, easy integration into existing approaches.

We compared our approach to the standard shape modeling framework [1] and state-of-the-art HDLSS approaches [2, 3]. Our approach outperforms these methods in terms of generalization ability and segmentation accuracy.

Acknowledgement. This work is funded by the DFG (EH 224/6-1).

References

1. Cootes TF, Taylor CJ, Cooper DH, et al. Active shape models-their training and application. Comput Vis Image Underst. 1995;61(1):38–59.
2. Cerrolaza JJ, Villanueva A, Cabeza R. Hierarchical statistical shape models of multiobject anatomical structures: application to brain MRI. IEEE Trans Med Imaging. 2012;31(3):713–24.

3. Cootes TF, Taylor CJ. Combining point distribution models with shape models based on finite element analysis. Image Vis Comput. 1995;13(5):403–9.

Kategorisierung der Beiträge

Autorenverzeichnis

Stichwortverzeichnis

Printed in the United States
By Bookmasters

Printed in the United States
By Bookmasters